15

CURRENT CLINICAL TOPICS IN INFECTIOUS DISEASES

15

CURRENT CLINICAL TOPICS IN INFECTIOUS DISEASES

Edited by

JACK S. REMINGTON, MD

Professor of Medicine
Division of Infectious Diseases and Geographic Medicine
Stanford University School of Medicine

Marcus A. Krupp Research Chair and
Chairman, Department of Immunology
and Infectious Diseases, Research Institute
Palo Alto Medical Foundation

MORTON N. SWARTZ, MD

Professor of Medicine
Harvard Medical School

Chief, James Jackson Firm
Medical Services
Massachusetts General Hospital
Infectious Disease Unit
Massachusetts General Hospital

Blackwell
Science

BLACKWELL SCIENCE

Editorial offices:

238 Main Street, Cambridge, Massachusetts 02142, USA
Osney Mead, Oxford OX2 0EL, England
25 John Street, London WC1N 2BL, England
23 Ainslie Place, Edinburgh EH3 6AJ, Scotland
54 University Street, Carlton, Victoria 3053, Australia
Arnette Blackwell SA, 1 rue de Lille, 75007 Paris, France
Blackwell Wissenschafts-Verlag GmbH, Kurfürstendamm 57, 10707 Berlin, Germany
Blackwell MZV, Feldgasse 13, A-1238 Vienna, Austria

Distributors:

North America
  Blackwell Science, Inc.
  238 Main Street
  Cambridge, Massachusetts 02142
  (Telephone orders: 800-215-1000 or 617-876-7000)

Australia
  Blackwell Science Pty Ltd.
  54 University Street
  Carlton, Victoria 3053
  (Telephone orders: 03-347-5552)

Outside North America and Australia
  Blackwell Science, Ltd.
  c/o Marston Book Services, Ltd.
  P.O. Box 87
  Oxford OX2 0DT
  England
  (Telephone orders: 44-865-791155)

Acquisitions: Victoria Reeders
Development: Coleen Traynor
Production: A. Maria Hight
Manufacturing: Kathleen Grimes
Typeset by Best-set Typesetter Ltd., Hong Kong
Printed and bound by Braun-Brumfield, Ann Arbor, MI

Library of Congress Cataloging in Publication Data

The Library of Congress has cataloged this
serial publication as follows:

Current clinical topics in infections diseases.
1-
  New York, McGraw-Hill Book Co.,
  c1980–1988
  Boston, Blackwell Science, Inc.
  c1989–
    v. ill. 25 cm
    Annual.
    Key title: Current clinical topics in
    infectious diseases, ISSN 0195-3842.
    I. Communicative diseases—
    Periodicals.
    DNLM: 1. Communicable Diseases—
    Periodicals. W 1 CU786T
  RC111.C87   616.9′05   80-643590
  ISBN 0-86542-397-0

To our fellows

Contents

Preface

As literature in the field of infectious diseases has increased in complexity and volume, a need has become evident for timely, concise summaries and critical commentaries on subjects pertinent to the student and practitioner of medicine, the specialist in infectious diseases, and those in allied fields. It is our intention that this series provide the reader with a true update of information in very specific areas of infectious diseases which require reevaluation.

Each author was requested to confine his/her chapter to a relatively narrow subject, to deal only with contemporary questions and problems, to gather and synthesize the information on recent advances which is often spread diffusely among numerous journals, to offer critical evaluation of this information, to place the information into perspective by defining its present status, and to point out deficiencies in the information and thereby indicate directions for further study. All of this was to be done within the most rigid deadlines to ensure that the chapters be written and published in less than a year. We are extremely grateful to the contributing authors, each of whom is a recognized authority in the particular field, for consenting to undertake such an admittingly difficult task.

Current Clinical Topics in Infectious Diseases: 15 is the fifteenth volume of a series which is published annually. Each text in the series consists of updates of a variety of subjects covering the wide scope of clinical infectious disease problems, including bacteriology, mycology, virology, parasitology, and epidemiology.

JACK S. REMINGTON
MORTON N. SWARTZ

Contributors

John G. Bartlett, MD
Stanhope Bayne-Jones Professor of Medicine, Chief, Division of Infectious Diseases, Johns Hopkins University School of Medicine, Baltimore, Maryland

Nesli Basgoz, MD
Assistant in Medicine, Infectious Disease Unit, Massachusetts General Hospital; Instructor in Medicine, Harvard Medical School, Boston, Massachusetts

Stephen L. Boswell, MD
Instructor, Harvard Medical School; Section Chief, HIV Clinical Services, Assistant Physician, Massachusetts General Hospital, Boston, Massachusetts

Timothy Francis Brewer, MD, MPH
Instructor in Medicine, Harvard Medical School; Associate Physician, Channing Laboratory, Brigham and Women's Hospital, Boston, Massachusetts

James DeMaio, MD
Division of Infectious Diseases, Department of Medicine, Johns Hopkins University School of Medicine, Baltimore, Maryland

Roland D. Eavey, MD
Associate Professor of Otology and Laryngology, Harvard Medical School; Director, Pediatric Otolaryngology Service, Massachusetts Eye and Ear Infirmary, Boston, Massachusetts

John E. Edwards, Jr., MD
Chief, Division of Infectious Diseases, Harbor/UCLA Medical Center; Professor of Medicine, UCLA School of Medicine, Torrance, California

Theodore Eickhoff, MD
Professor of Medicine, Division of Infectious Disease, University of Colorado
School of Medicine, Denver, Colorado

Scott G. Filler, MD
Division of Infectious Diseases, Assistant Professor of Medicine, Harbor/
UCLA Medical Center, Torrance, California

Pierce Gardner, MD
Associate Dean of Academic Affairs, Professor of Medicine, State University
of New York at Stony Brook, Stony Brook, New York

Larry J. Goodman, MD
Associate Professor of Medicine, Associate Dean, Rush Medical College,
Section of Infectious Disease, Rush-Presbyterian-St. Luke's Medical Center,
Chicago, Illinois

Lawrence H. Hanau, MD, PhD
Assistant Professor of Medicine, Albert Einstein College of Medicine;
Director, Infectious Diseases Clinic, Montefiore Medical Center, Bronx,
New York

H. Hunter Handsfield, MD
Professor of Medicine, University of Washington School of Medicine;
Director, Sexually Transmitted Disease Control Program, Seattle-King
County Department of Public Health, Seattle, Washington

James William C. Holmes, MD
Associate Professor of Clinical Surgery, Tulane University School of
Medicine, New Orleans, Louisiana

Stuart Levin, MD, FACP
James R. Lowenstine Professor and Chairman, Department of Internal
Medicine, Vice Dean, Rush Medical College; Senior Attending in Medicine,
Rush-Presbyterian-St. Luke's Medical Center, Chicago, Illinois

Jeanne M. Marrazzo, MD, MPH
Senior Fellow, Infectious Diseases, University of Washington School of
Medicine, Seattle, Washington

Joseph B. Nadol, Jr., MD
Walter Augustus LeCompte Professor and Chairman, Department of
Otology and Laryngology, Harvard Medical School; Chief, Department
of Otolaryngology, Massachusetts Eye and Ear Infirmary, Boston,
Massachusetts

Edward A. Nardell, MD
Assistant Professor of Medicine, Harvard Medical School; The Cambridge
Hospital, Tuberculosis Control Officer, Massachusetts Department of Public
Health, Boston, Massachusetts

Ronald Lee Nichols, MD
William Henderson Professor of Surgery, Professor of Microbiology, Tulane
University School of Medicine, New Orleans, Louisiana

Robert H. Rubin, MD
Associate Professor of Medicine, Harvard Medical School; Chief of Infectious
Disease for Transplantation and Director, Clinical Investigation Program,
Massachusetts General Hospital, Boston, Massachusetts

Frederick S. Southwick, MD
Professor of Medicine, University of Florida College of Medicine; Chief,
Division of Infectious Diseases, Shands Hospital, Gainesville, Florida

Neal H. Steigbigel, MD
Professor of Medicine, Albert Einstein College of Medicine; Head, Division
of Infectious Diseases, Montefiore Medical Center, Bronx, New York

Christine A. Wanke, MD
Assistant Professor of Medicine, Harvard Medical School; Division of
Infectious Diseases, New England Deaconess Hospital, Boston, Massachusetts

Mary E. Wilson, MD
Assistant Clinical Professor in Medicine, Harvard Medical School; Assistant
Professor, Departments of Population and International Health and
Epidemiology, Harvard School of Public Health; Chief, Infectious Diseases,
Mount Auburn Hospital, Cambridge, Massachusetts

Edward J. Young, MD
Professor of Medicine, Departments of Medicine and Microbiology and
Immunology, Baylor College of Medicine; Chief of Staff, Veterans Affairs
Medical Center, Houston, Texas

Other Volumes in the Series

Prophylaxis and Treatment of Malaria
Guillain-Barré Syndrome
Newer Antifungal Agents and Their Use, Including an Update on Amphotericin B and
   Flucytosine
Role of Ultrasound and Computed Tomography in the Diagnosis and Treatment of
   Intraabdominal Abscess
Treatment of Infections Due to Atypical Mycobacteria
Combination of Single Drug Therapy for Gram-Negative Sepsis
Deep Infections Following Total Hip Replacement
Treatment of the Child with Bacterial Meningitis
Diagnosis and Management of Meningitis Associated with Cerebrospinal Fluid Leaks
Prophylactic Antibiotics for Bowel Surgery
Infections Associated with Intravascular Lines
Diagnosis and Treatment of Cutaneous Leishmaniasis
Candida Endophthalmitis

CURRENT CLINICAL TOPICS IN INFECTIOUS DISEASES 4

Diagnosis and Management of Septic Arthritis
Kawasaki's Disease
A Critical Review of the Role of Oral Antibiotics in the Management of Hematogenous
   Osteomyelitis
When Can the Infected Hospital Employee Return to Work?
Endocardiography and Infectious Endocarditis
Orbital Infections
The Use of White Blood Cells Scanning Techniques in Infectious Disease
Antimicrobial Prophylaxis in the Immunosuppressed Cancer Patient
The Diagnosis of Fever Occurring in a Postpartum Patient
Management at Delivery of Mother and Infant When Herpes Simplex, Varicella-Zoster,
   Hepatitis, or Tuberculosis Have Occurred during Pregnancy
"Nonspecific Vaginitis," Vulvovaginal Candidiasis, and Trichomoniasis: Clinical Features,
   Diagnosis and Management
Radionuclide Imaging in the Management of Skeletal Infections
Comparison of Methods for Clinical Quantitation of Antibiotics
What Is the Clinical Significance of Tolerance to B-lactam Antibiotics?
A Critical Comparison of the Newer Aminoglycosidic Aminocyclitol
The Third Generation Cephalosporins

CURRENT CLINICAL TOPICS IN INFECTIOUS DISEASES 5

Prostatitis Syndromes
Staphylococcus epidermidis: The Organism, Its Diseases, and Treatment
Management of Nocardia Infections
Current Issues in Toxic Shock Syndrome
Isolation and Management of Contagious, Highly Lethal Diseases
Nutrition and Infection
Infections Associated with Hemodialysis and Chronic Peritoneal Dialysis
New Perspectives on the Epstein-Barr Virus in the Pathogenesis of Lymphoproliferative
   Disorders
Staphylococcal Teichoic Acid Antibodies
Current Status of Granulocyte Transfusion Therapy
Infections Associated with Intrauterine Devices
Hospital Epidemiology: An Emerging Discipline
The Viridians Streptococci in Perspective
Current Status of Prophylaxis for *Haemophilus influenzae* Infections
Acute Rheumatic Fever: Current Concepts and Controversies

CURRENT CLINICAL TOPICS IN INFECTIOUS DISEASES 6

The Acquired Immunodeficiency Syndrome
Health Advice and Immunizations for Travelers

CURRENT CLINICAL TOPICS IN INFECTIOUS DISEASES 14

15

CURRENT CLINICAL TOPICS IN INFECTIOUS DISEASES

When and How to Treat Serious Candidal Infections: Concepts and Controversies

SCOTT G. FILLER
JOHN E. EDWARDS, JR.

The rapid evolution of *Candida* species to their current prominence in clinical medicine has occurred mainly during the past decade. For this reason, there have been only limited therapeutic trials on most forms of candidal infections. Furthermore, the number of controlled trials comparing the efficacies of azoles and amphotericin B is small. Thus, most of the recommendations for therapy in this discussion are the opinions of the authors. These opinions are based both on limited therapeutic study data and on sentiments expressed by prominent clinical mycologists during discussions of these topics at national and international meetings. In this discussion, we have attempted to derive specific therapeutic strategies from available data and opinions. These strategies are certainly subject to change as results from ongoing and future clinical trials become available.

CANDIDEMIA

Should all patients with candidemia be treated with an antifungal agent?

Perhaps one of the most important developments in the treatment of candidal infections has been the agreement among clinical mycologists that it is impossible to accurately predict which patients with candidemia do not require antifungal therapy. There is little question that some patients with candidemia, especially when it has developed as a result of intravascular catheterization, are at low risk for serious complications from the fungemia. However, at present it is not possible to use any combination of signs, symptoms, and diagnostic tests to reliably distinguish this subgroup from those patients who will develop sequelae if a systemic antifungal agent is not administered. For instance, retrospective reviews have indicated that approximately 30% of patients with catheter-associated candidemia will have a complication related to the infection if the infection is not treated (1,2). Therefore, we consider that

1

the most prudent strategy for patients with candidemia, whether or not the candidemia is associated with an intravascular catheter and whether or not they are neutropenic, is to administer a systemic antifungal agent. The development of this consensus has been facilitated, in part, by the introduction of the newer azoles, which are significantly less toxic than amphotericin B and can be administered orally.

Which antifungal should be used and for how long in patients with candidemia?

A randomized comparative study of amphotericin B versus fluconazole has been conducted in patients who were not neutropenic. This study was a cooperative effort between Roerig Pfizer and the NIH-NIAID, Mycoses Study Group (3). It demonstrated that the efficacies of the two drugs were not significantly different. Because of these results, fluconazole is considered to be acceptable for treatment of candidemia in clinically stable non-neutropenic patients. Patients who develop the sepsis syndrome as a result of candidemia present a special problem. These patients should be treated with amphotericin B, either alone or in combination with 5-fluorocytosine or fluconazole. Monotherapy with 5-fluorocytosine should be avoided because both primary and secondary resistance to the agent have been reported for *Candida albicans* (4,5). Although data on the use of amphotericin B and fluconazole as combination therapy are limited, some clinical mycologists are administering both agents simultaneously to severely ill patients.

General guidelines for dosing of systemic antifungal agents are empiric at the present. The authors favor administering amphotericin B at 0.7 mg/kg/d and fluconazole at 400 mg/d. Adjustments in these dosages should be made according to the patient's clinical condition and renal function. Note that in the amphotericin B versus fluconazole trial, the fluconazole was administered intravenously for the first week of therapy and then orally for the remainder of therapy. When 5-fluorocytosine is used, serum levels should be measured to avoid bone marrow suppression. The serum level should be kept below 100 μg/mL; some investigators prefer to use 50 μg/mL as the maximum level for this drug. The duration of therapy for candidemia is also empiric. A reasonable approach is to treat for two weeks after signs and symptoms referable to the candidal infection have resolved.

A comparative study of fluconazole and amphotericin B in neutropenic patients has not been completed. Thus, it is not known, definitively, if fluconazole is as efficacious as amphotericin B in such patients, and whether the strategy of starting with amphotericin B and then finishing the course with fluconazole is an acceptable approach. We favor using fluconazole as primary therapy only in neutropenic patients who meet the following criteria: 1) clinically stable, 2) no evidence of hematogenous dissemination, 3) the candidemia has occurred in association with an intravascular catheter, 4) not receiving an azole on a prophylactic basis, and 5) infections with *Aspergillus* species are uncommon at that medical center. Amphotericin B should be used in all other cases, until further information about the efficacy of fluconazole in neutropenic patients is available.

Because primary resistance to fluconazole is common in *Candida krusei* (6,7) and *Torulopsis glabrata* can rapidly develop resistance to this drug (8), fluconazole should be used with caution in patients with either of these organisms in their blood. Strong consideration should be given to treatment with amphotericin B, whether or not neutropenia is present.

Ketoconazole should be not be used for the treatment of candidemia because it has been shown to be less efficacious than amphotericin B (9). In addition, there is no parenteral formulation of ketoconazole, and the bioavailability following oral administration is variable.

Data about the use of itraconazole in patients with candidemia are limited. In one small randomized study, 10 of 16 patients with neutropenia and candidal infections responded to oral itraconazole (200 mg twice a day) whereas 9 of 16 responded to amphotericin B with or without 5-fluorocytosine (10). However, the median duration of therapy was longer in the patients receiving itraconazole and subtherapeutic blood levels of the drug were seen in some of the patients who failed therapy. Like ketoconazole, itraconazole can only be given orally, and absorption requires the presence of food or acid in the stomach (11).

In patients with candidemia, should the intravascular catheters be changed or removed?

This question should be addressed by classifying patients into two separate groups: 1) intensive care unit (ICU) patients who do not have long-term, central venous lines tunneled under the skin, and 2) cancer patients with Hickman or Broviac catheters that will be used for long-term administration of therapeutic agents or for blood sampling.

ICU patients.   The recently completed study comparing the efficacies of amphotericin B and fluconazole referred to above showed that, in those patients in whom all intravascular catheters were changed at the time the patients were known to be candidemic, the duration of candidemia was shortened (3). Therefore, until further studies are completed, changing of all lines in the candidemic patient is the most appropriate strategy.

Cancer patients.   In this population, replacing a long-term indwelling central venous catheter may significantly diminish the patient's quality of life. Limited data have been presented in abstract form, indicating that some of these patients can be treated successfully with amphotericin B without removing the lines (12). In our opinion, central venous catheters in these patients should be changed whenever feasible. However, under circumstances where changing the catheter is an unacceptable option, amphotericin B should be administered.

Should certain noncandidemic patients be treated for suspected deep tissue candidal infection?

This question is raised most commonly in two situations. The first is a patient who is in the ICU, who has recently undergone major surgery, who has no obvious focal source of infection, in whom a species of *Candida* is cultured from several sites, and who remains febrile despite treatment with broad-spectrum antibacterial antibiotics. There has been a gradual lowering of the threshold for treating this type of patient over the last several years, even though their blood cultures never become positive. The basic reason has been the knowledge that the incidence of disseminated candidiasis diagnosed only at autopsy is unacceptably high and that the incidence of false negative blood cultures is substantial (13). Whether these patients should be treated with amphotericin B or fluconazole has not been studied. In our opinion, patients who are clinically unstable should be treated with amphotericin B, whereas patients who are febrile but clinically stable should be treated with fluconazole.

The second group of patients for whom empiric antifungal therapy is indicated are those who are neutropenic from cytotoxic chemotherapy and develop fevers that are unresponsive to antibacterial antibiotics. Substantial data from oncology centers indicate that early empiric treatment with amphotericin B reduces mortality from fungal infections in these patients (9,14–18). Because proper clinical studies are not available to guide the choice of an agent, strategies need to be devised for individual circumstances. We would use amphotericin B in situations where the patient has been receiving prophylaxis with fluconazole, when the patient is not clinically stable, when non-*albicans* species of *Candida* are recovered from sites other than the blood, and when *Aspergillus* species are a relatively common cause of infection in the susceptible patients at that medical center. In other circumstances, fluconazole is an acceptable alternative. Because of the problems of variable bioavailability and the lack of a parenteral formulation, itraconazole is a less attractive alternative in this situation. Ketoconazole should not be used.

In which patients does prophylactic antifungal therapy prevent hematogenously disseminated candidal infections?

Three general types of patients are candidates for prophylactic antifungal therapy because they are at high risk for developing hematogenously disseminated candidiasis. These categories are: 1) neutropenic patients, 2) burn patients, and 3) patients who have had major surgery.

Neutropenic patients. Several studies have indicated that neither oral nystatin nor ketoconazole prevents disseminated candidal infections in patients with leukemia (19–21). Fluconazole has been shown to significantly decrease candidal colonization and mucosal candidal infections in neutropenic cancer patients and patients who have undergone bone marrow transplantation (22–24). However, only in bone marrow transplant patients does the prophylactic use of fluconazole reduce the incidence of suspected or proven hematogenously disseminated candidal infections. Also, fluconazole prophy-laxis does not prevent infections by *Aspergillus* species and *C. krusel* (23–25).

Low-dose amphotericin B (0.1 mg / kg / d) has been shown to be superior to placebo in preventing invasive candidal infections in neutropenic cancer pa-tients (26). Although the prophylactic use of amphotericin B was associated with an improved survival in these patients, this survival benefit could not be attributed to a decrease in fatal fungal infections. Also, compared to placebo, there was a significant increase in infusion-related side effects in the patients receiving amphotericin B, but no difference in systemic toxicities.

Burn patients. There have been few studies on the efficacy of antifungal prophylaxis in patients who have had extensive burns. In one center, burn patients treated with oral and topical nystatin had a significant decrease in candidal colonization, wound infections, and fungemia compared to historical controls (27). The use of amphotericin B or azoles prophylactically has not been examined.

Postsurgical patients. The efficacy of antifungal prophylaxis in postsurgical or trauma patients who are not neutropenic is unclear. One group of investiga-tors found that there were no significant differences in the rates of candidal colonization or candidemia among surgical ICU patients who received clotrimazole, ketoconazole, nystatin, or no therapy (28). However, in another trial, treatment with ketoconazole significantly reduced the incidence of invasive candidal infections in postsurgical patients (29). A randomized study to determine if administration of fluconazole prevents candidal infections in postoperative patients is currently ongoing. Until the results of this study are known, we do not recommend routine systemic antifungal prophylaxis in patients who have undergone major surgery or trauma.

However, patients who have recently had an allograft of a solid organ, such as the liver, kidney, lung or heart, represent a special subset with an increased risk of developing both mucosal and disseminated candidal infections. Clotrimazole troches and nystatin appear to have similar efficacies in prevent-ing oropharyngeal candidiasis in patients who have undergone orthotopic liver transplantation (30). One center reported that three cases of invasive aspergillosis developed in liver transplant patients who were receiving amphotericin B (0.5 mg / kg / d) for candidemia (31). These data indicate that this dose of amphotericin B does not prevent infections with *Aspergillus* species in susceptible patients. Further studies on the use of antifungal prophylaxis in solid organ transplant patients need to be performed before firm recommenda-tions can be made. However, at present, we do not recommend the routine use of systemic antifungal agents on a prophylactic basis in these patients.

Are there risks associated with the prophylactic use of antifungal agents?
Several risks are associated with the routine prophylactic use of azole antifun-gal agents including: 1) emergence of azole-resistant organisms such as *C. krusei*

and *T. glabrata*, 2) high cost, 3) delayed recognition of disseminated fungal infection, 4) creating a false sense of security regarding protection from fungi not susceptible to the antifungal agent (such as *Aspergillus* species), and 5) potential drug toxicity (31–33). These risks need to be weighed against the potential benefits before antifungal prophylaxis is instituted.

Guiot et al. (34) retrospectively examined the charts of 341 consecutive patients who were admitted for treatment of leukemia, including some patients who underwent bone marrow transplantation, to identify risk factors for invasive fungal infections in this population. They found that patients with high-level candidal colonization and preceding bacteremia were predisposed to developing disseminated candidal infections. In addition, significantly more transplant patients with chronic graft versus host disease developed fatal infections with *Aspergillus* species. These data suggest that prospective studies are needed to determine which subset of neutropenic or postsurgical patients is at particularly high risk for developing disseminated fungal infections. Limiting antifungal prophylaxis to these extremely high-risk patients could significantly improve the risk–benefit ratio of this procedure.

ESTABLISHED DEEP CANDIDAL INFECTIONS

How should chronic hematogenously disseminated candidiasis be treated?
Formerly called hepatosplenic candidiasis, chronic hematogenously disseminated candidiasis is characterized by widespread micro- and macroscopic abscesses in the liver, spleen, kidneys, and lungs. This syndrome is usually identified in patients who are recovering from profound neutropenia and either remain or become febrile. Abdominal pain and an elevated serum alkaline phosphatase may be present. Computed tomography (CT) or ultrasonography of the abdomen reveal multiple filling defects in the liver, spleen, and kidneys (35–39). If possible, aspiration of one or more of these abscesses should be performed in an attempt to identify the infecting organism. Although *Candida* species can frequently be identified by histopathology, cultures from these lesions are often sterile.

Treatment of chronic hematogenously disseminated candidiasis requires long-term antifungal therapy. This syndrome is relatively rare; thus, no randomized trials on its treatment have been performed. The predominant experience is with amphotericin B. When this drug is used, the average total dose should be approximately 5 g and most clinical mycologists would also add 5-fluorocytosine (40,41). However, 35% to 40% of patients will not be cured with this regimen (42). Because of the considerable toxicity and diminished quality of life associated with a prolonged course of amphotericin B, fluconazole and liposomal formulations of amphotericin B have been used as alternatives (41,43,44). In retrospective studies, initial treatment with amphotericin B followed by a prolonged course of fluconazole resulted in a 91% response rate

(43,44). However, in one study, 3 of the 20 patients who responded to this regimen developed superinfection with *Aspergillus* species (43). For this reason, it is prudent to treat patients with chronic hematogenously disseminated candidiasis with an initial course of amphotericin B and 5-fluorocytosine. Subsequently, if resolution of the lesions does not occur or if there is unacceptable toxicity from amphotericin B, therapy can be continued with fluconazole. If the logistics of administering amphotericin B make it extremely difficult to use this drug, then early switching to fluconazole may be considered. The efficacy of therapy in all patients should be monitored by relatively frequent CT scans to assess the size of the lesion(s).

Peritoneal Candidiasis

Peritoneal infections with *Candida* species are seen in two types of patients. The first group includes patients who have either recently undergone intra-abdominal surgery or have had a perforation somewhere in their gastrointestinal tract. When a patient has developed peritonitis as a result of spillage of gastrointestinal contents, *Candida* species may be recovered as either a pure culture or mixed with one or more types of bacteria. The incidence of dissemination from an intra-abdominal infection is low in adults but is significantly higher in neonates (45). However, a search for evidence of dissemination, such as obtaining blood cultures using the lysis centrifugation technique and performing a careful physical examination, should be performed in all patients with candidal peritonitis.

There is a general consensus that all patients who have signs and symptoms of peritonitis and from whom *Candida* species grows in pure culture should receive systemic antifungal therapy. However, when a species of *Candida* is isolated from a patient as part of mixed culture, therapy must be individualized. If the patient has responded clinically to antibacterial antibiotics alone and any intra-abdominal abscesses have been drained, then it may not be necessary to administer antifungal therapy. Growth of *Candida* species from a drain should be considered to represent colonization and antifungal therapy should not be given for this circumstance alone. It is our opinion that fluconazole (400 mg/d) is adequate therapy for candidal peritonitis. However, if a non-*albicans* species of *Candida* is isolated or the patient is clinically unstable, then the use of amphotericin B may be indicated. In general, the threshold for treating patients whose peritoneal cultures grow *Candida* species is lowering among clinical mycologists. Reasons for this lowered threshold include the difficulty in diagnosing established candidal infections of the peritoneum, and the experience that a short course of fluconazole or amphotericin B has little long-term toxicity.

The second group of patients who may develop candidal peritonitis are those who are on chronic ambulatory peritoneal dialysis (CAPD). Because the incidence of dissemination is low in these patients, they can be treated by the addition of amphotericin B to the dialysis fluid to achieve a concentration of 2 to 4 µg/mL. Several reports have indicated that fluconazole is an acceptable alternative to amphotericin B (46–49). Fluconazole should be administered as a loading dose of 200 to 400 mg followed by 50 to 200 mg fluconazole daily (50). The peritoneal catheter should be removed whenever possible because inability to clear the infection and relapses are common if the catheter is left in place (50). One center advocates treating candidal peritonitis in CAPD patients with catheter removal alone (51).

Candidal Infections of Intra-abdominal Structures

Billary tract infections. Candidal cholecystitis, as well as fungus balls in the bile ducts and gallbladder have been reported (52,53). These conditions may respond to intravenous amphotericin B alone (53). However, the fungus balls should be removed surgically if they are large or do not respond to therapy. Bile concentrations of fluconazole equal or exceed serum levels; successful treatment of candidal cholecystitis with this drug has been reported (52).

Pancreatic abscesses. Pancreatic abscesses caused by *Candida* species are rare. The few cases of this disease have been treated with CT-guided percutaneous drainage and amphotericin B (54,55). The use of fluconazole has not been studied sufficiently to provide a clear picture of its utility. We would use amphotericin B initially and, in cases where toxicity of amphotericin B was prohibitive, finish therapy with fluconazole.

What should be done about candiduria?
Candiduria in a patient may represent colonization, candidal cystitis, or pyelonephritis that has developed from either hematogenous seeding or an ascending infection. It is difficult to distinguish these possibilities, especially in an ill patient with an indwelling Foley catheter (56,57). A large study to determine the significance and optimal treatment of candiduria is currently being conducted by the Mycoses Study Group of the NIAID, but the collection and analysis of data are incomplete at this time.

In patients with candiduria, evidence of urinary tract obstruction should be sought because it is a predisposing factor for dissemination (58). Urine should be examined carefully because the presence of white blood cell casts is indicative of renal involvement (59). In addition, the presence of pyuria makes it less likely that the bladder is merely colonized. However, virtually all cases of candiduria should be treated in patients who are neutropenic or have undergone renal transplantation, irrespective of their symptoms. If possible, the Foley catheter should be removed and all antibiotics should be discontinued. However, this practice is often not feasible.

Candidal cystitis should be treated for 2 to 3 days with either fluconazole (50 to 100 mg/d) or bladder irrigation with amphotericin B. Amphotericin B is commonly mixed to a final concentration of 50 mg/L (50 µg/mL) in sterile water or 5% glucose and administered as a continuous infusion through a three-way Foley catheter. This technique should cure 80% of patients (60). However, Sanford (56) advocates using amphotericin B at a concentration of 10 mg/L (1 µg/mL) to decrease local irritation. To achieve more even distribution of the drug, he suggests that, instead of continuous irrigation, 200 to 300 mL of amphotericin B should be infused into the bladder intermittently, after which the catheter should be cross-clamped for 60 to 90 minutes. We would use fluconazole instead of local amphotericin B as long as the organism is neither *T. glabrata* nor *C. krusel*.

If the candiduria does not respond to a short course of bladder irrigation or fluconazole, then it is likely that the patient has either an upper urinary tract infection or a fungus ball. Renal infections should be treated using systemic therapy with amphotericin B or fluconazole; fungus balls should be removed surgically.

Endophthalmitis

Candidal endophthalmitis has been found in 28% to 37% of nonneutropenic patients who have candidemia (61,62). Endophthalmitis is less commonly detected in neutropenic patients with cancer. There are two likely explanations for this difference. First, the retinal lesions are composed predominantly of neutrophils, so the low number of neutrophils results in few lesions that are small and poorly formed (63). Second, neutropenic patients have an increased incidence of infections caused by non-*albicans* species of *Candida* (64–66), and disseminated infections caused by these organisms are less commonly complicated by endophthalmitis (67).

Endophthalmitis should be treated aggressively with prolonged therapy to minimize visual impairment and because most patients with endophthalmitis have widespread infection in multiple organs (68). If the lesion is near the macula or the infection is caused by a non-*albicans* species of *Candida*, then the patient should be treated with amphotericin B (500 to 1000 mg total dose) and 5-fluorocytosine (69,70). Consultation with an ophthalmologist is imperative; vitrectomy may be beneficial in severe cases (71). When candidal endophthalmitis is associated with an intraocular lens implant, the prosthesis should be removed to prevent relapse (72). Fluconazole has been used successfully in the treatment of endophthalmitis caused by *C. albicans* (73). However, at this time we would consider using this drug only in cases where the lesions are small and not located near the macula, and when *C. albicans* is known to be the infecting organism.

Central Nervous System Infections

Infections of the meninges and brain parenchyma by *Candida* species may occur as a complication of hematogenously disseminated candidiasis (74,75) or due to direct inoculation via head trauma or a neurosurgical procedure (76). Candidal meningitis is occurring more frequently in neonates and children (77–80). Furthermore, patients with acquired immunodeficiency syndrome (AIDS) are at an increased risk of developing this disease (81–84). Initial treatment of meningitis or encephalitis should be with intravenous amphotericin B and 5-fluorocytosine (85,86). Any shunts should be removed. In refractory cases, either fluconazole or intrathecal amphotericin B can be tried.

Endocarditis

Candidal endocarditis is most commonly seen in association with prosthetic heart valves, intravenous drug abuse (especially when the drug is diluted in lemon juice) (87), neutropenia, prolonged use of central venous catheters, pre-existing valvular heart disease, and bacterial endocarditis (88,89). The disease is difficult to diagnose because associated candidemia is low grade and intermittent; blood cultures are frequently sterile. Once this disease is identified, the patient should be treated with amphotericin B and early valve replacement (90). Following surgery, the amphotericin B should be continued for 6 to 10 weeks to prevent relapse (91). Because relapses have occurred years after treatment, even with optimal therapy, patients with candidal endocarditis should be monitored periodically for at least two years. There are rare reports of long-term survival following treatment of endocarditis without valve replacement, and other physicians have reported the successful use of fluconazole for this infection (92,93). However, it is our opinion that this drug is best used in patients who require long-term suppressive therapy because valve replacement cannot be performed.

Candidal Infections of the Musculoskeletal System

Candidal osteomyelitis is usually the result of hematogenous dissemination. In adults, the axial skeleton is most frequently involved, whereas the long bones are the most common sites of infection in children. Because blood cultures are often negative, a needle aspirate of the lesion should be performed to identify the causative organism.

Candidal arthritis can develop from either hematogenous seeding or direct inoculation via trauma or intra-articular injections. There is a higher incidence of arthritis caused by non-*albicans* species, especially *Candida parapsilosis*, when infection is caused by direct inoculation (94).

Both candidal osteomyelitis and arthritis should be treated with amphotericin B and 5-fluorocytosine; the efficacy of fluconazole in these types of infections is unknown.

Infections of Prosthetic Devices

In most cases, prosthetic devices infected with *Candida* species should be removed. Because these organisms adhere avidly to most prosthetic surfaces (95), infection is difficult to eradicate with antifungal therapy alone. Rarely, patients have been successfully treated without removal of their prostheses, usually in situations where further surgery was not feasible (96–98). Such patients may require life-long therapy.

ORAL AND ESOPHAGEAL CANDIDIASIS

What is the best therapy for oral and esophageal candidiasis in patients with AIDS or chronic mucocutaneous candidiasis?
Oral candidiasis is frequently a significant problem in patients with defects in cell-mediated immunity, particularly those with AIDS or chronic mucocutaneous candidiasis. Oral fluconazole (100 mg once daily) and oral clotrimazole (10 mg 5 times daily) have shown to be equally efficacious in the treatment of oral candidiasis in AIDS patients (99). However, in this study, most patients relapsed once therapy was discontinued, and the relapses occurred sooner in the patients treated with clotrimazole. Although ketoconazole and fluconazole have similar efficacies in patients with oral candidiasis (100), fluconazole is superior for the treatment of esophageal candidiasis in AIDS patients (101). In addition, fluconazole is better absorbed and probably has a lower incidence of toxicity than ketoconazole.

Is it necessary to perform endoscopy in all AIDS patients who have esophageal symptoms?
Esophageal candidiasis should be considered in immunocompromised patients who have odynophagia. Many patients with oral candidiasis do not have esophageal candidiasis, and some patients with esophageal candidiasis do not have thrush (102). Furthermore, up to 43% of patients with esophageal candidiasis do not have esophageal symptoms (103). Because it is often not practical to perform endoscopy on all AIDS patients who have esophageal symptoms, it is reasonable to treat such patients empirically with fluconazole and to reserve endoscopy for patients who do not respond to such treatment (104). In one study of AIDS patients who underwent endoscopy because their symptoms did not resolve after treatment with fluconazole or ketoconazole, the most common cause of esophagitis was still *Candida* species, followed by herpes simplex, cytomegalovirus, peptic esophagitis, and Kaposi's sarcoma (105). Most of these patients responded to intravenous amphotericin B or fluconazole or specific antiviral therapy.

Does prophylaxis diminish the occurrence of thrush in patients with AIDS?
Relapses after successful therapy for oral or esophageal candidiasis are very common in patients with AIDS or chronic mucocutaneous candidiasis (99,106–108). For this reason, most patients require some form of long-term therapy to prevent recurrent infections. There is no doubt that prophylaxis with azoles,

and especially fluconazole, diminishes the incidence of thrush in AIDS patients. The preferred dose of fluconazole is 100 mg/d (109). However, some physicians are using 150 to 200 mg given as a single dose once a week (110). No controlled trials have compared the oral azoles with clotrimazole or nystatin for prophylaxis of candidal infections. However, either of these regimens is less well tolerated by the patients. Additionally, prophylactic azoles diminish the incidence of candidal esophagitis. Suppression therapy with fluconazole is thought to reduce the incidence of cryptococcal meningitis (109). Data are insufficient to suggest that the incidence of other systemic fungal infections is reduced with the use of prophylactic fluconazole in AIDS patients.

Are there risks to treating AIDS patients with prophylactic azoles?
A number of studies have now demonstrated clinical failure of the azoles in AIDS patients to whom azoles have been administered either as primary treatment or as prophylaxis for mucosal candidal infections. Some isolates from these patients have remained susceptible to the azole used, whereas other isolates have demonstrated azole resistance in vitro (111–114). In general, the patients in whom relapses occur while on therapy have low CD4 counts (less than 50) and have received azoles for a prolonged period of time (111,112). Whether those patients who have isolates that are resistant to fluconazole can be treated with itraconazole is under investigation. Although toxicities to fluconazole have been manifested by skin rashes (including toxic epidermal necrolysis) (115) and abnormal liver function tests (99,100), most AIDS patients tolerate the agent well. Patients with severe oral/esophageal candidiasis who have failed azole therapy will respond to a short course of low-dose intravenous amphotericin B (116). Once the infection is cleared with amphotericin B, some of these patients can be successfully maintained on fluconazole.

SERODIAGNOSIS

Are there any serodiagnostic tests that are available for making a diagnosis of hematogenously disseminated candidiasis or monitoring therapy?
Despite extensive investigation on the development of a serodiagnostic test to differentiate disseminated candidiasis from colonization, there is no commercially available test that is widely accepted. Candida precipitins, D-arabinatol, and enolase, just to name a few, have been investigated. With the exception of the Candidtec test for candidal antigen, these tests are not available commercially at this time. The Candidtec test has been criticized for its lack of sensitivity. Most clinical mycologists do not use any serodiagnostic tests to either diagnose hematogenous dissemination or to follow patients at this time. The topic has been extensively reviewed by Reiss and Morrison (117). It is likely that in the future a panel of tests will be developed to determine the probability that a deep infection is present and to monitor the response to therapy.

IMMUNOMODULATORS

What is the role of immunomodulators in preventing or treating deep-seated candidal infections?

Because *Candida* species are opportunistic pathogens that cause infections mainly in patients with some form of immunosuppression, the use of cytokines to reduce the level of immunosuppression in these patients is an attractive treatment strategy. However, there are few clinical studies on the efficacy of cytokines in the prevention or treatment of candidal infections. Granulocyte colony-stimulating factor (G-CSF) and granulocyte-macrophage colony-stimulating factor (GM-CSF) have been shown to reduce the duration of granulocytopenia in cancer patients and patients undergoing bone marrow transplantation (119,120). Although the ability of these agents to reduce the incidence or severity of fungal infections in granulocytopenic patients has not yet been studied, it is highly likely that their use is beneficial in this group of patients. Whether G-CSF, GM-CSF, or macrophage colony-stimulating factor (M-CSF) is useful in preventing or treating candidal infections in non-neutropenic patients remains to be determined. Interferon-γ improved resistance to hematogenously disseminated candidiasis in nonneutropenic mice (121) and it was found to be helpful in treating a child with chronic granulomatous disease and a candidal hepatic abscess (122). However, the efficacy of this cytokine in other patient groups has not been studied. In the future, as clinical data on the use of various cytokines become available, it is likely that these agents will be used routinely in combination with antifungal agents.

REFERENCES

1 Fraser VJ, Jones M, Dunkel J, Storfer S, Medoff G, Dunagan WC. Candidemia in a tertiary care hospital: epidemiology, risk factors, and predictors of mortality. Clin Infect Dis 1992;15:414–421.

2 Lecciones JA, Lee JW, Navarro EE, et al. Vascular catheter-associated fungemia in patients with cancer: analysis of 155 episodes. Clin Infect Dis 1992;14:875–883.

3 Rex JH, Bennett JE, Sugar AM, et al. A randomized trial comparing fluconazole with amphotericin B for the treatment of candidemia in patients without neutropenia. N Engl J Med 1994;331:1325–1330.

4 Stiller RL, Bennett JE, Scholer HJ, et al. Susceptibility to 5-fluorocytosine and prevalence of serotype in 402 *Candida albicans* isolated from the United States. Antimicrob Agents Chemother 1982;22:482–487.

5 Bennett JE. Flucytosine. Ann Intern Med 1977;86:319–322.

6 Fisher MA, Shen S, Haddad J, Tarry WF. Comparison of in vivo activity of fluconazole with that of amphotericin B against *Candida tropicalis, Candida glabrata,* and *Candida krusei.* Antimicrob Agents Chemother 1989;33:1443–1446.

7 Dermoumi H. In vitro susceptibility of yeast isolates from the blood to fluconazole and amphotericin B. Chemotherapy 1992;38:112–117.

8 Warnock DW, Burke J, Cope NJ, Johnson EM, von Frauhoffer NA, Williams EW. Fluconazole resistance in *Candida glabrata.* Lancet 1988;ii:1310.

9 Walsh TJ, Rubin M, Hathorn J, et al. Amphotericin B vs. high-dose ketoconazole for empirical antifungal therapy among febrile, granulocytopenic cancer patients. A prospective, randomized study. Arch Intern Med 1991;151:765–770.

10 **Van't Wout JW.** Itraconazole in neutropenic patients. Chemotherapy 1992; 38(suppl 1):23–26.

11 **Heykants J, Van Peer A, Van de Velde V, et al.** The clinical pharmacokinetics of itraconazole: an overview. Mycoses 1989; 32(suppl 1):67–87.

12 **Kulak K, Maki DG.** Treatment of Hickman catheter-related candidemia without removing the catheter. In: Programs and Abstracts of the 32nd Interscience Conference on Antimicrobial Agents and Chemotherapy, Atlanta. Washington, DC: American Society for Microbiology 1992: 249. Abstract 831.

13 **Jones JM.** Laboratory diagnosis of invasive candidiasis. Clin Microbiol Rev 1990;3:32–45.

14 **Sugar AM.** Empiric treatment of fungal infections in the neutropenic host. Review of the literature and guidelines for use. Arch Intern Med 1990;150:2258–2264.

15 **Stein RS, Kayser J, Flexner JM.** Clinical value of empirical amphotericin B in patients with acute myelogenous leukemia. Cancer 1982;50:2247–2251.

16 **Stein RS, Greer JP, Ferrin W, Lenox R, Baer MR, Flexner JM.** Clinical experience with amphotericin B in acute myelogenous leukemia. South Med J 1986; 79:863–870.

17 **Pizzo PA, Robichaud KJ, Gill FA, Witebsky FG.** Empiric antibiotic and antifungal therapy for cancer patients with prolonged fever and granulocytopenia. Am J Med 1982;72:101–111.

18 **EORTC International Antimicrobial Therapy Cooperative Group.** Empiric antifungal therapy in febrile granulocytopenic patients. Am J Med 1989;86:668–672.

19 **De Gregorio MW, Lee WMF, Ries CA.** Candida infections in patients with acute leukemia: ineffectiveness of nystatin prophylaxis and relationship between oropharyngeal and systemic candidiasis. Cancer 1982;50:2780–2784.

20 **Hansen RM, Reinerio N, Sohnle PG, et al.** Ketoconazole in the prevention of candidiasis in patients with cancer. A prospective, randomized, controlled, double-blind study. Arch Intern Med 1987;147:710–712.

21 **Meunier F.** Prevention of mycosis in immunocompromised patients. Rev Infect Dis 1987;9:408–416.

22 **Bodey GP, Samonis G, Rolston K.** Prophylaxis of candidiasis in cancer patients. Semin Oncol 1990;17:24–28.

23 **Winston DJ, Chandrasekar PH, Lazarus HM, et al.** Fluconazole prophylaxis of fungal infections in patients with acute leukemia. Results of a randomized placebo-controlled, double-blind, multicenter trial. Ann Intern Med 1993; 118: 495–503.

24 **Goodman JL, Winston DJ, Greenfield RA, et al.** A controlled trial of fluconazole to prevent fungal infections in patients undergoing bone marrow transplantation. N Engl J Med 1992;326:845–851.

25 **Quabeck K, Muller KD, Beelen DW, et al.** Prophylaxis and treatment of fungal infections with fluconazole in bone marrow transplant patients. Mycoses 1992;35:221–224.

26 **Perfect JR, Klotman ME, Gilbert CC, et al.** Prophylactic intravenous amphotericin B in neutropenic autologous bone marrow transplant recipients. J Infect Dis 1992; 165:891–897.

27 **Desai MH, Rutan RL, Heggers JP, Herndon DN.** Candida infection with and without nystatin prophylaxis. A 11-year experience with patients with burn injury. Arch Surg 1992;127:159–162.

28 **Savino JA, Agarwal N, Wry P, Policastro A, Cerabona T, Austria L.** Routine prophylactic antifungal agents (clotrimazole, ketoconazole, and nystatin) in nontransplant/nonburned critically ill surgical and trauma patients. J Trauma 1994;36:20–25.

29 **Slotman GJ, Burchand KW.** Ketoconazole prevents Candida sepsis in critically ill surgical patients. Arch Surg 1987;122:147–151.

30 **Ruskin JD, Wood RP, Bailey MR, Whitmore CK, Shaw BW.** Comparative trial of oral clotrimazole and nystatin for oropharyngeal candidiasis prophylaxis in orthotopic liver transplant patients. Oral Surg Oral Med Oral Pathol 1992;74:567–571.

31 **Singh N, Mieles L, Yu VL, Gayowski T.** Invasive aspergillosis in liver transplant recipients: association with candidemia and consumption coagulopathy and failure of prophylaxis with low-dose amphotericin B. Clin Infect Dis 1993; 17:906–908.

32 **Wingard JR, Merz WG, Rinaldi MG, Johnson TR, Karp JE, Saral R.** Increase in *Candida krusei* infection among patients with bone marrow transplantation and neutropenia treated prophylactically with

fluconazole. N Engl J Med 1991;1274–1277.

33 Borg-von Zepelin M, Eiffert H, Kann M, Ruchel R. Changes in the spectrum of fungal isolates: results from clinical specimens gathered in 1987/88 compared with those in 1991/92 in the University Hospital Gottingen, Germany. Mycoses 1993;36:247–253.

34 Guiot HFL, Fibbe WE, Van't Wout JW. Risk factors for fungal infection in patients with malignant hematologic disorders: implications for empirical therapy and prophylaxis. Clin Infect Dis 1994;18:525–532.

35 Haron E, Feld R, Tuffnell P, Patterson B, Hasselback R, Matlow A. Hepatic candidiasis: an increasing problem in immunocompromised patients. Am J Med 1987;83:17–26.

36 Lewis JH, Patel HR, Zimmerman HJ. The spectrum of hepatic candidiasis. Hepatology 1982;2:479–487.

37 Tashjian LS, Abramsom JS, Peacock JE Jr. Focal hepatic candidiasis: a distinct clinical variant of candidiasis in immunocompromised patients. Rev Infect Dis 1984;6:689–703.

38 Bodey GP, Anaissie EJ. Chronic systemic candidiasis. Eur J Clin Microbiol Infect Dis 1989;8:855–857.

39 Grunebaum M, Ziv N, Kaplinsky C, Kornreich L, Horev G, Mor C. Liver candidiasis. The various sonographic patterns in the immunocompromised child. Pediatr Radiol 1991;21:497–500.

40 Pizzo PA, Walsh TJ. Fungal infections in the pediatric cancer patient. Semin Oncol 1990;17:6–9.

41 Blade J, Lopez-Guillermo A, Rozman C, et al. Chronic systemic candidiasis in acute leukemia. Ann Hematol 1992;64:240–244.

42 Bodey GP. Azole antifungal agents. Clin Infect Dis 1992;14 (suppl 1):S161–S169.

43 Anaissie E, Bodey GP, Kantarjian H, et al. Fluconazole therapy for chronic disseminated candidiasis in patients with leukemia and prior amphotericin B therapy. Am J Med 1991;91:142–150.

44 Kauffman CA, Bradley SF, Ross SC, Weber DR. Hepatosplenic candidiasis: successful treatment with fluconazole. Am J Med 1991;91:137–141.

45 Johnson DE, Conroy MM, Foker JE, et al. Candida peritonitis in the newborn infant. J Pediatr 1980;97:298–300.

46 Huang TC, Chung WK. Fluconazole in the treatment of candida peritonitis in continuous ambulatory peritoneal dialysis: report of a case. J Formos Med Assoc 1993;92:190–191.

47 Chan TM, Chan CY, Cheng SW, Lo WK, Lo CY, Cheng IK. Treatment of fungal peritonitis complicating continuous ambulatory peritoneal dialysis with oral fluconazole: a series of 21 patients. Nephrol Dial Transplant 1994;9:539–542.

48 Mehes M, Mohai L, Szollosy G. Candida peritonitis: successful treatment with CAPD in two patients. Int Urol Nephrol 1992;24:665–672.

49 Levine J, Bernard DB, Idelson BA, Farnham H, Saunders C, Sugar AM. Fungal peritonitis complicating continuous ambulatory peritoneal dialysis: successful treatment with fluconazole, a new orally active antifungal agent. Am J Med 1989;86:825–827.

50 Hoch BS, Namboodiri NK, Banayat G, et al. The use of fluconazole in the management of Candida peritonitis in patients on peritoneal dialysis. Perit Dial Int 1993;13(suppl 2):S357–S359.

51 Nagappan R, Collins JF, Lee WT. Fungal peritonitis in continuous ambulatory peritoneal dialysis—the Auckland experience. Am J Kidney Dis 1992;20:492–496.

52 Bozzette SA, Gordon RL, Yen A, Rinaldi M, Ito MK, Fierer J. Biliary concentrations of fluconazole in a patient with candidal cholecystitis: case report. Clin Infect Dis 1992;15:701–703.

53 Schreiber M, Black L, Noah Z, et al. Gallbladder candidiasis in a leukemic child. Am J Dis Child 1982;136:462–463.

54 Keiser P, Keay S. Candidal pancreatic abscesses: report of two cases and review. Clin Infect Dis 1992;14:884–888.

55 Howard JM, Bieluch VM. Pancreatic abscess secondary to Candida albicans. Pancreas 1989;4:120–122.

56 Sanford JP. The enigma of candiduria: evolution of bladder irrigation with amphotericin B for management—from anecdote to dogma and a lesson from Machiavelli. Clin Infect Dis 1993;16:145–147.

57 Wong-Beringer A, Jacobs RA, Guglielmo B. Treatment of funguria. JAMA 1992;267:2780–2785.

58 Ang BS, Telenti A, King B, Steckelberg JM, Wilson WR. Candidemia from a urinary tract source: microbiological

aspects and clinical significance. Clin Infect Dis 1993;17:662–666.

59 **Gregory MC, Schumann GB, Schumann JL, et al.** The clinical significance of Candida casts. Am J Kidney Dis 1984; 4:179–184.

60 **Jacobs LG, Skidmore EA, Cardoso LA, Ziv F.** Bladder irrigation with amphotericin B for treatment of fungal urinary tract infections. Clin Infect Dis 1994; 18:313–318.

61 **Brooks RG.** Prospective study of Candida endophthalmitis in hospitalized patients with candidemia. Arch Intern Med 1989;149:2226–2228.

62 **Parke DWI, Jones DB, Gentry LO.** Endogenous endophthalmitis among patients with candidemia. Ophthalmology 1982;89:789–796.

63 **Henderson DK, Hockey LB, Vukalcic LJ, Edwards JE Jr.** Effect of immunosuppression on the development of experimental hematogenous Candida endophthalmitis. Infect Immun 1980;27:628–631.

64 **Meunier F, Aoun M, Bitar N.** Candidemia in immunocompromised patients. Clin Infect Dis 1992;14(suppl 1):S120–S125.

65 **Wingard JR, Merz WG, Saral R.** *Candida tropicalis*: a major pathogen in immunocompromised patients. Ann Intern Med 1979;91:539–543.

66 **Meunier-Carpentier F, Kiehn TE, Armstrong D.** Fungemia in the immunocompromised host. Changing patterns, antigenemia, high mortality. Am J Med 1981;71:363–370.

67 **Joshi N, Hamory BH.** Endophthalmitis caused by non-*albicans* species of *Candida*. Rev Infect Dis 1991;13:281–287.

68 **Edwards JE Jr, Foos RY, Montgomerie JZ, Guze LB.** Ocular manifestations of Candida septicemia. Review of seventy-six cases of hematogenous Candida endophthalmitis. Medicine 1974;53:47–75.

69 **Cohen M, Montgomerie JZ.** Hematogenous endophthalmitis due to *Candida tropicalis*: report of two cases and review. Clin Infect Dis 1993;17:270–272.

70 **McQuillen DP, Zingman BS, Meunier F, Levitz SM.** Invasive infections due to *Candida krusei*: report of ten cases of fungemia that include three cases of endophthalmitis. Clin Infect Dis 1992; 14:472–478.

71 **Barrie T.** The place of elective vitrectomy in the management of patients with Candida endophthalmitis. Arch Clin Exp Ophthalmol 1987;225:107–113.

72 **Kauffman CA, Bradley SF, Vine AK.** Candida endophthalmitis associated with intraocular lens implantation: efficacy of fluconazole therapy. Mycoses 1993;36:13–17.

73 **del Palacio A, Cuetara MS, Ferro M, et al.** Fluconazole in the management of endophthalmitis in disseminated candidosis of heroin addicts. Mycoses 1993;36: 193–199.

74 **Walsh TJ, Hier DB, Caplan LR.** Fungal infections of the central nervous system: comparative analysis of risk factors and clinical signs in 57 patients. Neurology 1985;35:1654–1657.

75 **Treseler CB, Sugar AM.** Fungal meningitis. Infect Dis Clin North Am 1990; 4:789–808.

76 **Sugarman B, Massanari RM.** Candida meningitis in patients with CSF shunts. Arch Neurol 1980;37:180–181.

77 **Flynn PM, Marina NM, Rivera GK, Hughes WT.** *Candida tropicalis* infections in children with leukemia. Leuk Lymphoma 1993;10:369–376.

78 **Glick C, Graves GR, Feldman S.** Neonatal fungemia and amphotericin B. South Med J 1993;86:1368–1371.

79 **Buchs J.** Candida meningitis: A growing threat to premature and full-term infants. Pediatr Infect Dis 1985;4:122–124.

80 **Goldsmith LS, Rubenstein SD, Wolfson BJ, Faerber EN, Fisher MC.** Cerebral calcifications in a neonate with candidiasis. Pediatr Infect Dis J 1990;9:451–453.

81 **Ehni WF, Ellison RT, III.** Spontaneous *Candida albicans* meningitis in a patient with the acquired immune deficiency syndrome. Am J Med 1987;83:806–807.

82 **Spencer PM, Jackson GG.** Fungal and mycobacterial infections in patients infected with the human immunodeficiency virus. J Antimicrob Chemother 1989;23(suppl A):107–125.

83 **Bruinsma-Adams IK.** AIDS presenting as *Candida albicans* meningitis: a case report. AIDS 1991;5:1268–1269.

84 **Scheld WM.** Treating systemic fungal infections in AIDS patients. Prolonging life against the odds. Postgrad Med 1990; 88:97–104.

85 **Calderone RA, Scheld WM.** Role of fibronectin in the pathogenesis of candidal infections. Rev Infect Dis 1987; 9(suppl 4):S400–S403.

86 Smego RA, Perfect JR, Durack DT. Combined therapy with amphotericin B and 5-fluorocytosine for Candida meningitis. Rev Infect Dis 1984;6:791–801.

87 Bisbe J, Miro JM, Latorre X, et al. Disseminated candidiasis in addicts who use brown heroin: report of 83 cases and review. Clin Infect Dis 1992;15:910–923.

88 Moyer DV, Edwards JE Jr. Fungal endocarditis. In: Kaye D, ed. Infective Endocarditis, 2nd ed. New York: Raven Press, 1992:299–312.

89 Hallum JL, Williams TW Jr. Candida endocarditis. In: Bodey GP, ed. Candidiasis: Pathogenesis, Diagnosis and Treatment, 2nd ed. New York: Raven Press, 1993:357–369.

90 Reyes MP, Lerner AM. Endocarditis caused by Candida species. In: Bodey GP, Fainstein V, eds. Candidiasis. New York: Raven Press, 1985:203–209.

91 Galgiani JN, Stevens DA. Fungal endocarditis: need for guidelines in evaluating therapy. J Thorac Cardiovasc Surg 1977;73:293–296.

92 Czwerwiec FS, Bilsker MS, Kamerman ML, Bisno AL. Long-term survival after fluconazole therapy of candidal prosthetic valve endocarditis. Am J Med 1993; 94:545–546.

93 Hernandez JA, Gonzalez-Moreno M, Llibre JM, Aloy A, Casan CM. Candidal mitral endocarditis and long-term treatment with fluconazole in a patient with human immunodeficiency virus infection. Clin Infect Dis 1992;15:1062–1063.

94 Cuende E, Barbadillo C, E-Mazzucchelli R, Isasi C, Trujillo A, Andreu JL. Candida arthritis in adult patients who are not intravenous drug addicts: report of three cases and review of the literature. Semin Arthritis Rheum 1993;22:224–241.

95 Rotrosen D, Calderone RA, Edwards JE Jr. Adherence of Candida species to host tissues and plastic surfaces. Rev Infect Dis 1986;8:73–85.

96 Seelig MS, Speth CP, Kozinn PJ, Taschdjian CL, Toni EF, Goldberg P. Patterns of Candida endocarditis following cardiac surgery: importance of early diagnosis and therapy (an analysis of 91 cases). Prog Cardiovas Dis 1974;XVII:125–160.

97 Koch AE. Candida albicans infection of a prosthetic knee replacement: a report and review of the literature. J Rheumatol 1988; 15:362–365.

98 Walsh TJ, Bustamente CI, Vlahov D, Standiford HC. Candidal suppurative peripheral thrombophlebitis: recognition, prevention, and management. Infect Control 1986;7:16–22.

99 Pons V, Greenspan D, DeBruin M, The Multicenter Study Group. Therapy for oropharyngeal candidiasis in HIV-infected patients: a randomized, prospective multicenter study of oral fluconazole versus clotrimazole troches. J Acquir Immune Defic Syndr 1993;6:1311–1316.

100 Barchiesi F, Giacometti A, Arzeni D, et al. Fluconazole and ketoconazole in the treatment of oral and esophageal candidiasis in AIDS patients. J Chemother 1992;4:381–386.

101 Laine L, Dretler RH, Conteas CN, et al. Fluconazole compared with ketoconazole for the treatment of Candida esophagitis in AIDS. A randomized trial. Ann Intern Med 1992;117:655–660.

102 Pennazio M, Arrigoni A, Spandre M, et al. Endoscopy to detect oral and oesophageal candidiasis in acquired immune deficiency syndrome. Ital J Gastroenterol 1992;24:324–327.

103 Lopez-Dupla M, Mora Sanz P, Pintado Garcia V, et al. Clinical, endoscopic, immunologic, and therapeutic aspects of oropharyngeal and esophageal candidiasis in HIV-infected patients: a survey of 114 cases. Am J Gastroenterol 1992;87:1771–1776.

104 Porro GB, Parente F, Cernuschi M. The diagnosis of esophageal candidiasis in patients with acquired immune deficiency syndrome: is endoscopy always necessary? Am J Gastroenterol 1989;84:143–146.

105 Parente F, Cernuschi M, Rizzardini G, Lazzarin A, Valsecchi L, Bianchi Porro G. Opportunistic infections of the esophagus not responding to oral systemic antifungals in patients with AIDS: their frequency and treatment. Am J Gastroenterol 1991;86:1729–1734.

106 Korting HC, Blecher P, Froschl M, Braun-Falco O. Quantitative assessment of the efficacy of oral ketoconazole for oral candidosis in HIV-infected patients. Mycoses 1992;35:173–176.

107 Marriott DJ, Jones PD, Hoy JF, Speed BR, Harkness JL. Fluconazole once a week as secondary prophylaxis against oropharyngeal candidiasis in HIV-infected patients. A double-blind placebo-controlled study. Med J Aust 1993;158:312–316.

108 **Rosenblatt HM, Stiehm ER.** Therapy of chronic mucocutaneous candidiasis. Proceedings of a symposium on new developments in therapy for the mycoses. Am J Med 1983;74(1B Jan suppl):20–22.

109 **Stevens DA, Greene SI, Lang OS.** Thrush can be prevented in patients with acquired immunodeficiency syndrome and the acquired immunodeficiency syndrome-related complex. Randomized, double-blind, placebo-controlled study of 100 mg oral fluconazole daily. Arch Intern Med 1991;151:2458–2464.

110 **Leen CL, Dunbar EM, Ellis ME, Mandal BK.** Once-weekly fluconazole to prevent recurrence of oropharyngeal candidiasis in patients with AIDS and AIDS-related complex: a double-blind placebo-controlled study. J Infect 1990;21:55–60.

111 **Reynes J, Mallie M, Andre D, Janbon F, Bastide JM.** Traitement et prophylaxie secondaire par fluconazole des candidoses oropharyngees des sujets VIH +. Analyse mycologique des echecs. Pathol Biol (Paris) 1992;40:513–517.

112 **Bruatto M, Marinuzzi G, Raiteri R, Sinicco A.** Susceptibility to ketoconazole of *Candida albicans* strains from sequentially followed HIV-1 patients with recurrent oral candidosis. Mycoses 1992; 35:53–56.

113 **Heinic GS, Stevens DA, Greenspan D, et al.** Fluconazole-resistant Candida in AIDS patients. Report of two cases. Oral Surg Oral Med Oral Pathol 1993;76:711–715.

114 **Sanguineti A, Carmichael JK, Campbell K.** Fluconazole-resistant *Candida albicans* after long-term suppressive therapy. Arch Intern Med 1993;153:1122–1124.

115 **Azon-Masoliver A, Vilaplana J.** Fluconazole-induced toxic epidermal necrolysis in a patient with human immunodeficiency virus infection. Dermatology 1993;187:268–269.

116 **Medoff G.** Controversial areas in antifungal chemotherapy: short-course and combination therapy with amphotericin B. Rev Infect Dis 1987;9:403–407.

117 **Reiss E, Morrison CJ.** Nonculture methods for diagnosis of disseminated candidiasis. Clin Microbiol Rev 1993; 6:311–323.

118 **Antman K, Griffin J, Elias A, et al.** Effect of recombinant human granulocyte-macrophage colony stimulating factor on chemotherapy-induced myelosuppression. N Engl J Med 1988;319:593–598.

119 **Gabrilove J, Jakubowski A, Scher H, et al.** Effect of granulocyte colony-stimulating factor on neutropenia and associated morbidity due to chemotherapy for transitional-cell carcinoma of the urothelium. N Engl J Med 1988;318: 1414–1422.

120 **Brandt S, Peters W, Atwater S, et al.** Effect of recombinant human granulocyte-macrophage colony stimulating factor on hematopoietic recognition after high-dose chemotherapy and autologous bone marrow transplantation. N Engl J Med 1988;318:869–876.

121 **Kullberg BJ, Van't Wout JW, Hoogstraten C, Van Furth R.** Recombinant interferon-gamma enhances resistance to acute disseminated *Candida albicans* infection in mice. J Infect Dis 1993; 168:436–443.

122 **Hague RA, Eastham EJ, Lee RE, Cant AJ.** Resolution of hepatic abscess after interferon gamma in chronic granulomatous disease. Arch Dis Child 1993;69:443–445.

An Approach to Acute Fever and Rash (AFR) in the Adult

STUART LEVIN
LARRY J. GOODMAN

In approaching the problem of acute fever and rash (AFR) in the adult, we have benefited from previous outstanding articles on the same subject written by many authors. Special credit must be given to Dr. James D. Cherry and Dr. Herbert A. Wenner, pediatricians who have made monumental contributions to this extensive and deceptively complex subject. With a few exceptions, we have purposely eliminated the category of local and regional inflammation of the skin, believing that to be more appropriately covered as a separate review subject. We have decided to use eight categories of skin rash and have chosen to put each illness in its most characteristic (and most unique) category whenever possible (1,2). Ideally, a picture atlas of skin rashes due to infection would be a useful adjunct to this chapter.

BACKGROUND

Historically the recognition and accurate description of the black plague due to *Pasteurella pestis* and spotted fever epidemics due to *Neisseria meningitides*, as well as the numbering of common febrile exanthems from first through sixth disease (measles, scarlet fever, rubella, unknown illness, erythema infectiosum, and roseola) speak to the obvious interest of pre-twentieth century physicians in the combination of fever and rash (3–5).

Most recent review articles about the AFR syndrome are either limited to the pediatric age group or have not separated the adult experience from the more common pediatric one (1,2).

In the best of circumstances, rashes associated with fever can be suggestive of an etiology but are usually not diagnostic and are often so nondescript that only knowledge of the entire clinical syndrome, season, recent and past travel history, local epidemic information, environmental and human contacts, and simultaneous associated organ system involvement can lead to an appropriate diagnosis. A serious potential error that may be made in the AFR patient is failure to notice the rash or specific lesions because of inattention.

The specialty of dermatology stresses the careful observation and accurate description of skin lesions. The infectious disease specialist must pay attention to such details as the plane of the skin involved, size, shape, texture, color, arrangement, distribution, extent, symmetry, and depth of the lesion. However, the patient with AFR requires a greater integration of the complete illness with the description of the rash than is often necessary for the correct diagnosis of many chronic skin conditions. Complicating the diagnosis are the rapidly changing characteristics of many common febrile exanthems. In the more serious AFR condition, the characteristic or more diagnostic rash may not appear in optimal time to help the clinician begin specific therapy or institute appropriate public health measures.

In the adult, the classification of organisms commonly associated with a high percentage of skin manifestations in symptomatic individuals include viral groups, rickettsia, and spirochetes. On the other hand, chlamydia, legionella, most bacteria, mycobacteria, fungi, and most protozoa are not usually associated with disseminated rashes in normal hosts. However, many exceptions exist to these useful generalizations.

Common Exanthem Patterns

There are approximately eight patterns that the infectious disease specialist should look for in attempting to master the interesting and occasionally urgent clinical problem of the AFR (see Table 2.1). They include the following: macular–papular rashes centrally distributed; macular–papular rashes with acral or peripheral distribution, including erythema multiforme; macular–papular rashes with a larger, earlier, more advanced single eschar with or without regional adenitis (herald lesion or tache noire); diffuse confluent bright erythema; pustular, vesicular, or bullous rashes; disseminated nodules including erythema nodosum; urticarial rashes; and petechial or hemorrhagic rashes (2). If diagnosticians can accurately characterize the sometimes rapidly changing skin rash into one of these categories, the differential diagnosis of the AFR in the adult can become somewhat more focused.

It must be understood that there is considerable overlap among all these syndromes, and that while one agent may cause many syndromes, many agents may also cause a single similar syndrome. We expect that new information and wiser insights will lead to modifications of this approach in the future.

Decreasing Classical Exanthems

With the institution of national immunization programs for rubella and measles and the soon to be released varicella vaccine, plus the extensive use of antimicrobial therapy for streptococcal infections resulting in fewer cases of scarlet fever, literally millions of patients with febrile exanthems who would previously have been seen on a yearly basis are now happily eliminated from the clinical experience of physicians.

Thus, classical first, second, and third diseases have now become quite rare. Similarly, as smallpox has been eradicated and smallpox vaccination eliminated, the local, regional, and systemic complication of smallpox vaccination with the vaccinia virus will also no longer be seen.

"New" AFR in Normal Hosts

There are a number of newly recognized or etiologically solved AFR. Parvovirus B19 is now an established cause of classical fifth disease or erythema infectiosum, whereas sixth disease (roseola or exanthema subitum) has been shown to be caused by the newly discovered herpes virus 6 (HSV-VI). The newly described tick-borne intracellular pathogen, *Ehrlichia chaffeensis*, may cause a febrile, diffuse, centrally located rash in up to 30% of cases and can mimic Rocky Mountain spotted fever (RMSF). A new indigenous strain of classical typhus has caused human disease in the southeast United States. The source of this is the flying squirrel. Lyme disease is another recently characterized illness of great notoriety and is caused by the tick-transmitted spirochete *Borrelia burgdorferi*. Thirty percent of patients with the initial tick bite-induced erythema chronicum migrans lesion will develop multiple widespread erythematous macules. *Pseudomonas aeruginosa* is a cause of nonfebrile, diffuse folliculitis in otherwise healthy individuals exposed to contaminated heated whirlpools and hot tubs. Toxic shock syndrome due to *Staphylococcus aureus* and the even more dangerous *Streptococcus pyogenes* can be differentiated from both scarlet fever and the mucocutaneous lymph node syndrome (Kawasaki syndrome).

"New" AFR in Immunocompromised Hosts

A number of clinical syndromes have been described in the new human immunodeficiency virus (HIV) pandemic, including an acute fever macular rash syndrome that is seen as an initial HIV clinical illness in one-third of new cases and may be predictive of a shorter incubation period for acquired immunodeficiency syndrome (AIDS). The etiologic agents associated with cat scratch disease, *Rochalimaea henselae* and *Rochalimaea quintana* have been shown to cause disseminated bacillary angiomatosis in HIV patients.

Unfortunately, the graft-versus-host reaction (GVHR) has become an important illness in patients receiving blood transfusions (rarely) and in patients undergoing transplant (more commonly). GVHR is characterized by fever, a specific rash, and multiorgan involvement. The disseminated nodule and fever syndrome is an important problem in leukopenic patients receiving immunosuppressive therapy and is often caused by fungi and mycobacteria. These are truly illnesses of recent medical progress, and the lesions demand early biopsy and appropriate processing of the specimen to identify these pathogens in a timely manner. Localized *ecthyma gangrenosum* lesions characterize another recently described syndrome seen in neutropenic patients. These lesions are primarily caused by *P. aeruginosa, Aeromonas hydrophilia,* and *Candida* species.

Noninfectious Causes of the AFR

Drug reactions are the major noninfectious mimics of the AFR presentation. These allergic rashes may manifest any of the described patterns and should be part of the differential diagnosis for many of the situations described in this chapter. In fact, in all difficult diagnostic problems, the consultant must return to drug reactions as a possible cause.

The collagen vascular diseases of unknown etiology, such as juvenile rheumatoid arthritis (JRA), vasculitis, and thrombotic thrombocytopenia purpura often manifest the symptoms of rash and fever, but the course of the rash is almost always subacute to chronic Kawasaki syndrome, and

Table 2.1.   Types of Rashes and Associated Causes in the Adult with AFR

Rash type	Associated Diseases/Organisms
Maculopapular (reticular) rash-central	Rubeola
	Rubella
	Enteroviruses
	Erythema infectiosum
	Roseola
	Rickettsial prowazekii (endemic typhus)
	Rickettsial typhi (murine typhus)
	Ehrlichiosis
	Leptospirosis
	Arboviruses
Acral or peripheral macular-papular skin rash	Rocky Mountain spotted fever
	Secondary syphilis
	Erythema multiforme
	Atypical measles
	Hand-foot-and-mouth syndrome
	Streptobacillus moniliformis
	Acrodermatitis enteropathica
Diffuse skin rash with eschar and regional adenitis	Rickettsial pox
	Scrub typhus
	Boutonneuse fever
	Queensland fever
	North Asia fever
	Oriental spotted fever
	Spirillum minus
	Lyme disease
	Trypanosomiasis
	Pityriasis rosea

Table 2.1. *Continued*

Rash type	Associated Diseases/Organisms
Diffuse confluent erythema	Scarlet fever
	Staphylococcal toxic shock syndrome
	Streptococcal toxic shock syndrome
	Staphylococcal scalded skin syndrome
	Kawasaki syndrome
Vesicular-bullous rash	Chickenpox
	Disseminated herpes simplex
	Disseminated herpes zoster
	Smallpox
	Vaccinia
	Monkeypox
	Vibrio vulnificus
Disseminated nodules and fever syndrome	Candida sp.
	Coccidioidomycosis
	Sporotrichosis
	Cryptococcus
	Histoplasmosis
	Fusaria sp.
	Mycobacteria
	Disseminated necrotic macronodules
	Factitious panniculitis
	Erythema nodosum
Diffuse urticarial rash and fever	Acute hepatitis B and urticaria
	Enterovirus infections (coxsackie A-9)
	Acute schistosomiasis
	Strongyloides stercoralis
	Loiasis
	Trichinosis
	Onchocerciasis
Petechial—hemorrhagic rash—AFR	Acute meningococcemia—chronic meningococcemia
	Echo-9 and other enterovirus
	Viral hemorrhagic fevers

eosinophilia myalgia syndrome can also mimic the febrile exanthem of infections. Although a specific diagnosis can eventually be made with correct serologic tests or biopsy results, on rare occasion these illnesses may present in an acute form.

Some classical dermatologic illnesses may present with the signs of fever and rash and resemble infectious syndromes. These conditions include Fabry's disease, Sweet's disease, acrodermatitis enteropathica, dermatitis herpetiformis, and acute intermittent porphyria. Pyoderma gangrenosum, a regional skin ulceration, does not fulfill the criteria of a diffuse rash, but surely presents infectious disease specialists with a puzzle unless they are familiar with the many presentations of this illness.

MACULAR–PAPULAR (RETICULAR) RASHES—CENTRALLY LOCATED

The central macular–papular rash is the most common of the eight skin rash patterns. A significant number of respiratory and enteric viral pathogens such as influenza, parainfluenza, mumps, rhinovirus, adenovirus, reovirus, and rotavirus, are rarely considered as causes of febrile exanthems, but these pathogens do result in a central macular–papular rash in 1 to 5% of cases, mostly in the pediatric population (6–8). In these circumstances, the particular rashes add no additional diagnostic information, but their presence might lead the confused physician to rule out the correct diagnosis. Additionally, illnesses such as those caused by Epstein-Barr virus (EBV), cytomegalovirus (CMV), *Toxoplasma*, and HIV, which on occasion are the sole cause of an AFR, are much more likely to have associated acute febrile rashes because of their unique propensity to drug reactions (9–11). For patients infected with CMV and EBV, ampicillin is the chief culprit; in the case of HIV infection, many drugs such as trimethoprim, sulfonamides, dapsone, and others can do this. Brucellosis, tularemia, Q fever, psittacosis, and plague will also cause the development of diffuse central macular rashes in a small number of cases, although they have no reputation for this association (12–15).

Measles (Rubeola)—First Disease

The rash of measles usually is first noted on the second or third day of illness (10 to 14 days after exposure) and is the finding that separates the initial presentation of fever and coryza from a common viral cold. The exanthem begins on the back of the head, behind the ears, and at the hair line and spreads centrifugally to involve most of the body. The palms and soles are spared. The rash is an erythematous macular–papular one, with areas of confluence at the sites involved initially. The erythema blanches on pressure. The rash lasts at least 3 days and then begins to fade. As it fades, the blanching erythema darkens and appears as a nonblanching brownish "stain" that fades entirely over the next several days. Many patients have mild desquamation of the superficial skin at this time. By the time the rash fades, fever, cough, and coryza should be nearly gone. If not, a secondary bacterial infection should be suspected. Koplik's spots are small white raised dots (1 to 2 mm) seen opposite the lower molars on the buccal mucosa. They are first seen 1 to 2 days before the rash and are pathognomonic of measles. Electron microscopic study suggests that both Koplik's spots and the exanthem of measles are due to direct infection of the epithelia by the virus (16).

Two variants of this classical presentation occur in vaccine recipients. The first, atypical measles, is found almost exclusively in recipients of the killed measles vaccine, which has not been distributed since 1967. Between 1963 and 1967, nearly 2 million doses of killed vaccine were administered. First described in 1965, atypical measles begins with a macular–papular rash on the distal extremities, which moves centripetally (17). Vesicle formation, pruritus, and purpura may be seen (18). A hemorrhagic, purpuric, petechial rash mimicking meningococcemia is a second type of rash in the atypical measles syndrome (19). Koplik's spots are not part of the presentation. Coryza is absent or minimal, but fever and respiratory symptoms frequently persist for 10 days or more. Respiratory symptoms and chest x-ray abnormalities are common and help differentiate this disease from RMSF, which also is characterized by a centripetal rash. A more difficult clinical differentiation to make is the vesicular rash and pulmonary presentation of atypical measles from chickenpox.

A second syndrome in vaccinated individuals is the so-called vaccine-modified mild measles. Most patients vaccinated with the live virus vaccine have long-term persistence of antibody and presumed protection. However, outbreaks in highly vaccinated populations suggest that this protection is incomplete in some cases (20). Mild measles is usually characterized by a rash illness (similar to classic measles) with a fourfold or greater change in complement fixation or hemagglutination titers with negative IgM titers. Coryza, conunctivitis, and cough are present in fewer than half the cases. These patients do not appear to be contagious. This syndrome is particularly common in adolescents and young adults.

In the immunocompromised patient, pulmonary involvement with giant cell pneumonia is a common and serious complication of measles, which can develop in the absence of a rash (21).

Rubella (Third Disease)—German Measles

The rash of rubella (German measles/3-day measles) is maculopapular and begins on the face and spreads to cover most of the body. Forscheimer spots (petechiae on the soft palate) are a supportive but not diagnostic finding. Patients usually have malaise and adenopathy of the posterior neck. Fever may be present for the first day of illness, and most patients have coryza. The rash rarely lasts beyond 5 days and may clear with a mild desquamation. Severe illness and bacterial superinfection are rare. Despite the transient and mild clinical illness, patients are infectious from 10 days prior to the rash to 2 weeks after its onset. Congenital rubella, resulting from infection of a pregnant woman and transmission to the fetus, has been associated with multiple congenital defects (mental retardation, deafness, glaucoma, heart disease). Treatment of infected pregnant women with immune globulin does not appear to prevent viremia and subsequent fetal infection (22). Arthritis that begins with the onset of the rash may persist for months after the other manifestations of rubella have cleared. This complication resolves over months and may be seen in up to one-third of women who become infected (23). For unknown reasons, a smaller percentage of men develop arthritis.

Enteroviruses

Enteroviruses are believed to be responsible for the majority of rash illnesses in children. They produce a wide variety of syndromes which, with the exception of herpangina and hand-foot-and-mouth disease, are not distinctive by their appearance. Although adults are less frequently infected, when infection occurs, it is more severe. Most enterovirus infections mimic the skin manifestation of rubella (echovirus 2, 4, 9, 11, 19, 25 and coxsackie virus A9). However, other enteroviruses may resemble roseola (echovirus 11, 16, and 25 and coxsackie virus B1 and B5) or chickenpox (coxsakie virus A4).

Erythema Infectiosum—Fifth Disease

Erythema infectiosum, or fifth disease, is another diffuse maculopapular rash syndrome. The rash begins on the face with a bright erythema suggesting "slapped cheeks." Unlike erysipelas, scarlet fever, or the toxic shock syndromes, the rash of erythema infectiosum begins after the fever has abated. Patients are not particularly toxic but may have an associated sore throat, headache, or generalized malaise. Later, a diffuse erythematous maculopapular rash develops over the body. In about 15% of cases, a lacy erythema will fade and recur over the next 3 or more weeks (24).

Roseola

Like erythema infectiosum, the rash of roseola infantum (exanthem subitum) presents following a period of fever when the patient is clinically improved. However, the rash is usually confined to the body (sparing the face) and fades within days without sequelae. Although diffuse erythema has been reported, it is typically a maculopapular eruption. Human herpesvirus 6 is the cause of this infection (25). A similar clinical picture is seen with echovirus 16 (the Boston exanthem).

Rickettsial Infections

Rickettsia prowazekii (Epidemic Louse-borne Typhus, Classical Typhus)   Classical louse-borne epidemic typhus is now a rare disease in the United States and the rest of the world, except in the mountainous areas of the Andes in South America, the Himalayas, and the mountainous regions of North Africa. However, at the end of World War I, 30 million cases occurred in eastern Europe in a 4-year period. The conditions of war, natural disaster, and extreme cold weather with inadequate housing fostered the conditions necessary for the spread of human body lice that transmit this disease.

The clinical syndrome in typhus consists of fever, headache, and a central macular–papular rash involving the trunk and extremities and rarely involving the face, palms, or soles. There is no eschar. The rash will often evolve from a blanching pink macular rash to a confluent dense rash with petechiae. Pathologically, a diffuse vasculitis affects many organs, and a mortality rate of 10 to 40% in untreated patients can be seen. The diagnosis of typhus depends on knowledge of local conditions of places on the patient's travel itinerary and specific complement fixation (CF) serology, or a positive Weil-Felix OX-19 titer. Recently, polymerase chain reaction (PCR) has been used to make the diagnosis (26,27). A single dose of doxycycline is curative.

Recrudescent *Rickettsia prowazekii* (Brill-Zinsser Disease)   Brill-Zinsser disease is a mild form of epidemic typhus caused by a relapse of an infection acquired as many as 30 to 50 years before. The rash is similar in distribution to classical typhus, but it is more evanescent. The diagnosis is made by an occasionally positive low titer OX-19. More specifically, the diagnosis is made using the CF test for *R. prowazekii*. In these patients only IgG antibodies are present, as opposed to the presence of IgM antibodies in acute classical typhus (28).

***Rickettsia prowazekii*—Typhus Indigenous to the United States**   The indigenous typhus strain in the United States is a variant of the classical epidemic typhus strain. Recently 15 cases have been described in human beings in the southeastern United States, and the flying squirrel is considered to be a reservoir. The method of spread is not yet determined, but squirrel lice or fleas are the chief suspects. Indigenous typhus is significantly milder than classical typhus, and the typical central rash seen in typhus is more evanescent in this illness. However, as many as 40% of patients have had serious central nervous system (CNS) symptoms in addition to headache. All of the patients have recovered. Eighty percent of the cases occurred in the winter months when RMSF is rarely seen (29).

Murine Typhus—Endemic Typhus—*Rickettsii typhi*   Murine typhus is observed throughout the world and is usually spread from rat fleas to human beings. However, recent epidemiology suggests that the cat flea, which also inhabits skunks, racoons, and opossums, may be the vector of murine typhus in the Rio Grande area of southern Texas. This area is now the major source of murine typhus in the United States. Outside of the Texas Rio Grande area, the illness is seen much more commonly in the United States in urban environments rather than rural environments (30).

Severe headache, myalgia, fever, and a central rash seen mostly on the trunk and proximal extremities characterize this illness. There is no eschar. A rash is seen in 70 to 80% of patients and rarely effects the palms and soles. The illness is milder in children than adults, and it is much less severe than classical typhus. There are fewer CNS symptoms and far fewer complications involving the cardiorespiratory or renal systems. A rapid lysis of fever occurs with tetracycline (30,31). The central rash distribution, urban location, and serology help differentiate murine typhus from RMSF. Serologic studies will eventually show a positive OX-19 titer and a variable but lower OX-2 titer. Tetracycline is the drug of choice.

Q Fever and Rash   Q fever is a worldwide disease caused by the rickettsia, *Coxiella burnetii*. The illness is acquired by inhalation of infectious aerosols and is usually seen in animal slaughterhouse workers. The most common clinical syndromes include a self-limited febrile illness, pneumonia, hepatitis, and endocarditis. Traditionally the differences between Q fever and other rickettsia were a negative Weil-Felix reaction throughout the course of the illness, the absence of an insect vector, and the absence of a rash. However, in two recent studies, a centrally located macular papular rash was seen in 6% and 21% of patients with acute Q fever, and a petechial rash was seen in 37% of patients with chronic Q fever endocarditis (32–34). The diagnosis of Q fever is made by serology. Tetracycline is the therapy of choice for the acute pneumonia.

***Ehrlichia chaffeensis*—Ehrlichiosis**   Ehrlichiosis is a recently described tick-borne illness most commonly seen in the mid-Atlantic and central southwestern United States (35–37). *E. chaffeensis* is a very small obligate intracellular bacteria that is leukotropic and goes through the three stages of development similar to the *Chlamydia* species.

The clinical illness of ehrlichiosis is similar to rickettsial infections. The chief symptoms are fever, headache, abdominal pain, and arthralgia. A rash is seen in about 40% of patients and is central in distribution.

Leukopenia, lymphopenia, and thrombocytopenia are characteristic of acute ehrlichiosis. The illness is usually differentiated from typical RMSF because there is either no rash in ehrlichiosis or there is a central macular–papular rash, which occurs in 10 to 30% of cases. The rash almost never involves the extremities or the palms or soles of the feet. The diagnosis of ehrlichiosis is made by serology, and tetracycline is the current drug of choice. The illness is much less serious than RMSF.

Zoonotic, Spirochetes, and AFR

Tick-borne Relapsing Fever—*Borrelia recurrentis*   The spirochete, *Borrelia recurrentis*, is acquired in the western mountains of the United States from a tick bite. Three to seven days after the tick bite (usually not noticed), there is a sudden onset of chills, fever, headache, prostration, severe weakness, myalgias, backache, and arthralgias. Nausea, vomiting, diarrhea, abdominal pain, cough, and dyspnea may also appear. Physical examination reveals an ill-appearing patient with splenomegaly, lymphadenopathy, and hepatic tenderness. Jaundice can appear in one-third of patients. A central macular–papular rash is seen in 5 to 50% of patients. The rash can be petechial. Rarely, a tiny 2-mm pruritic eschar can be seen.

The attack lasts 3 to 7 days; however, the most characteristic part of this illness is the relapsing course that ensues. In the absence of antibiotic therapy, an average of three attacks occur with up to 13 attacks having been recorded in some patients. The afebrile episodes can last between one and 60 days, and the subsequent attack is generally milder and shorter than the preceding one. All symptoms and signs disappear with resolution of fever and generally return with its appearance. Therapy is successful with tetracycline or doxycycline. The Jarisch-Herxheimer reaction is consistently seen in patients who receive therapy for this disease. In the United States, death from the tick-borne relapsing fever syndrome is rare. Microscopic diagnosis is made from the peripheral blood smears, looking for the extracellular large spirochetes (38–41).

Leptospirosis—AFR Leptospirosis is acquired from contaminated water containing the spirochete *Leptospira interrogans*. This spirochete can penetrate through the oral mucosa or through cutaneous lesions. The highly variable symptoms of this disease include headache, myalgia, nausea, and vomiting. Physical findings of conjunctivitis and occasional scleral hemorrhages and a central macular–papular rash are seen in 20 to 50% of cases. Other laboratory abnormalities include cerebral spinal fluid (CSF) lymphocytic pleocytosis, elevated blood, urea, nitrogen (BUN) and bilirubin levels, and thrombocytopenia. Tetracycline therapy becomes relatively limited in efficacy if the illness is not treated within the first 5 days. Tetracycline prophylaxis has been found to be successful, and penicillin therapy has also been found to be efficacious. The diagnosis is made on clinical grounds (the hepatorenal syndrome) using the combination of conjunctivitis, myalgia, and aseptic meningitis. Urine and blood cultures are occasionally positive, and serologic titers can be used to confirm the diagnosis at a later date. This disease in its most fulminant course is called ictero hemorrhagic fever (Weil's disease). Leptospirosis is one of the zoonotic infections that can be acquired in an urban setting, with many sick patients acquiring it from dog urine transmitted to the owner during the winter (42,43).

Arbovirus and AFR

West Nile fever (seen on three continents) and classical dengue fever (seen on five continents) are caused by flaviviruses and are the most widespread common cause of AFR syndrome due to arboviruses. Both viruses cause a central macular–papular rash with polyarthralgia. Dengue virus is the prototypic member of the arbovirus AFR group, and any one of dozens of the arboviruses in which fever and diffuse rash (AFR) are present is said to be dengue-like. The classical presentation of dengue virus includes abrupt onset of fever, chills, headache, myalgia, arthralgia, back pain, conjunctivitis, pharyngitis, lymphopenia, thrombocytopenia, increased bands, leukopenia, and central rash (44–46).

More than 100 arboviruses may infect human beings. Initial febrile rashes seen in the first two days of illness may be replaced by more dense macular–papular rashes by the end of the first week of illness. Up to now, only a few other arboviruses such as the Bunyaviridae-like agents Bangui, Bwamba,

Dugbe, and Tataguine, and other viruses including Usutu, Orungo, and Zika from Africa, Chandipura from India, and Kunjin from Australia have been found to be causes of the AFR (47).

In the United States none of the mosquito-borne encephalitis illnesses— Eastern, Western, St. Louis, California, and Venezuela—or the tick-borne encephalitis illnesses due to Powassan virus have been associated with rashes (48). However, Colorado tick fever rarely causes encephalitis but does cause a central rash in 5 to 12% of cases (49,50). Internationally, many important arbovirus infections, including Japanese encephalitis, Rift Valley fever, sandfly fever, Murray Valley fever, Ilhéus fever, and Semliki Forest fever do not cause the development of rashes (47).

On each inhabited continent except North America, mosquito-borne arbovirus infections cause a significant number of nonspecific AFR. Although rash is not universal, it is characteristic of the following five alpha viruses: chikungunya and O'nyong-nyong of East Africa, Majora of South America, Ross River of Australia and the South Pacific, and the relatively infrequent but widely distributed Sinbis virus of Asia, Africa, and Europe. These five viruses typically induce multiple tender swollen joints, fever, and a macular–papular rash centrally located (51–53).

Typhoid Fever

Typhoid fever caused by *Salmonella typhi* has several associated skin rashes. "Rose spots" are centrally distributed erythematous macules and papules. They are painless, rarely seen on the extremities or face, measure 2 to 4 mm in diameter, and blanche on pressure. Cultures of skin biopsy yield organisms in over 50% of cases (54). These lesions are suggestive but not diagnostic of typhoid fever. They are also usually seen in brucellosis, leptospirosis, psittacosis, and rat bite fever. Erythema typhosum (a diffuse erythema) and erythema nodosum have also been seen in patients with typhoid fever.

ACRAL OR PERIPHERAL MACULAR–PAPULAR SKIN RASH

This pattern contains a diverse variety of pathogens and clinical syndromes that generally induce dissimilar clinical pictures. The unifying theme in this classification is the concentration of the early rash on the palms and soles and dorsum of feet and hands, with extension of the rash centrally. This is in contrast to the majority of diffuse macular–papular rashes that start centrally on the proximal extremities or on the chest or back and were described above. The final stages of both pattern I and pattern II rashes can rarely exactly mimic each other.

The major conditions in this "peripheral" group are secondary syphilis, RMSF, erythema multiforme, or the more severe Stevens-Johnson syndrome, and hand-foot-and-mouth disease. Specific dermatologic manifestations of endocarditis, particularly acute staphylococcal endocarditis, can concentrate macules or large hemorrhagic lesions on the fingers, toes, palms, and soles.

Non-infectious disorders associated with multiple peripheral cyanotic or gangrenous changes (blue toes syndrome) include atheroembolism, cholesterol or platelet emboli, myxoma, mural thrombi, hyperviscosity syndromes, primary and secondary hypercoagulable syndromes, vasculitis, vasospastic disorders, and drug reactions.

Another group of impressive acral rashes is seen with the bright palm and sole erythema of the toxic shock syndromes, Kawasaki syndrome and acute graft-versus-host disease (GVHD).

Rocky Mountain Spotted Fever

Rocky Mountain spotted fever caused by tick-borne *Rickettsia rickettsii* is the most common rickettsial infection in the United States and its incidence is apparently increasing. It is also the most serious of all tick-borne rickettsial infections in the world. It presents one of the most difficult dilemmas to the infectious disease specialists of the United States. As in most rickettsial infections the classical triad of rash, fever, and headache is typical, but the complete triad is present in only two-thirds of cases. Symptoms of fever and myalgia usually begin about 4 days after the tick bite, a history of which is obtainable in less than 50% of patients. In 20% of patients no rash is seen until after the sixth day of constitutional symptoms, and 5% of the patients will not develop a rash until after the tenth day of illness, with 2 to 5% of patients never demonstrating any observable rash. In approximately 66 to 80% of patients, the rash will begin around the wrists and ankles, eventually involving the palms and soles and spreading to the rest of the body. In approximately 50% of patients the rash is petechial. In the other half, it is a nonspecific macular–papular rash. In 15 to 25% of the patients the rash will start on the trunk or appear to start everywhere at once (55,56).

Rocky Mountain spotted fever is notorious for the potential to form a petechial purpuric rash that can mimic fulminant meningococcemia. In many patients, the rash can become fully hemorrhagic leading in about 5% of these cases to severe skin necrosis that requires multiple skin grafts if the patient survives (57,58). Features similar to meningococcemia include the sudden onset of severe constitutional symptoms, petechial rash, thrombocytopenia, severe headache, meningeal symptoms, a relatively high frequency of disease in otherwise very healthy young adults, and the potential for death if the correct therapy is not given very early in the course of the illness. In patients with RMSF, the white blood cell (WBC) count is generally normal or slightly elevated, with mild lymphocytosis, whereas in patients with meningococcemia, the WBC is generally very high and there is a profound left shift. The poorly named RMSF is usually seen in the southeast United States, particularly in the Carolinas and the surrounding states. There is a second focus of RMSF in the southwest central states, particularly centered in Oklahoma. Less than 1 to 2%

of the total cases per year in the United States are actually seen in the Rocky Mountain states. The disease may be more common in New York City than in Montana (59).

A delayed diagnosis can lead to a fatal outcome, and untreated RMSF has mortality rates of 15 to 40% (60). If an early diagnosis can be made within the first 2 to 3 days, when a relatively innocuous looking pale macular pink rash may be present, then appropriate therapy can lead to a very rapid resolution of all symptoms and little or no residual effect (61). Unfortunately, cases in the endemic area can be seen as early as April and as late as December, which are far beyond what many consider the classical tick season (55,56). Many patients can present with any combination of acute abdominal pain; renal, cardiac, or pulmonary failure; musculoskeletal pain; and CNS and ophthalmic complications (62,63). Any of these may confuse the usual classical systemic presentations of RMSF. RMSF has been confused with thrombotic thrombocytopenia purpura (64). Culture is rarely available, and where culture is available, results are not rapid enough. The Weil-Felix reactions OX-2 and OX-19 are insensitive, being positive in less than 50% of proven cases. Only the direct identifications of the organism by PCR and immunofluorescence can provide an early diagnosis (65). Unfortunately, these procedures are not available in most centers.

Empirical therapy with tetracycline or chloramphenicol is necessary in many situations, with an obvious necessity to overtreat by many fold so that the fewest possible number of cases of RMSF are missed (66). In the worst cases of RMSF, patients present with shock, encephalopathy, rash, and fever, which mimics not only meningococcemia, but also mimics severe leptospirosis (Weil's disease) and diffuse hemorrhage, atypical measles in the immunocompromised patient, black measles in the malnourished patient, and the typical severe presentations of toxic shock due to staphylococci or streptococci. The classical conundrum of whether it is RMSF or meningococcal disease is generally best answered by beginning intravenous chloramphenicol or several antibiotics, including tetracycline and a β-lactam, to treat both illnesses simultaneously until a final answer is available.

Secondary Syphilis

Secondary syphilis in the adult is the classical disease to consider when macular lesions are seen on the palms and soles. The rapid plasma reagin (RPR) or another nontreponemal serologic test is mandatory in any patient with an unknown macular–papular rash on the palms and soles. The initial syphilis lesion, the chancre, may still be present in 10% of patients when the diffuse rash appears. In a minority of cases, characteristics of secondary syphilis can mimic the classical tache noire rashes of the tick-borne rickettsial spotted fever group. There is often a transitory rubelliform rash in secondary syphilis that disappears after 24 to 48 hours and then evolves into the more well-known macular–papular rash. The rash may become papular–nodular, but never becomes vesicular or bullous (67).

In addition to the dry, slightly contagious macular–papular skin lesions, there are moist, highly infectious papules called condyloma latum, which are often seen around the genitals, umbilicus, anus, axilla, submammary folds, and the interdigital spaces of fingers and toes. Oral mucus patches, thinning eyebrows, focal alopecia, and local involvement of almost any organ can accompany the highly suggestive rash. Meningovascular syphilis is usually the most serious organ system involved during the secondary syphilis stage. Patients may have severe constitutional symptoms requiring hospitalization, or constitutional symptoms may be nonexistent. The nontreponemal serologic tests are 100% sensitive particularly if blocking antibodies are eliminated.

Appropriate doses and duration of therapy lead to cure in nearly 100% of cases. The Jarisch-Herxheimer reaction will exacerbate skin lesions in 50% of patients with secondary syphilis, as is commonly seen in the rashes of the other spirochetes causing leptospirosis, Lyme disease, and relapsing fever (68). Although palm and sole lesions are not always seen, they are the rule and are the most characteristic finding of the skin rash of secondary syphilis. Vesicles and bullae literally rule out this diagnosis in the adult. The skin lesions of the nonsyphilitic treponemas, which cause yaws, pinta, and bejel, may be ulceronodular, erythematous macules, or patches of vitiligo. However, these are usually afebrile chronic problems and are not the subject of this review.

Erythema Multiforme

Erythema multiforme and its more severe variant, the Stevens-Johnson syndrome, consistently result in the appearance of numerous lesions on the palms and soles very early in the disease. This illness is easily diagnosed with careful observation because of the definitive "target" or "bulls-eye" or "iris" lesions containing clear to hemorrhagic central bullae. The illness is thought to be immunologically mediated. High levels of circulating immune complexes are often seen. Erythema multiforme has been attributed to a large number of infectious illnesses and allergic drug reactions (69).

The most well established infectious agents leading to erythema multiforme are herpes simplex type 1 (HSV-1) and *Mycoplasma pneumoniae* (70). Most recurrent episodes of erythema multiforme are due to HSV-1 (71). *Pasteurella tularensis*, *Yersinia enterocolitica*, histoplasmosis, and coccidioidomycosis also have been consistently associated with erythema multiforme reactions (70). Among many identified drugs, long-acting sulfas, and sulfapyrimethamine are the most well known provocative agents leading to both erythema multiforme and the more severe Stevens-Johnson syndrome. The oral ulcerations of Stevens-Johnson syndrome are very painful, and the patient is generally incapable of swallowing water or food. Most patients with Stevens-Johnson syndrome appear quite toxic. Untreated cases have a mortality rate as high as 5 to 15% (72). In recovered patients, blindness can ensue because of the ophthalmic complications (73).

Even when the characteristic bull's-eye lesions represent only a small percentage of the total multiforme lesions, the diagnosis of erythema multiforme or Stevens-Johnson syndrome is still established. Often the "target" lesions are seen on the palms, and the two characteristic findings grouped together make the diagnosis relatively straightforward, even if the cause remains to be determined.

There is an apparent relationship between erythema multiforme and erythema nodosum in some patients. Histoplasmosis and yersinia bacteria can produce both syndromes in the same patient. Erythema multiforme and toxic epidermal necrolysis (a classical drug-induced serious skin eruption) have also been seen in the same patients and are thought to share some similarities in pathogenesis.

Mycoplasma pneumoniae—**Erythema Multiforme**   In approximately 15% of cases of *Mycoplasma pneumoniae*, a rash will be present, and *M. pneumoniae* should be strongly considered whenever both pneumonia and erythema multiforme or Stevens-Johnson syndrome are present. Other diffuse rashes are also seen with *M. pneumoniae* infections. These include the full gamut of maculopapular, vesicular, petechial, urticarial, and confluent rashes. These rashes are usually but not always present after the fever has begun. Vesicular enanthems and conjunctivitis are also common with *M. pneumoniae* (70).

Atypical Measles

Atypical measles (previously described above) is a now rare disease that is described here because of its remarkable resemblance to the hemorrhagic skin pattern of RMSF. Patients with atypical measles develop a hemorrhagic vesicular rash, peripherally distributed, with swollen hands and feet, severe pneumonia, laryngeal involvement, high-grade fever, and prostration. There should be very few remaining individuals who were immunized with this vaccine in the early 1960s and who have not yet either already developed measles or been protected with the live vaccine (19).

Hand-Foot-and-Mouth Syndrome (Coxsackie A16)

Hand-foot-and-mouth syndrome is one of the most distinctive of all enteroviral syndromes and is usually caused by coxsackie A16 or by enterovirus 71. Other coxsackie A and B viruses have occasionally caused the same syndrome. Following a very short period of fever, multiple oral vesicular lesions form and rapidly ulcerate to form shallow yellow or gray ulcers with surrounding erythema. These lesions occur anywhere in the mouth and can be painful. Simultaneously, small papules, 1/4 cm in size, appear on the dorsum and less commonly on the flexor surfaces of the fingers and feet. Oval vesicles develop within these erythematous lesions and tend to be asymmetrical and flame shaped. The vesicles number between a few and up to 10 to 30 in the adult. Aseptic meningitis or pericarditis can be seen in complicated cases. These diagnostic skin lesions are seen as commonly in the adult population as in children. This is quite different from the other coxsackie and echo virus AFR, where rashes usually appear only in the pediatric age group.

No therapy is available, but eventually the diagnosis can be made either by culture of the vesicles, throat washings, or stool culture, or if the right antigens are available in the laboratory, by convalescent serum antibodies. Although hand-foot-and-mouth syndrome is a vesicular rash, we have included it in this section because of the concentration of the dermal lesions on the hands and feet. This distribution, together with the involvement of the oral mucosa and the asymmetrical flame shape of the skin vesicles with surrounding erythema, resembles no other conditions and become a strong clue for the enteroviral etiology (74).

Rat Bite Fever—Haverhill Fever—*Streptobacillus moniliformis*

Streptobacillus moniliformis is a filamentous gram-negative rod that is a commensal of the oral pharynx of rodents. It is one of the two causes of rat bite fever, but disease often comes from drinking contaminated raw milk. A severe migratory polyarthritis, fever, and erythematous macules, papules, vesicles, pustular and petechial lesions, as well as fully developed scabs characterize the clinical syndrome. The erythematous rash is usually concentrated on the hands, feet, palms, and soles. An eschar is usually absent in rat bite cases because the bite wound has usually healed by the time the rash and fever begin. The diagnosis is generally confirmed by positive blood cultures, and penicillin therapy is effective (75). This organism occasionally causes endocarditis, and skin lesions can be prominent.

Acrodermatitis Enteropathica

Acrodermatitis enteropathica may present, with a reddened ichthyotic plaque-like dermatitis diffusely or limited to involvement of the palms or areas near orifices. It is a chronic syndrome that may be inherited or acquired. Involved skin may be superinfected with bacteria or *Candida* species. Most patients have diarrhea, but fever, toxicity, and mucus membrane involvement are rare. The disease is caused by zinc deficiency, and symptoms are reversed by zinc supplementation (76,77).

DIFFUSE SKIN RASH WITH ESCHAR AND REGIONAL ADENITIS

The third pattern of diffuse macular–papular rashes consists of a combination of a local bite lesion, the eschar, or tache noire or its equivalent, and a diffuse, often centrally located, rash. Diagnosis of the syndromes in this group depends on knowledge of geographically limited infectious agents (78). Many of the eschar-diffuse rash syndromes will resemble each other clinically.

The usual pattern of these cases consists of an insect or animal bite (history known in about half the cases) that evolves over a 2- to 5-day period into a black eschar, usually 1 to 3 cm in size, and often associated with tender regional adenopathy. In some of these illnesses, only a larger macule will indicate the initial lesion. After a few days, a diffuse rash evolves, with the constitutional symptoms of fever, myalgia, and fatigue. Rash variations can be urticarial, petechial, or chickenpox-like. The eschar can rarely present without a rash and there may be a rash without any observable initial bite papule. A careful search for the eschar should be made in all cases in which a history consistent with this pattern is obtained. On occasion, the presence of more than one eschar suggests that there was more than one bite at the same time.

Rickettsialpox

In the United States, the only endemic rickettsial infection in the rash-eschar group is the relatively rare rickettsialpox, caused by *Rickettsia akari*, transmitted by a mouse mite bite that is usually seen in an urban rather than rural setting and is usually not recognized. Approximately 24 to 48 hours after the bite, an asymptomatic erythematous papule evolves, which develops a central clear vesicle that eventually becomes cloudy. The papule then dries up into a central dark brown or black eschar with a larger 1- to 3-cm surrounding area of erythematous induration. At this time the patient generally develops fever and tender regional adenopathy without lymphangitis. In rickettsialpox, the eschar is found in up to 95% of cases and can persist for up to 4 weeks. Fever and frontal headache are found in most cases. The diffuse rash is generally composed of small papules, 0.2 to 1 cm, that develop central clear vesicle fluid and may become pustular. The total number is between 4 and 100, and the lesions are usually seen on the face, trunk, and extremities, with infrequent spread to the oral mucosa, palms, and soles. Many of these cases resemble chickenpox, and only the eschar and regional adenopathy will be a strong clue against the much more common varicella. Diagnosis is made by CF, or more specific microimmunofluorescence (MIF), or indirect immunofluorescent antibody (IFA) tests to *R. akari*. Tetracycline is an effective therapy (79,80).

Scrub Typhus

Scrub typhus due to *Rickettsia tsutsugamushi* is the most common, widespread, and serious of the tache noire rickettsial group. The mortality rate is 5 to 10% without therapy, and there is an extensive prolonged morbidity from the illness unless therapy is started early. The illness is transmitted by mite bites and is uncommon in travelers returning to the United States. It is, however, endemic and common throughout Southeast Asia, India, Nepal, China, Australia, and Indonesia. The incubation period from the bite to the eschar is approximately 1 to 3 weeks. Regional adenopathy, constitutional symptoms with fever, and a macular rash on the trunk begin shortly after the eschar has developed. Confirmatory diagnosis is by the relatively insensitive Weil-Felix OX-K reaction, which is positive in less than 50% of the cases, or by more sensitive and specific CF or IFA serology. A single 200-mg dose of doxycycline is often curative, and most patients will respond rapidly. An absence of rash or eschar is seen in 50% of patients proven to be recently infected by this agent. Pneumonia is much more common in this group than had been originally recognized. In one series from Thailand, 12.5% of 75 patients had meningitis or encephalitis (81). Travelers who have been in the "scrub bush" environments, with potential insect exposure, and develop pneumonia or the above AFR should be investigated and treated for scrub typhus (82–86).

Other Tick-borne Rash/Eschar Rickettsial Infections

Boutonneuse Fever, Queensland Fever, North Asia Fever, and Oriental Spotted Fever   Boutonneuse fever is the best known member of this group and is a relatively benign spotted fever syndrome associated with an eschar or tache noire. It is distributed through the entire Mediterranean basin and most of Africa. This tick-borne disease is due to *Rickettsia conorii*. Queensland fever of Australia is due to *Rickettsia australis*, North Asian fever is due to *Rickettsia sibirica*, and the newly described Oriental spotted fever is due to *Rickettsia japonica* (87). All four agents have a similar clinical presentation and prognosis.

R. conori is the most common rickettsial infection imported into the United States and has an incubation period of approximately 6 to 10 days from tick bite to onset of the developing eschar followed by a period of 5 days until fever, regional adenitis, and rash develop. The rash begins on the proximal extremities and spreads to the face, body, and then to the hands and soles (88,89).

Rickettsia australis has a 5-day incubation period from the bite to the development of the eschar and another 5-day period until the constitutional symptoms, regional adenitis, and macular–papular rash occur (84).

In both of these illnesses, the rash can rarely be petechial or vesicular (chickenpox-like), and in both illnesses, a small number of cases have been described in which the patient was ill but no rash was evident (90–92). The eschar is seen in up to 75% of patients with boutonneuse fever and in one-third to two-thirds of patients with Queensland fever.

The diagnosis of the entire group is by Weil-Felix OX-2 and OX-19 tests, which are relatively insensitive, or more specifically by MIF or CF antibody titers. A few deaths have been reported recently (93). Because there are such similarities in clinical manifestations, it would be impossible to clinically differentiate among scrub typhus, Queensland fever, murine typhus, and the occasional Q fever with a rash when an individual has an AFR syndrome and has just returned from Australia, where all of these diseases can be acquired. Similar problems will arise in travelers from other parts of the world. Serologic tests would be necessary for a specific diagnosis, but therapy with tetracycline is effective for all of the rickettsia infections (84).

Spirillum minus

One of the causes of rat bite fevers, *Spirillum minus* has a dermatologic presentation similar to that of boutonneuse fever. There is a local papule that evolves 1 to 4 weeks after the initial bite lesion is well healed. The papule then evolves into an eschar, with lymphangitis and tender regional adenopathy. A diffuse central reddish to purplish rash develops, which often dramatically and spontaneously fades within 3 to 5 days. Even without therapy, however, the rash may return with fever with each recrudescence of the spirochetal infection. Each recurrence may last 3 to 5 days. The entire course may last up to a month, and even longer courses have been described. The differences between this rat bite fever and that due to the gram-negative bacillus *S. moniliformis* include: 1) *Spirillum* has a central erythematous rash and *Streptobacillus* develops an acral and foot rash and sepsis (75); 2) *Streptobacillus* has an associated arthritis; and 3) the rash of *Spirillum* begins with an eschar. Classical relapsing fever due to *B. recurrentis* does not have an eschar and regional adenitis, and the rash is central in location.

Lyme Disease

Lyme disease due to the spirochete *B. burgdorferi* can occasionally mimic the eschar rash pattern. The initial erythema chronicum migrans (ECM) lesion at the site of the tick bite at first looks like the early papules of other illnesses in this group and is seen in 70 to 80% of infected patients. The nodule, however, rapidly evolves into a large, flat, annular lesion that can be as large as 20 to 70 cm in size. In 5 to 50% of patients with ECM, secondary multiple lesions up to 50 in number will develop, and thus can mimic the initial big lesion followed by diffuse rash pattern of this group. However, the lesions of the initial ECM and its secondary satellites are individually much larger than in other illnesses listed and generally demonstrate a characteristic central clearing. Usually, the rash and original ECM lesion are diagnostic. Vesiculation and pustulation are rare.

Systemic symptoms of fever, chills, myalgia, arthralgia, fatigue, nausea, vomiting, and headache are common during these early phases of the skin rash in Lyme disease (94).

Diagnosis is generally made by clinical examination. The less-than-optimal serologic examinations presently available provide adjunctive but rarely definitive proof of etiology. More specific diagnoses can be made with difficulty by biopsy of skin lesions with appropriate staining and by culture. Such techniques are not yet available to most physicians.

The dermatologic complications of Lyme disease are rare in the United States and include acrodermatitis chronicum atrophicans and benign borrelia lymphocytoma. These effects appear years later and are chronic afebrile skin conditions.

As in other spirochetal infections, exacerbation of the intensity of the skin lesions or the Jarisch-Herxheimer reaction can occur in 10% of the cases after initial antibiotic therapy. This is more commonly observed in patients with large multiple lesions and probably correlates with the number of spirochetes in the lesions. In retrospect, this disturbing reaction can occasionally be used as a diagnostic clue.

Trypanosomiasis

African Trypanosomiasis   Approximately 5 to 15 days after the tsetse fly bite, there is a painful circular, rubbery, indurated, red papule 2 to 5 cm in size. The papule will eventually resolve spontaneously in 2 to 3 weeks without therapy. It is much more commonly seen in non-Africans and much more likely to be seen with *Trypanosoma rhodesiense* than with *Trypanosoma gambiense* infections. Within a few hours of the onset of the chancre, a high-grade fever ensues, which will last between 1 and 7 days. African *T. gambiense* has a much more indolent onset. About the time of the onset of the fever, an irregular circinate evanescent rash will appear on the trunk, shoulders, and thighs. This is much more easily seen in light-skinned individuals. The individual lesions are scattered, oval, pinkish, quite large (at 6 to 10 cm), and demonstrate central clearing. Additionally, there may be pruritus and painful edema of the hands, feet, and other joints. At this stage, the diagnosis depends on puncture of the chancre to demonstrate the motile trypanosoma forms by wet preparation. A thick and thin peripheral blood smear may also demonstrate flagellar forms at this time of heavy parasitemia (95,96).

American Trypanosomiasis   South American trypanosomiasis also demonstrates an inoculum site in approximately 50% of patients. If the reduviid bug material is rubbed into the eye, then Romana's sign will be demonstrated. This is a 2- to 4-week period of bipalpebral unilateral edema. If the initial inoculum is through abraded skin, the chagoma chancre will be seen. An aspirate of the chagoma and wet preparation microscopic examination will often demonstrate organisms. Fever will be present in many patients with South American trypanosomiasis for a short period of time. Most patients who develop this disease, however, are asymptomatic. In some of the patients, chagoma and an evanescent erythematous rash will be seen at the same time.

Pityriasis Rosea

Pityriasis rosea is a dermatologic condition of unknown etiology that might be infectious in origin and tends to occur most commonly in late summer and fall and is always without fever or any other constitutional sign. There is an acute onset of the widespread macular lesions preceded 20 days earlier by a much larger usually asymptomatic plaque (herald patch or moth patch). The diffuse macular–papular lesions follow the line of skin cleavage, particularly on the chest and back in what is described as a Christmas tree pattern. Because of the initial large herald patch, this illness may occasionally be confused with mild secondary syphilis, rickettsialpox, or any of the above-mentioned tick-borne rickettsial infections.

Bacterial and Eschar Rash Syndromes

Many bacteria, but particularly those with an inoculum from trauma followed by sepsis with secondary metastatic lesions to the skin, will resemble the eschar diffuse rash syndrome. Secondary syphilis, with an initial chancre, or disseminated herpes simplex, with an original skin vesicle complex still present, will occasionally resemble the eschar diffuse rash pattern. A few other causative agents to consider include *S. aureus*, endocarditis from an initial auto-inoculation with the primary lesion still present, *Erysipelothrix* from a fish, or an animal bone inoculation with endocarditis and the original lesions still unhealed. Tularemia, melioidosis, and leptospirosis can all occur secondary to insect bites, inoculums from soil-contaminated injuries, or rat bites. In all cases, a diffuse systemic disease with a central macular–papular rash and the continued presence of the original lesion causing the disease can lead to an eschar diffuse rash syndrome.

In immunocompromised hosts, particularly cirrhotic hosts, various vibrio bacteria, particularly *Vibrio vulnificus* and yersinia organisms, can receive a local traumatic lesion from a seawater injury or seafood injury and then develop a rapidly evolving initial abscess, bacteremia, and multiple metastatic abscesses and vesicles and grossly resemble the inoculum and diffuse skin rash syndrome.

In many illnesses an eschar and a systemic disease with or without a rash are characteristic. These include all of the tick-borne rickettsia infections except RMSF, rickettsialpox, scrub typhus, relapsing fever, rat bite fever from *S. minus*, other spirochetal infections including syphilis, leptospirosis from animal bites, South American trypanosomiasis, African trypanosomiasis, visceral leishmaniasis and leishmaniasis due to *Leishmania tropica* with systemic spread, dracunculosis, and oncherca volvulus.

Any member of the eschar rash group can present with rash but no eschar. The differential diagnosis of the entire eschar rash group must also include RMSF, typhus, rubella, rubeola, meningococcemia, disseminated gonorrhea, parvovirus, fifth disease, *Borrelia* relapsing fever, and some alpha and flavi arboviruses, coxsackie, and echo viruses.

DIFFUSE CONFLUENT ERYTHEMA

Diffuse erythroderma may be seen in scarlet fever, *Arcanobacterium haemolyticum*, staphylococcal toxic shock syndrome, streptococcal toxic shock syndrome, staphylococcal scalded skin syndrome, Kawasaki disease, JRA, and a number of viruses, particularly enteroviruses. The major clinical clues that are useful in differentiating these processes include the timing of the onset of the rash in comparison to the rest of the illness, the presence of any associated enanthem, the age of the patient, the duration and evolution of the rash, the severity of the illness, and the degree of involvement of other organ systems.

Scarlet Fever (Second Disease)

Scarlet fever is caused by the group A streptococcus. The rash usually appears 1 to 2 days after the development of sore throat, fever, and headache and is caused by the elaboration of an exotoxin (erythrogenic or pyrogenic exotoxins A, B, C, and D) (97). The rash is a diffuse erythema that begins on the face and spreads to the trunk and extremities. Several findings are characteristic of this illness. These include sparing of the area around the mouth (circumoral pallor), blanching of the rash on pressure, small rough elevations of the skin in involved areas producing a "sandpaper" quality, an enanthem consisting of a bright red tongue with enlarged papillae producing a "strawberry" appearance, a pronounced linear erythema in the axilla and other skin folds that also occurs after applying pressure by a tourniquet (termed Pastia's lines, these are caused by petechiae associated with capillary fragility), and a desquamation of the skin during the second week of the illness.

Formerly called *Corynebacterium haemolyticum*, *A. haemolyticum* causes a pharyngitis and scarlatiniform rash in young adults that is clinically indistinguishable from scarlet fever (98).

Staphylococcal Toxic Shock Syndrome

Staphylococcal toxic shock syndrome is characterized by fever (usually greater than 102°F), multisystem involvement (including renal failure, alterations in level of consciousness, diarrhea, thrombocytopenia, heart failure or heart block, pulmonary edema, and rash) (99,100). The rash is a diffuse erythroderma often involving the palmar surfaces. Most patients have a bright erythema of mucous membrane surfaces and a nonpurulent conjunctivitis. Although changes consistent with a "strawberry tongue" have been reported, this is an uncommon finding. Petechiae, maculopapular changes, and a positive Nikolsky's sign are occasionally seen. Beginning approximately on the seventh day of illness and peaking on the tenth day, desquamation begins, ranging from a powdery dandruff-like appearance to a full-thickness peeling skin loss. Over the next 60 days, hair and nail loss in previously involved areas may be seen (100). This syndrome is caused by a *Staphylococcus* species that elaborates toxic shock syndrome toxin (TSST) and acts as a superantigen, stimulating this dramatic host response (101). Blood and skin cultures are usually negative, but the organism can be found in typical sites of "colonization" such as the vagina, nasopharynx, or a surgical wound. First associated with the use of highly absorbent tampons, today nonmenstrual cases represent about half the reported cases. Antimicrobial therapy may decrease the rate of relapse.

Streptococcal Toxic Shock Syndrome

Streptococcal toxic shock syndrome produces a similar clinical picture, except bacteremia (often with no obvious source) or a localized area of cellulitis is frequently present. The 30% mortality rate is higher than the 2 to 5% rate found in staphylococcal toxic shock syndrome (97). Patients are younger and more likely to have no underlying illness than patients with other invasive streptococcal infections. The streptococcal M protein and streptococcal pyrogenic exotoxins appear to act as superantigens initiating this illness. Patients may have a mild nonspecific prodrome illness, after which shock with multiorgan system failure occurs. Early antimicrobial therapy should include coverage for streptococcus, staphylococcus, and the possibility of community-onset gram-negative rods. The severity of illness, multiorgan system involvement, and rapid pace of the toxic shock syndromes separate these illnesses from scarlet fever.

Staphylococcal Scalded Skin Syndrome

Staphylococcal scalded skin syndrome, first described by Ritter in 1878, begins as a diffuse erythema over the whole body, including the circumoral area. The erythematous areas are tender, mimicking a sunburn. Over the next several days, bullae form in these areas. Nearby apparently normal skin will frequently demonstrate a positive Nikolsky sign (wrinkling or bullae formation with gentle rubbing or pressure). Involved skin eventually sloughs and desquamates. Staphylococcus is frequently isolated from the skin but rarely from blood. This syndrome is uncommon in adults.

Kawasaki Syndrome

Both scarlet fever and Kawasaki syndrome are associated with a strawberry tongue and desquamation. However, in Kawasaki syndrome there is usually an associated conjunctivitis and adenitis (typically involving a single tender, enlarged node in the cervical chain). Erythema and fissuring of the lips, profound erythema of the palms and soles, and fever are seen in most patients (102,103). The rash may be scarlatiniform, maculopapular, or similar to erythema multiforme. Kawasaki syndrome is primarily a disease of children, with a peak incidence at one year of age. It is rare after the age of 8 years. Although it has characteristics of a vasculitis, with a unique predilection for coronary artery involvement, steroids are not recommended. Aspirin and immunoglobulin therapy appear to be beneficial (104).

Depending on the location, Kawasaki syndrome may mimic the early phase of other diffuse erythema diseases. Erysipelas is a cutaneous infection due to group A streptococcus. The involved skin is erythematous and edematous secondary to lymphatic involvement. Patients are toxic and the leading edge of the involved skin may visibly progress over hours. The demarcation from the involved to uninvolved area is usually quite obvious. Erysipelas is a focal process, but because it is often on the face, it may mimic early scarlet fever, toxic shock syndrome, erythema infectiosum, or the "butterfly" rash of systemic lupus erythematosus.

VESICULAR–BULLOUS RASH

The varicella-zoster virus and the herpes simplex virus are among the most common causes of vesicular skin lesions with an infectious cause. Disseminated herpes simplex, disseminated herpes zoster, hand-foot-and-mouth disease, rickettsialpox, atypical measles, staphylococcal scalded skin syndrome, and *V. vulnificus* each may cause vesicular lesions. The distribution of the lesions and the underlying host status are helpful in distinguishing these syndromes.

Local diseases such as impetigo, milker's nodules, and orf (bovine pustular stomatitis) may be confusing with the early phases of this group of rashes. Gram stain of vesicles (impetigo) and the lack of dissemination are key differential points. Gram stain, trunk smear, and viral and bacterial culture are indications for this group.

Chickenpox—Varicella

Chickenpox infects approximately 3 million Americans annually, most of whom are under the age of 14. The virus is acquired by direct exposure to infected respiratory secretions or a varicella or zoster lesion. Chickenpox occurs year-round, but the peak incidence is in the spring. The first symptom may be malaise or fever followed by the rash, which may begin anywhere on the body. It is pruritic and consists of clear vesicles on an erythematous base. Over the next 4 to 6 days, lesions crust over. Lesions in various stages of evolution (new to crusted) are seen, which was a critical differential point separating chickenpox from smallpox, an illness characterized by lesions evolving together in phase. Rickettsialpox may also mimic chickenpox, but the former is much less common, has an eschar and regional adenopathy, and is found primarily in urban areas of the United States, particularly New York City.

Bacterial superinfection of the skin, purpura fulminans, cerebellitis (a usually benign self-limited complication in children characterized by ataxia and vomiting), Reye's syndrome, and pneumonia are the most common complications of chickenpox (40). Adults with chickenpox are more likely to develop symptomatic pneumonia or a severe encephalitis.

Disseminated Herpes Simplex and Disseminated Herpes Zoster

The individual lesions of herpes simplex and zoster are virtually indistinguishable from chickenpox. However, these infections are usually localized to the genital or oral area in the case of simplex and a dermatome in the case of zoster. The Tzanck smear will not distinguish these infections but will confirm that the etiology is a herpesvirus. Dissemination of zoster and simplex may occur, particularly in the immunocompromised host with a defect in cell-mediated immunity. Herpes simplex may also disseminate in patients with severe eczema. Patients with disseminated herpes simplex usually have visceral involvement. Fulminant hepatitis is particularly common in this infection and is a useful clinical clue suggesting the etiology. The fatality rate of disseminated herpes simplex is higher than disseminated herpes zoster. Acyclovir therapy may be lifesaving, but even with therapy many patients do not survive. The lesions of herpes simplex and zoster are more painful than pruritic and, in the case of zoster, the pain may persist after the lesions have cleared (postzoster neuralgia). The trunk smear will show intranuclear inclusions and giant cells in herpes simplex and varicella-zoster.

Smallpox (Variola)

The last indigenous case of smallpox occurred in 1977. The rash of smallpox progresses centripetally from macules to vesicles to scabs, with all lesions at approximately the same stage of eruption at any given time (unlike chickenpox). Effective vaccination programs have eradicated this disease.

Vaccinia

Generalized vaccinia and eczema vaccinatum are diffuse vesicular rash syndromes following vaccination with vaccinia virus (cowpox). This complication may be seen in vaccinated patients with underlying eczema or immunodeficiency states. It may also be acquired by close contact with a vaccine recipient. Visceral involvement is uncommon.

Monkeypox

Monkeypox is a rare cause of a disseminated vesicular rash acquired in central and west Africa from riftail monkeys. Most reported cases are from Zaire. The appearance and evolution of the rash and clinical illness are similar to smallpox. Most cases have occurred in children, and vaccination against smallpox provides protection against monkeypox.

Vibrio vulnificus

Vibrio vulnificus is the only bacteria that has bullae as part of its characteristic presentation. *V. vulnificus* has been associated with a bacteremic septic shock syndrome. Cellulitis with large hemorrhagic bullae is seen as a manifestation of metastatic infection in up to 75% of bacteremic patients (105). Patients with liver disease are at particular risk for systemic bacteremic infection after exposure. Saltwater fish (e.g., raw clams and oysters) and seawater are common vehicles.

DISSEMINATED NODULES AND FEVER SYNDROME

This section will stress the need for skin nodule biopsy for stain and culture. Even a single nodular lesion without any of the interesting diffuse patterns described below must be considered of great importance in the appropriate clinical setting of acute fever and immunosuppression, particularly with leukopenia. Although some controversy exists in the literature, we believe strongly that biopsy is important in such circumstances (106).

Acute Disseminated Nonnecrotic Maculonodules (Leukopenic and Small [0.3- to 0.5-cm] Papules)

Leukemia patients with leukopenia provide the most common setting for the sudden eruption of disseminated erythematous maculonodules. The most common isolate is a *Candida* organism. These patients are often receiving antibacterial agents and intravenous fluids. Over a period of several hours to several days, dozens to hundreds of 0.3- to 0.5-cm papules will erupt over the trunk and, less intensely, on the extremities. These nodules are part of a triad of fever, myalgia, and multiple eruptive skin nodules consistently described in the literature as suggesting disseminated candidiasis (107–111). Skin involvement is seen in approximately 5 to 20% of all disseminated candidiasis cases established in life or at autopsy and may be somewhat more common in patients with disseminated *Candida tropicalis* than in dissemination of other *Candida* species (112).

The lesions may begin as pink papules but then develop into lesions variously described as maculopapular or maculonodular. Less typically, large erythematous plaques or hemorrhagic nodules (usually associated with significant thrombocytopenia) are seen. There is generally no scale or crust over the lesions and lesions are asymptomatic. Less common are the necrotic pustules and ulcerative plaques that mimic pseudomonas-induced erythema gangrenosum (113). Purpura fulminans and flaccid hemorrhagic bullae have also been described under the same conditions due to the same organisms, but the most common lesions are the small maculonodular lesions (114).

When this syndrome occurs under fluconazole prophylaxis, it strongly suggests fluconazole-resistant *Candida krusei* or *Torulopsis glabrata*. If the patient is receiving amphotericin B, the clinician must suspect the consistently amphotericin-resistant *Candida lusitanaei* or the occasionally resistant *Candida albicans* or *C. tropicalis* (115–117). The diagnosis is made by smear and aspiration of lesions or more often by biopsy with appropriate stains and cultures. The smear of the skin biopsy can be diagnostic in culture-negative cases and vice versa. Retinal involvement and arthralgias are often associated findings.

Muscle pain is usually in the lower extremities and can be quite profound. Muscle biopsy may be diagnostic if the skin lesions are not.

Disseminated Nonnecrotic Macronodules—Fungal Nonleukopenic Immunocompromised and Large Nodules (0.5 to 3 cm)

Multiple macronodules and fever have been described in a large variety of nonleukopenic immunocompromised hosts, including patients with AIDS, alcoholics, and intravenous drug abusers. These lesions may be eruptive and pustular or noneruptive and more subcutaneous. The lesions may resemble the classical disseminated candidiasis lesions described in the leukopenic patient, but these macronodules are larger, 0.5 to 3 cm in size, and they tend to be pustular or, less commonly, pustulonecrotic (118,119). A diagnostic syndrome of extremely painful multiple erythematous subcutaneous scalp macronodules due to candida and numbering up to 200 has been described in a large group of intravenous brown heroin abusers. These patients had diluted the heroin in lemon juice, a good culture media for candida (120).

Noneruptive (for the most part) multiple disseminated subcutaneous macronodules have also been caused by sporotrichosis, coccidioidomycosis, cryptococcosis, and histoplasmosis in many clinical settings in immunosuppressed hosts (121). Deep skin biopsies are necessary to prove the etiology of these organisms.

Disseminated Macroulcerated Nodules—Mycobacteria

Macronodular skin lesions of disseminated *Mycobacterium chelonae*, a rapid growing mycobacteria, can arise in a variety of leukopenic immunocompromised patients. The diagnosis is made by biopsy and culture of the lesions. Erythromycin has been found to be effective for this illness (122).

A relatively new syndrome of macroulcerative lesions (0.5 to 2 cm) has recently been ascribed to *Mycobacterium haemophilum* (123). Most of the cases have arisen in AIDS patients or bone marrow transplant patients. The lesions are raised, violaceous, and fluctuant and then become pustular and eventually draining serosegmenous material. The distribution of these lesions differs from that of the disseminated candidal infections because in disseminated *M. haemophilum* the greatest concentration of lesions is on the extremities rather than on the trunk as it is in systemic candidiasis. Culture and biopsy of these lesions is usually diagnostic. In addition, the *M. haemophilum* lesions tend to involve areas over the joints where the temperature of the subcutaneous tissues is somewhat lower. Direct invasion of joint and bone lesions is also common and can be a source of positive culture. Other mycobacteria such as *Mycobacterium marinum* and *Mycobacterium avium* complex can rarely cause the same disseminated macroulcerative skin lesions in AIDS patients.

Disseminated Necrotic Macronodules—Fusaria Fungi

These skin nodules are not only ulcerative but are also necrotic and therefore the majority of lesions will differ from the previous groups. *Fusaria* species are the major cause of this syndrome, although on occasion a small number of disseminated *Aspirgilla*, *Mucor*, and *Mycobacteria* species may cause the same necrotic macronodules. In burn, leukemia, lymphoma, and particularly bone marrow transplant patients, fever and myalgia are followed by an eruption of tender erythematous macronodules over one extremity. These 0.3- to 3-cm lesions will vesiculate and rapidly develop black necrotic centers, while the opposite extremity will begin to develop the same lesions. Similar rashes are also seen in the orbital facial and nasal areas. The trunk will exhibit only a small number or no lesions. Nasal lesions are usually quite necrotic. Blood cultures are usually positive for fusaria in approximately 75% of cases. This concentration of skin nodules on the extremities differentiates the fusaria syndrome from systemic candidiasis and other fungal syndromes. Although the concentration of skin lesions is similar to the distribution of *M. haemophilum*, there is not the similar concentration of lesions over the joints as there is in the mycobacterium infection, and evolution to necrosis is uncommon with the mycobacterium. Even though aspirgilla and mucor classically involve blood vessels and lead to necrosis in the tissues that they invade, dissemination of these two organisms by the hematogenous route into the skin is relatively uncommon and generally produces just a single or small number of lesions (124–127).

Factitious Panniculitis and Dermatitis

This condition occurs in young, healthy individuals, usually female, who have a relationship to the health care industry. The skin lesions are often chronic and nonhealing and can be associated with a large number of unusual bacteria that rarely occur in community skin infections. Biopsy may reveal foreign material with birefringent crystals under polarized light. The patients often appear to be in a normal psychological state, and might angrily deny the possibility of self-mutilation when the issue is raised. However, the patients often generally sign out of the hospital or remove themselves from care of the accuser. Most of these patients appear to be healthy and afebrile. These self-induced skin conditions are chronic, but a few individuals present with fever and acute multiple lesions due to secondary infection. In this setting, the illness can mimic the AFR syndrome (128–130).

Erythema Nodosum

This immunologically mediated illness consists of a variable number of relatively large tender erythematous subcutaneous inflammatory nodules generally concentrated over the extensor or shin surfaces of the lower extremities. The nodules can turn into large plaques. The nodules eventually turn purple after a few weeks, but generally heal up with minimal scarring at the end of 4 to 6 weeks. Microscopically these are septal panniculitis without vasculitis. High levels of circulating immune complexes are present. Erythema nodosum can be triggered by a wide variety of infectious and noninfectious antigens. Erythema nodosum often follows an upper respiratory infection but is usually of unknown etiology even after intense investigation. In general, except for erythema nodosum leprosum of lepromatous leprosy, no new active lesions will exist after the sixth week. On occasion, lesions can be seen over the arms, face, or anywhere that there is subcutaneous fat, and thus widespread dissemination can be seen with erythema nodosum. Fever and symmetrical ankle or knee pain is common in erythema nodosum.

The major diagnosed etiology of erythema nodosum in Great Britain has been found to be sarcoidosis; in Scandinavia, *Yersinia enterocolitica*; in Southwest United States, coccidioidomycosis; and in the midcentral United States, histoplasmosis.

In general, diffuse rashes are uncommon following bacterial infections. Two exceptions are the postinfectious complications of *S. pyogenes* (reviewed above) and those of *Y. enterocolitica*. *Y. enterocolitica* is a gram-negative bacillus that together with *Yersinia pseudotuberculosis* causes intestinal infections that result in diarrhea or pseudoappendicitis due to mesenteric adenitis and fever. Erythema nodosum is not limited to the lower extremities in yersiniosis. Less commonly, erythema multiforme is also seen in this disease and both erythema multiforme and erythema nodosum may be seen in the same patient. Occasionally patients demonstrate other types of rashes including diffuse erythematous vesicles, erythema marginatum, or erythema figuratum. Arthritic syndromes, including a migratory polyarthritis similar to rheumatic fever and rat bite fever, a symmetrical ankle or knee arthritis as seen with erythema nodosum, a typical Reiter's syndrome, axial skeleton and large joint or an arthritis are also seen following *Yersinia* infections. *Yersinia* infections are relatively rare in the United States but are quite common in northern Europe. The diagnosis is made either by stool culture or serologic examination (131–133).

Other etiologic agents of erythema nodosum include all of the other diphasic yeast fungi such as cryptococcosis, sporotrichosis, and blastomycosis, and many intracellular pathogens such as tularemia, *Lymphogranuloma venereum*, psittacosis, leptospirosis, infectious mononucleosis, CMV, the cat scratch agents, *Campylobacter fetus*, tuberculosis, and leprosy. In the past, streptococcal pharyngitis was though to be a major trigger (134,135).

Erythema nodosum can be an early sign of solid tumor, leukemia, or lymphoma. Erythema nodosum is strongly associated with many illnesses of unknown etiology that demonstrate immunologic features including, most importantly, sarcoidosis, ulcerative colitis, Crohn's disease, and Behcet's syndrome. Drug reactions to sulfa, penicillins, and birth control pills have all been associated with secondary erythema nodosum. Bilateral hilar adenopathy is common and though typical for sarcoidosis, this can be seen in erythema nodosum associated with other etiologies.

Rarely, an infectious agent such as histoplasmosis has been demonstrated within the apparent erythema nodosum lesion. *Leptospira autumnalis*, the cause of Fort Bragg fever, has caused an outbreak of large (1 to 5 cm) pretibial erythematous, subcutaneous nodules. Hematogenous spread in immuno-compromised hosts of rapidly growing *Mycobacterium fortuitum* has produced similar pretibial lesions; however, these are culture positive for the mycobacteria and do not have the pathology of erythema nodosum.

Noninfectious dermatologic conditions such as Weber Christian syndrome, Sweet's syndrome, and lupus erythematosus profundus can resemble erythema nodosum by physician examination, but these illnesses are otherwise quite different clinically and pathologically. In AIDS patients, the smooth dome-shaped purple lesions of disseminated bacillary angiomatosis due to *Rochalimaea* organisms and the lesions of Kaposi's sarcoma can have, on occasion, the same distribution as classical erythema nodosum lesions, but the observation of individual lesions should not allow confusion with the classical erythematous subcutaneous lesions of erythema nodosum.

DIFFUSE URTICARIAL RASH AND FEVER (SERUM SICKNESS)

Urticaria (hives) is the result of intradermal edema just as angioedema is the result of subcutaneous edema. A number of categories are associated with the causation of urticaria including cold, light, heat, physical trauma, heredity, food, and desensitization reactions that are generally not associated with signs of inflammation (136). The serum sickness variant of urticaria demonstrates fever, chills, urticarial rash, and other constitutional symptoms. Although the etiology of afebrile acute urticaria is often never determined, with the syndrome of urticaria and fever, there is a much greater chance that an etiology will be determined. Drug reactions are the major determinable cause of fever and an urticarial rash.

Urticaria can be seen with collagen vascular diseases such as systemic lupus erythematosus and malignancies such as Hodgkin's disease. The combination of fever and urticarial rash in these syndromes can be confusing until the underlying serious pathology is determined.

On rare occasions, urticaria has been reported associated with active infection of a large number of infectious agents, such as *Shigella, Pseudomonas pseudomallei,* amoeba, giardia, *Trichomonas,* cat scratch disease, EBV, CMV, mumps, coxiella, *Yersinia,* and *Neisseria* (137–139). However, the causal relationship between these agents and urticaria remains suspect. In other cases, the internal migration of parasitic organisms such as hookworm, ascaris, filaria, schistosomiasis, and on rare occasion, the sudden traumatic release of antigenic material in cysts of echinococcal disease can also be associated with an urticarial rash, fever, bronchospasm, and even shock. A few of these will be discussed in further detail.

In the adult, the bites or infestation of ectoparasites such as scabies, cercarial dermatitis (swimmer's itch), flies, maggots, scabies, brown recluse spider, no-ceums, maggots, mites and chiggers, bedbugs, bees and wasps, and even ticks can all lead to a diffuse erythematous or urticarial rash (140–146). In some cases the systemic reaction is severe and is associated with chills, fever, and other systemic reactions including shock. Most of these causes will be self-evident because of the history, the local changes at the site of the bite, or the typical signs of infestation. However, on occasion, unrecognized invasion of normal orifices as in myiasis or the absence of local changes at the site of the bite as is typical of the tick can make the problem difficult to unravel.

Acute Hepatitis B and Urticaria

Approximately 5 to 25% of patients with acute hepatitis B will develop a serum sickness-like reaction 2 to 20 days prior to the onset of clinically obvious hepatitis. Typically in these cases there will be fever, polyarthralgia, and polyarthritis. A diffuse exanthem that is usually urticarial or macular–papular will be found in 50% of cases. Activation of both the classical and alternative complement pathways lead to hypocomplementemia. This serum sickness reaction will generally disappear in 1 to 2 weeks with the onset of the clinical hepatitis, but in some cases the serum sickness reaction will last much longer. This syndrome is the best established urticarial serum sickness reaction associated with a nonparasitic infectious agent (147).

The Gianotti-Cresti syndrome, usually due to hepatitis B in children, is an erythematous rash syndrome called papular acrodermatitis, with localization to the extremities and face. It is thought to be caused by hepatitis B and probably other viruses. The syndrome is rare in the United States and not yet described in adults (148–150).

Urticarial and Enterovirus Infections (Coxsackie A9)

The classical presentation of an exanthem of the coxsackie and echovirus group is the morbilliform rash with or without an enanthem that presents simultaneously with fever, chills, and perhaps local symptoms, depending on whether or not any other organ system is involved. Pharyngitis, meningitis, tracheobronchitis, pleurodynia, and myocarditis are among the more notorious complications.

A smaller number of enterovirus-infected patients develop a herpetiform eruption, a pattern characteristic of classical roseola, or an even less common hemorrhagic rash, as is seen in echo 9 and sometimes coxsackie A9 infections.

Coxsackie A9 has also been associated with multiple outbreaks of a syndrome of fever and a diffuse urticarial rash. The importance of this rash, as in most other enterovirus rashes, is the potential confusion the rash brings to the clinician if the association of the rash and enterovirus infection is unrecognized. In these coxsackie A9 infections, the rash does look hivelike or urticarial in appearance. However, there is very rarely any pruritus or angioedema, there is no response to antihistamines, and there is no response to subcutaneous adrenalin. The diagnosis depends on viral culture and serology, which will only be useful in retrospect in a given patient. A common cause of confusion is a possible drug reaction to an antibiotic inappropriately given for the initial fever syndrome (151).

Acute Schistosomiasis

The acute schistosomiasis (Katayama fever) reaction is seen most commonly with *Schistosoma japonicum*, somewhat less commonly with *Schistosomiasis mansoni*, and very rarely with *Schistosomiasis haematobium*. Approximately 2 weeks to 2 months after a first exposure to cercarial-contaminated waters, symptoms of fevers, sweats, abdominal pain, myalgia, diarrhea, cough, lymphadenopathy, hepatosplenomegaly, angioedema, perioral edema, and urticaria will arise in the most severe cases. Recovery usually occurs within 2 to 3 weeks without therapy, but some patients have died of the more severe serum sickness that this represents. This acute schistosomiasis syndrome is thought to be mediated through circulating immune complexes. The reaction is related to both the recent deposit of large numbers of schistosome eggs and release of antigens because of migration of the worms. Although more than a half million U.S. citizens currently have schistosomiasis, Katayama fever will only be seen in patients never before exposed who have recently been infected. Marked eosinophilia is almost universal in this reaction and helps in the differential diagnosis of this infrequently seen illness. Stool examination is negative at the beginning of this reaction. At a later date, stool examination and serology can confirm the diagnosis. Therapy is still controversial, but some experts suggest therapy with praziquantel with or without steroids (152,153).

Schistosomiasis dermatitis (swimmer's itch) is acquired throughout the world, including in the United States, particularly in the Great Lakes area. This is probably a type I allergic reaction caused by previous sensitization due to cercariae of bird schistosomes after bathing in contaminated waters. In the full syndrome, there is an initial immediate pruritus at the site of cercarial penetration, which disappears within a few minutes. This is followed by a diffuse erythematous rash, which also disappears. However, within 24 hours, an intensely pruritic urticarial rash appears, which can last up to 7 to 10 days. Fever is uncommon. These bird cercaria cannot invade further in the human being. Human schistosomes acquired in other parts of the world can also cause this syndrome.

Strongyloides stercoralis

Strongyloides stercoralis is a highly infectious soil-transmitted nematode that resides in the small intestine. The classical triad is abdominal pain, urticaria, and eosinophilia. Recurrent and increasingly severe symptoms are not uncommon and are due to the unusual life cycle of successful autoinoculation. Rash, urticaria, and pruritus may be seen in 15% of the patients, and cough and wheezing are seen in 10%. Eosinophilia is common and sometimes is the only sign of infection with strongyloides. The illness is endemic to the tropics and subtropics of the Americas, Europe, and Asia. The most severe infestations come from Southeast Asia. The diagnosis is very difficult to make by stool examination because the filariform worms reside in the submucosa of the duodenum and jejunum and not in the lumen of the bowel. Repeated stool examination, the swallowed string and capsule test (Enterotest), as well as serology can help diagnose the condition. Recurrent attacks of urticaria due to *S. stercoralis* have been recorded over a 65-year period in a single patient. Chronic urticaria on both the abdomen and perineum, but also on the wrists or ankles has also been associated with this organism (154–156). Infections of great notoriety occurred in prisoners of war building the Thailand-China railroad during World War II. Recurrent urticaria was reported in 100% of such persons over many years.

Many cases of recurrent pulmonary eosinophilia syndromes with fever have been reported and are due to large numbers of larvae migrating through the lung. Any type of pruritic rash can be seen with strongyloides, but there is a pathognomonic rash called larva currens (racing worm) because of observable subcutaneous migration at a speed of 2 to 4 inches an hour. The pathway is marked by an intensely pruritic urticarial wheal and can be observed over days to weeks. These clinical findings are diagnostic and are generally seen over the perineum or abdomen. Cutaneous larva migrans in human beings due to cat and dog hookworm moves only 1/2 inch per day, and compared to larva currens, is a true "creeping" eruption. Thiabendazole is usually effective as therapy, although Ivermectin is now being studied as a potential substitute.

Loiasis

Loiasis is a filarial infestation secondary to bites by tanabid flies. This illness is characterized by transient noninflammatory subcutaneous swellings due to subcutaneous edema. The lesions are called Calabar swellings and are often associated with pruritus and pain and occasionally fever. Half of the patients will develop diffuse urticaria or other pruritic rashes. Moderate eosinophilia is characteristic, and asthma is seen in some patients. On occasion the adult worms are noticed crossing under the skin or the conjunctiva of the patient during the migratory phase. The diagnosis is established by finding the microfilaria in direct blood smears of daytime blood. These urticarial rash attacks are only seen in newly exposed individuals to this filaria and are not seen in the population of chronically infected individuals. Similar attacks of rash and hives have been described in newly exposed nonimmune individuals infected with *Bancroftian filariasis* and onchocerciasis (157–161).

Trichinosis

Trichinosis in human beings is a result of ingesting undercooked meat that is contaminated with the infective larva of *Trichinella spiralis*. Heavy exposure in the nonimmune host can lead to symptoms of fever, periorbital edema, muscle pain, abdominal pain, diarrhea, weakness, and less commonly, a central maculopapular or urticarial pruritic rash in up to 20% of patients. Eosinophilia is seen in more than 90% of patients. Conjunctival hemorrhages and splinter hemorrhages mimicking endocarditis are also seen in 10% of such cases (162,163). The diagnosis is made by the clinical presentation and the history of suspect food ingestion. It can be confirmed by a rising antibody titer or, if necessary, by a biopsy of a swollen painful muscle group.

Onchocerciasis

Onchocerciasis is a filarial infection transmitted by black flies to the human host with three central features: subcutaneous nodules containing adult worms, diffuse pruritic dermatitis, and sclerosing keratitis that can progress to blindness. Dermatologic variations include an erysipelas syndrome or a regional unilateral pruritic papular rash with massive regional adenopathy. Diagnosis is made by recognition of the clinical presentation skin snips or, less commonly, by a provocative massone test. The illness is usually afebrile, but occasionally there are diffuse erythematous rashes and fever (164).

The reports of an urticarial rash associated with a large number of infectious agents including EBV, CMV, mumps, cat scratch disease, *Shigella*, *Mycoplasma*, *Yersinia*, *Coxiella*, and *N. meningitides* are mostly anecdotal but are important in the sense that if no other cause can be found for the urticaria, and the underlying illness is otherwise established, one can attribute individual cases of uncommon rash to an unusual reaction to a common condition.

PETECHIAL—HEMORRHAGIC RASH—AFR

The presentation of an acute onset of fever and a petechial rash should suggest some of the most serious and life-threatening infectious diseases. Although these fulminant diseases must be considered initially, there is a subset of patients with illnesses such as enterovirus, rubella, rubeola, and scarlet fever who will ultimately exhibit a very benign course and yet will demonstrate a petechial rash (165). Nonetheless, the petechial rash should immediately bring to mind illnesses that leave the physician no time to be wrong and require rapid decision-making with regard to hospitalization and the ordering of empiric treatment and diagnostic tests. Because of this appropriate concern, many of these cases will receive empiric therapy prior to the determination of the specific etiology. Some patients with variants of idiopathic disseminated vasculitis will present with a diffuse petechial rash, and only biopsy will eventually settle the diagnosis.

Acute Meningococcemia—*Neisseria meningitidis*

Neisseria meningitidis is an encapsulated gram-negative diplococcus with sufficient virulence factors to cause the vascular damage that leads to the characteristic hemorrhagic skin lesions and internal organ system dysfunction, shock, and death.

Acute meningococcemia is one of the most virulent of all infections acquired by healthy adults in the United States. In most acute cases, a typical upper respiratory infection is suddenly followed by symptoms of rigors, fever, vomiting, headache, and then stupor, diffuse hemorrhagic rash, and shock. These findings may peak within a 2- to 4-hour period from the onset of the initial symptoms. In other meningococcal rash cases, the illness evolves over 24 to 72 hours and most of the findings may be limited to the CNS, with nuchal rigidity and encephalopathy, while the petechial rash may be barely noticed. In the latter situation, the rash is useful in predicting the etiology.

A diffuse macular or macular–papular rash (or rarely an urticarial rash) may precede the petechial skin lesions in a minority of patients. This diffuse rash may completely disappear or dramatically evolve into the typical petechial rash. Initially, a few petechiae may be barely evident or they may be "hidden" in the flexor surfaces, groin, and axilla, or on the ankles, or may be even more sequestered in the conjunctiva, sclera, or oral mucosa. In some patients, a few to a few dozen petechial lesions may blossom into hundreds to thousands of large lesions in an extremely short period of time, literally under the eyes of the observer. In early cases, the petechial lesions are small and slightly raised, but these can enlarge into peripheral lesions with a vesicular center. The distribution of the rash is usually not symmetrical initially and may be found anywhere on the body. Most lesions are seen on the trunk and extremities. Palm and sole lesions, as well as hemorrhages on the back of the hands and feet, will be found in some patients with meningococcemia mimicking RMSF. Extensive ecchymotic lesions and gangrenous lesions typical of disseminated intravascular coagulation are present in the most severe cases. Signs of shock will rarely be seen in meningococcemia in the absence of extensive cutaneous hemorrhages. Laboratory findings of a large percentage of band form in the peripheral smear, the classical CSF findings of acute purulent meningitis, a positive gram stain of the CSF, smears of serum from skin lesions or the buffy coat of peripheral blood, a positive latex agglutination of the CSF, and eventually, positive CSF and blood cultures, all differentiate acute meningococcal disease from its other mimics.

The differential diagnosis of this presentation includes disseminated *Strepto-coccus pneumoniae, Haemophilus influenzae*, gonorrhea, RMSF, typhus, enterovi-rus, leptospirosis, and subacute and acute endocarditis. Even when only the early findings are present, such as a petechial rash with leukocytosis in the absence of meningeal signs, it is generally recommended to treat for acute meningococcal disease (166).

When the clinical picture and history are compatible with RMSF, therapy may consist of two drugs such as intravenous tetracycline and a cephalosporin, or one drug such as intravenous chloramphenicol, which should be instituted immediately to treat these two serious diseases.

Chronic Meningococcemia

There is a rare chronic meningococcemia syndrome with many of the character-istics of a chronic relapsing vasculitis. Skin lesions may vary from small petechia, macules, papules, and vesicles, to large nodules, sometimes with hemorrhage. The rash is usually associated with low-grade fever, myalgia, arthralgia, cephalgia, and nuchal rigidity. The rash and all other symptoms may simultaneously disappear and reappear in 3- to 7-day cycles. Such a recurrent pattern may be seen over periods of 2 to 6 months. This specific mimicry of subacute vasculitis can be supported by skin biopsy and thus lead to inappropriate and dangerous steroid therapy for a suspected vasculitis. If steroids are given (and even in many cases if they are not), the illness may suddenly evolve after one of these mild episodes into a fulminant hemorrhagic meningococcemia with shock or into acute purulent meningitis.

Antibiotic therapy in the chronic phase is curative, and in most cases no host factors have been found to easily explain the chronic form of this otherwise acute fulminant illness (167).

Echo 9 and Other Enterovirus Petechial Rash

Enterovirus infections, particularly echo 9 and coxsackie 9, can present with fever with disseminated petechial lesions on the skin and occasionally on the oral mucosa. Occasionally these dermatologic signs with fever are associated with a simultaneous aseptic meningitis syndrome, therefore allowing echo 9 and its associates to completely mimic mild acute meningococcemia. The pe-ripheral WBC count in the CSF of patients with enterovirus infections is usually typical of an acute viral or aseptic meningitis picture and the disease is basically much less severe and much less progressive than the vast majority of cases of acute meningococcal disease. However, there are patients whose CSF is com-patible with an early bacterial infection and whose clinical presentation may appear to be sufficiently threatening so that the physician will appropriately begin immediate antibiotic therapy for a suspected meningococcemia. Al-though we have found the peripheral WBC count and smear to be helpful in this decision, "unnecessary" therapy would be considered a minor sin in such a clinical situation. Diagnosis of enteroviral infections depends on throat washings or stool cultures and convalescent serologic tests. These results will not be available for many days to weeks and therefore will have no effect on the decision-making of the physician (168).

Viral Hemorrhagic Fever Group

At least 12 accepted geographically confined viral agents can cause viral hemorrhagic fever (VHF) characterized by fever, shock, and hemorrhage. The hemorrhage is usually from the nose or the gums and gastrointestinal tract, with the worst prognosis existing with upper gastrointestinal tract bleeding. Microscopic and occasionally gross hematuria are also commonly seen. The initial symptoms of this group include sore throat, fever, headache, myalgia, abdominal pain, vomiting, and diarrhea. Physical findings are usually limited to conjunctivitis and a quite impressive purulent or erythematous pharyngitis. A sore throat is often the major initial symptom in these cases and should be considered a clue in the appropriate setting of a travel history and constitutional symptoms. Thrombocytopenia and mild leukopenia with lymphocytosis are typical (169,170).

Skin lesions of any type are very rare in VHF caused by Lassa fever, Kyasanur Forest fever, Omsk hemorrhagic fever, Rift Valley fever, and yellow fever. In the latter illness, the common severe fulminant hepatitis is often associated with scleral and dermal icterus. In the United States, the recently discovered Hantaan virus infection (Hantavirus muerte canyon) associated with an acute respiratory distress syndrome (ARDS) picture and a 60% mortality has not yet demonstrated either skin rash or pharyngitis (171).

The skin lesions of Argentine, Bolivian, Venezuelan, and hantavirus (HFRS—hemorrhagic fever and renal syndrome) hemorrhagic fevers are usually limited to an axillary petechial rash. These four conditions usually have an associated thrombocytopenia that is, however, not the mechanism of the petechiae or mucosal hemorrhage (172,173).

In Congo-Crimean hemorrhagic fever, a petechial rash is generally displayed, which rapidly evolves in many cases around the third to sixth day into very large ecchymosis, particularly on the trunk and extremities. Of all the so-called hemorrhagic fever groups, this is the one illness in which large cutaneous hemorrhages can dominate the clinical presentation and where the dermatologic picture lives up to the name hemorrhagic fever. Congo-Crimean hemorrhagic fever is a tick-borne disease acquired in the Mediterranean, eastern Europe, and most of Africa and is one of the potentially contagious illnesses of this group along with Lassa fever, Marburg virus, and Ebola virus that threatens the medical support team caring for the sick patient (174–176).

Dengue hemorrhagic fever, Ebola virus, and Marburg virus are the only members of this group that initially demonstrate a classical macular–papular rash. This rash is generally seen between the fifth and seventh day of illness, and the rash may fade completely after the tenth day, leading to desquamation.

A relatively unimpressive petechial rash in the axilla may also be seen in this trio.

These illnesses must be considered in patients who have arrived within 3 weeks from the geographically limited areas in which these viruses reside and who have symptoms of abrupt fever, pharyngitis, conjunctivitis, severe malaise, weakness, thrombocytopenia, and any evidence of mucosal hemorrhage. The skin lesions are in general an adjunct rather than an important diagnostic clue to determining the possible etiology of these cases.

Public health decisions, including extremely careful isolation of the patients, are important for the Ebola, Marburg, Lassa, and Congo-Crimean agents. The guidelines of the Centers for Disease Control and Prevention (CDC) must be followed, and the CDC will always enthusiastically offer help in suspected cases. There is no evidence of person-to-person spread in any of the other cases of VHF. Ribavirin therapy appears to be successful for Lassa fever (177–179).

The differential diagnosis in patients who have recently traveled to other parts of the world includes malaria, rickettsial infections, meningococcemia, leptospirosis, and other bacterial sepsis syndromes. Obviously, peripheral blood smears, the Weil-Felix reaction, skin biopsy, leptospiral serologies, and blood cultures are necessary. Coagulation studies may be instructive. Much milder VHF cases may mimic the arthropod-borne flavivirus and alpha virus groups in which petechiae are occasionally seen along with the more typically seen diffuse macular–papular rashes.

NONINFECTIOUS CAUSES OF THE AFR

Collagen Vascular Diseases

Collagen vascular diseases can manifest the combination of fever and skin rash and, intermittently, may demonstrate acute episodes of disease activity. These illnesses include the systemic vasculitis group, such as periarteritis nodosa, giant cell arteritis, hypersensitivity vasculitis, and variants such as essential mixed cryoglobulinemia and Henoch-Schönlein purpura as well as the vasculitides associated with other collagen diseases. In addition to the notorious classical organ system involvement seen in these illnesses, including arthritis and nephritis, the skin is commonly involved. The typical patterns are vasculitis skin lesions of the palpable purpuric type usually seen on the lower extremities, livedo reticularis, necrotic lesions, infarcts of the tips of digits, and chronic lower extremity ulcers. Diffuse urticaria is occasionally seen in this group. Other diffuse rashes are uncommon and rare at initial presentation. The skin lesions of the granulomatous vasculitis group such as Wegener's have the usual vascular palpable purpuric lesions on the lower extremities.

Collagen diseases in which the diagnosis is supported by serology, such as systemic lupus erythematosus, Sjögren's syndrome, mixed connective tissue disease, the "overlap" syndromes, and rheumatoid arthritis, rarely demonstrate diffuse erythematous rashes during their acute disease exacerbations.

Dermatomyositis commonly has a characteristic rash seen in more than 90% of the cases. The electromyogram, aldolase, creatine phosphokinase (CPK), and muscle biopsy can help establish the diagnosis. Along with muscle weakness and pain, a characteristic rash demonstrates a scaly, erythematous eruption, with dermal atrophy over the knuckles, elbows, knees, forehead, face, neck, and upper torso. This pattern is said to be pathognomonic of dermatomyositis (180).

Other etiology-unknown illnesses with potential AFR include the rash of antiphospholipid syndrome (usually livedo reticularis), Behcet's disease (erythema nodosum or palpable purpura), and the rash in polychondritis and thrombotic thrombocytopenia purpura (a vascular purpura) (181–186). The only rash commonly seen in familial Mediterranean fever is a characteristic erysipeloid rash over the ankles that progresses either very slowly or not at all.

The reactive hemophagocytic syndrome has recently been described and is characterized as a subacute to chronic syndrome with an acute onset with hepatosplenomegaly, lymphadenopathy, fever, pancytopenia, and rash in 10 to 30% of cases. The rash can be maculopapular, nodular, vasculitic, or petechial. The cause can be familial and is associated with known collagen vascular diseases, such as systemic lupus erythematosus, solid tumor, immunodeficiency states, and bone marrow transplantation. However, the majority of cases are due to lymphoma or intracellular infectious agents such as EBV, CMV, Q fever, brucella, tuberculosis, histoplasmosis, cryptococcosis, leishmaniasis, and endocarditis of unknown etiology (187). The diagnosis is established conveniently by bone marrow aspiration or more sensitively by lymph node or splenic aspiration.

Eosinophilia–Myalgia Syndrome AFR

The newly described and now disappearing eosinophilia–myalgia syndrome secondary to contaminated tryptophane commonly has a chronic, macular–papular, pruritic, erythematous, centrally located rash with extension to face, neck, and extremities. Eosinophilia is seen early in the course. The illness is chronic in nature and is associated with peripheral edema, severe myalgia, severe painful neuropathy, and bouts of fever and pneumonitis (188,189). The slow development of systemic symptoms and the diffuse rash that lasts for many months usually separate this illness from the AFR under discussion. New episodes of this illness should no longer be seen because the offending drug is no longer being used or marketed. The toxic-oil syndrome and eosinophilic fasciitis are variants of this syndrome (190,191).

Juvenile Rheumatoid Arthritis—AFR

Juvenile rheumatoid arthritis in the adult can mimic the acute febrile rash syndrome. It often presents with an acute onset of pharyngitis, very high-grade spiking fever, leukocytosis, and very early in the course, a diffuse macular–papular salmon pink rash, usually over the trunk and proximal extremities. The rash can be mildly pruritic, and the most important characteristic of the rash is the daily appearance in the evening along with the peak of the fever and the rapid disappearance of the rash by the morning, only to reappear each day with the peak of fever. This evening rash can also be seen in JRA patients who remain afebrile but symptomatic. Associated lymphadenopathy and hepatosplenomegaly confuse the picture, but eventually the symmetrical diffuse or pauciarticular arthritis dominates the clinical picture. Unfortunately, serologic studies and biopsies are not helpful in confirming a diagnosis in this disease. The diagnosis is made clinically by ruling everything else out, recognizing the clinical importance of the intermittent rash that is seen in 80% of the cases, and following the course of the patient (192).

In summary, very few of the collagen vascular diseases and their variants actually present initially with the characteristics of acute febrile rash syndrome. When rashes do occur, they are in the context of already diagnosed collagen vascular diseases. Lower extremity vascular purpura is the most common rash of this group and lends itself easily to diagnostic biopsy. Livedo reticularis and chronic leg ulcers are usually not part of the AFR. Dermatomyositis has a chronic scaling rash not consistent with the AFR, and muscle biopsy, CPK, aldolase, and chronicity will aid in the differential diagnosis.

Juvenile rheumatoid arthritis can present a difficult diagnostic problem at the onset of the illness and early in its course under any circumstances. Dermatomyositis and the reactive hemophagocytic syndrome can be proven by biopsy of appropriate material.

Any systemic illness that resembles a collagen vascular disease that cannot be proven must be considered as probably being caused by drug therapy, including medications taken over a long period.

Classical Dermatologic Skin Conditions in AFR

Occasionally, the infectious disease specialist must deal with diagnostic mysteries in patients with unusual skin lesions. Sweet's syndrome (neutrophilic dermatosis) is an erythematous plaque, fever, arthritis syndrome that becomes easily diagnosed with a skin lesion biopsy and rapidly responds to steroids. Occasionally, fever accompanies acute exacerbation of acute intermittent porphyria, Fabry's disease, dermatitis herpetiformis, pemphigus, Weber-Christian syndrome, and acrodermatitis enteropathica. The skin lesions are extremely localized in all of these conditions, and their chronicity again separates patients with these illnesses from typical AFR patients.

A small group of rare diseases presents with sterile epidermal neutrophilic pustules, including pustular psoriasis, palmoplantar pustulosis, subcorneal pustular dermatosis, Sweet's syndrome, and erythema multiforma (193,194). Acne fulminans is one of the most important dermatologic conditions in this group and classically presents with systemic reactions including fever, weight loss, anemia, leukocytosis, myalgias, myositis, osteoarthritis, arthritis, and osteolytic lesions (195,196). This condition is mainly seen in young men. The pustules are sterile and nonresponsive to antibiotics, but usually respond to steroid therapy. Acne fulminans is characterized by inflammatory tender ulcerative encrusted lesions on the back, chest, and face and is one of the most scarring acute dermatologic conditions seen in young individuals. The association of high fever and marked leukocytosis as well as polyarthrylgia often lead to antibiotic therapy, but if used alone antibiotics are consistently ineffective unless steroid therapy is also given.

Another recently described illness is acute generalized exanthematous pustulosis, usually precipitated by antibiotic therapy. This illness is best described as a diffuse toxic erythema that begins around the face, disseminates within a few hours and is associated with nonfollicular small pustules, often more than a hundred in number. The illness can be self-limited. Antibiotic therapy is usually given as a therapy, but as a matter of fact, in more than 80% of cases, antibiotics seem to be the provocative cause (197).

Impetigo herpetiformis is an illness of pregnancy that generally spontaneously remits in the puerperium. It is relatively rare and is thought to be a form of pustular psoriasis generally occurring in the last trimester. Antimicrobial therapy is often given because of the pustular appearance but is usually ineffective and steroid therapy is generally helpful. The illness may present in an acute fashion, but generally lasts for many months until the delivery of the baby (198).

The most common and important member of this group of patients with strange regional skin lesions and fever are the individuals with self-induced disease because of psychiatric illness. Pyoderma gangrenosum has baffled more than one infectious disease specialist and its association with fever due to undiagnosed inflammatory bowel disease or underlying hematologic malignancy guarantee the need for infectious disease specialists to maintain a high index of suspicion (199).

AFR AND SPECIFIC SYNDROMES

AFR and Hepatitis or Jaundice

The most common cause of this triad of rash, fever, and jaundice seen in the United States would be related to hypersensitivity reactions to drugs such as dilantin, sulfa agents, pyrimethamine, trimethoprim, clavulanate acid (given with amoxicillin), quinidine, and quinine.

Other very important causes of fever, rash, and acute hepatic disease include secondary syphilis, relapsing fever, leptospirosis (usually associated with renal involvement), cat scratch disease, and disseminated herpes simplex. Infrequently, Q fever, RMSF, typhus, psittacosis, *V. vulnificus* septicemia in cirrhotics, *Clostridia perfringens* gas gangrene, staphylococcal sepsis, infectious mononucleosis, CMV, gonococcemia, coxsackie B, varicella, measles, Marburg disease, Lassa fever, and Ebola virus are rare causes of rash, fever, and liver involvement (200,201). In immunocompromised hosts, disseminated herpes simplex, acute GVHD in liver transplant patients, disseminated histoplasmosis and toxoplasmosis in AIDS patients, and disseminated candidiasis in leukopenic patients can also result in the same combination of fever, disseminated rash, and clinical liver involvement.

Any patient with underlying liver disease, usually cirrhosis, who develops any acute cause of AFR syndrome could easily present with an acute febrile rash and jaundice due to stress on the already diseased liver.

Pneumonia and AFR

The differential diagnosis of pneumonia and diffuse rash includes *M. pneumoniae*, psittacosis, adenovirus, atypical measles, echo and coxsackie-viruses (particularly coxsackie A9), coccidioidomycosis, histoplasmosis, blastomycosis, Q fever, scrub typhus, classical typhus, and RMSF.

Polyarthritis and AFR

Rubella virus, parvovirus, arbovirus, hepatitis B, and much more rarely, measles and varicella, are viruses that can cause rash and symmetrical polyarthritis with a typical rheumatoid arthritis metaphalangeal and proximal interphalangeal joint distribution that sometimes lasts 3 to 4 weeks, particularly in the adult population (202,203). The previous described arbovirus Ross River, Sinbis, Majora, Q'nyong-Nyong and chikungunya cause rash and true polyarthritis and Dengue and West Nile cause polyarthralgias and rash.

Yersinia enterocolitica, disseminated gonococcemia, meningococcal disease, *S. moniliformis*, secondary syphilis, Lyme disease, endocarditis, and a variety of collagen vascular diseases can demonstrate fever, rash, and a polyarthritis syndrome. Erythema marginatum and polyarthritis can, rarely, be seen at the same time in acute rheumatic fever. JRA, leukocytoclastic angiitis, and other collagen vascular diseases also can cause polyarthritis and various types of skin manifestations.

Central Nervous System Disease and AFR

The majority of patients with AFR and CNS involvement present with a central rash, fever, and acute meningoencephalitis caused by coxsackievirus, echovirus, measles, rubella, EBV, HIV, and chickenpox. The previously listed causes of AFR in the hemorrhagic fever group and arbovirus group can also cause these symptoms. All of the rickettsia, systemic spirochete, ehrlichia, psittacosis, mycoplasma, toxic shock syndrome, and all causes of endocarditis must be considered in the differential diagnosis. Invasive bacteria, particularly the meningococcus, as well as tularemia, brucellosis, plague, cat scratch fever, and listeria, and *Tropheryma whippelli*, the cause of Whipple's disease. Parasitic infections would include strongyloides (often with secondary bacterial infection), schistosomiasis, trichinosis, gnathostomiasis, and rarely, toxoplasmosis.

The noninfectious causes include Kawasaki, eosinophilia, myalgia, vasculitis, antiphospholipid antibody syndrome, erythrophagocytosis syndrome, thrombocytic thrombocytopenic purpura, and drug reactions, particularly the Stevens-Johnson syndrome. This enormous list of possibilities obviously demands that the clinician possess great skill and knowledge of this syndrome when treating a patient difficult to diagnose.

SPECIFIC HOSTS

The Patient with HIV Infection

Abnormalities of the skin, both infectious and noninfectious, are common in patients infected with the HIV. In fact, the skin may be the most commonly affected organ in this disease. A complete summary of the myriad dermatologic manifestations and complications seen in the HIV-infected patient is beyond the scope of this review. The reader is referred to other sources for more complete discussion (204–206).

HIV

Acute infection with HIV is often associated with a mononucleosis-like illness with rash. The rash is noted within several weeks following exposure and may last up to 3 weeks (207). It is an erythematous macular eruption on the face, trunk, and extremities. Antibodies to HIV may be negative during this phase of infection and, therefore, should be repeated several weeks to 6 months later.

Eosinophilic pustular folliculitis is characterized by diffuse pustular lesions that are pruritic and sterile. Infiltration of the hair follicle with eosinophils and neutrophils eventually destroys the hair. Patients may have leukocytosis or eosinophilia but are without systemic toxicity. Skin biopsy reveals an intercellular edema (spongiosis) with cellular infiltration but negative stains for organisms and cultures. Although the illness may wax and wane, ultraviolet B phototherapy has been reported to be effective (208).

An unusual manifestation of toxin-producing staphylococcus has been reported in patients with AIDS. This illness is similar to classic toxic shock syndrome in that patients have episodes of hypotension and multiorgan system dysfunction. Reported cases of this toxic shocklike syndrome recurred over a mean of 50 days, leading to the term recalcitrant erythematous desquamating disorder or RED (209).

Folliculitis due to *Staphylococcus* species and dermatophytosis, common ailments in the non-AIDS patient, may be particularly unresponsive to therapy in this population. Botryomycosis is a severe bacterial folliculitis that mimics mycetoma (210). Staphylococcus and gram-negative rods may cause this disease. Pustular drainage with granules is seen, and the granules are made up of clumps of bacteria. Seborrheic dermatitis and psoriasis are more common in AIDS patients and may be less responsive to therapy. Severe pustular psoriasis and a presentation suggesting chronic Reiter's syndrome have also been described. The differential diagnosis of diffuse hyperkeratosis with crusting and peeling of skin includes hyperkeratotic (Norwegian) scabies, an illness characterized by involvement of most areas of the skin and a very large parasitic load. This usually occurs in an immunocompromised patient and has been reported in AIDS patients (211).

Syphilis can produce a variety of skin manifestations, as previously noted. In the patient coinfected with HIV, two syndromes are particularly noteworthy. Biopsy-proven cases of seronegative secondary syphilis have been reported in HIV-infected persons, further supporting the role of biopsy in patients with unexplained rash as well as the importance of appropriate barrier precautions in the examination of patients with skin lesions (212,213). Lues maligna is a rare manifestation of secondary syphilis characterized by an ulcerating necrotizing vasculitis with pustular, nodular, and ulcerating skin lesions. In the past, severe malnourishment was the main risk factor for this manifestation of syphilis, which appears to be more dependent on the underlying health status of the host than on an organism factor. The debilitation seen in advanced AIDS appears to be a similar risk factor for this presentation (214).

Other sexually transmitted infections may have atypical courses in patients infected with HIV. Persistent genital or anal ulcers are frequently due to herpes simplex virus. Although originally appearing as crops of vesicles on an erythematous base, these lesions may coalesce to form one or more large ulcers measuring several centimeters in diameter with clean borders and rare drainage or superinfection. The differential diagnosis includes pressure sores for the bedridden patient; however, herpetic lesions are rarely located at pressure points. Extension of lesions beyond the genital area may create confusion with some of the diffuse vesicular syndromes. Chronic acyclovir or other antiherpes medications may control this infection, but the development of resistance limits efficacy for many patients (215). Herpetic whitlow (ulceration of a finger at the terminal phalanx due to herpes simplex, typically acquired from auto-inoculation from a genital site) may also have a severe, persistent course in AIDS patients compared to a recurrent course in the immunocompetent individual (216). The differential diagnosis of perianal or genital ulcers includes CMV in the patient with AIDS. This is from spread of colonic disease to the perianal area with fissures and ulcerations. Quale et al. have reported data on a patient presenting with a painful penile ulcer with superinfection and subsequent development of ulcerated areas at distant sites (extremities) persisting for months. Cultures and response to therapy in this case was consistent with *Haemophilus ducreyi* (chancroid) (217). Ulcerated lesions confined to a dermatome are usually due to herpes zoster.

Focal persistent lesions, whether nodular, macular, erythematous, plaquelike, or ulcerating should be carefully evaluated for the possibility of malignancy or opportunistic infection. Several processes have been particularly notable in patients with AIDS. Mycobacterial species, particularly *M. tuberculosis* and *M. avium* complex are common pathogens in patients with HIV infection. Lupus vulgaris and tuberculosis cutis orificialis are two manifestations of cutaneous tuberculosis. Lupus vulgaris is a granulomatous lesion, usually found on the face or neck area, related to nearby draining infection. Tuberculosis cutis orificialis is a syndrome of ulcerations in the mouth and other mucocutaneous areas, usually confined to debilitated hosts with miliary disease, and is due to dissemination from the respiratory or gastrointestinal area. *M. haemophilum* is especially associated with skin involvement in AIDS patients and may be missed by routine mycobacterial culture methods. This organism grows slowly, requires iron supplementation, and grows best at 37°C. *M. haemophilum* causes nodular, pustular, necrotic lesions, more common on the extremities over bone or joints. Underlying joint effusions or bony infection are often present. The lesions are usually painful (123,128). Biopsy shows granuloma formation and assists in the differentiation from Kaposi's sarcoma, fungal infection, or bacillary angiomatosis; however, the distribution of the lesions on the extremities, possibly due to the impaired growth of the organism at warmer temperatures, is a clue.

Fungal infections frequently involve the skin and mucous membranes of patients with AIDS; however, most produce only local findings. Chronic dermatophytid infection, persistent *Candida* vaginitis, and oral thrush are all findings that should suggest a cell-mediated immunodeficiency. Oral hairy leukoplakia, associated with EBV, usually appears as an asymptomatic whitish plaque on the lateral aspect of the tongue and may mimic a fungal infection. Patients with AIDS are 10 to 15 times more likely than normal hosts to develop disseminated disease due to *Histoplasma capsulatum* (219). An erythematous papular rash of the upper body has been reported in some cases of disseminated histoplasmosis and is frequently smear and culture positive on biopsy (220). Although skin involvement is also uncommon in disseminated cryptococcal disease, umbilicated papules on the face and upper body, resembling molluscum contagiosum, have been described (221).

Bacillary angiomatosis is characterized by a diffuse distribution of subcutaneous and cutaneous vascular lesions that are palpable and show vessel proliferation on biopsy. Organisms (bacilli) may be seen on Warthin-Starry stain of the tissue. Recently *Rochalimaea henselae* and *Rochalimaea quintana* have been identified as the likely pathogens in this syndrome and the related peliosis hepatis (222). The presentation of bacillary angiomatosis may be indistinguishable from Kaposi's sarcoma. Clinical clues that can assist in making this distinction include the recognition that bacillary angiomatosis is more friable, with a greater likelihood of bleeding with trauma, erythema suggestive of cellulitis is often at the base of the lesions, the lesions are painful, and underlying bony disease may be present (223). Even with these characteristics, suspicious lesions should be biopsied. Another infection that may present with diffuse purplish papules or nodules is cutaneous pneumocystosis, with the external auditory canal a particularly common site of involvement (224). This same presentation, with or without ulceration of the lesions, may also be seen in infection due to acanthamoeba and leishmaniasis (225,226).

In addition to the many infectious and malignant skin diseases seen in AIDS, a number of unusual inflammatory and allergic syndromes are also seen. These include a high incidence of rash after exposure to trimethoprim-sulfamethoxazole, leukocytoclastic vasculitis, telangiectasias, photosensitivity, and increased reaction to insect bites.

Porphyria cutanea tarda, manifest by facial hypertrichosis, hyperpigmentation, photosensitivity, and bullae after sun exposure have also been reported (227).

Graft-versus-Host Disease

Graft-versus-host disease is a serious complication for the transplant recipient. The presence of a macular rash in a febrile patient during the posttransplant period generally brings to mind many conditions, but most importantly, acute GVHD. The only possibility for immediate diagnosis is a skin biopsy. The skin biopsy will show focal epithelial cell necrosis with basal cell vacuolization. The differential diagnosis of these pathologic lesions includes GVHD, toxic epidermal necrolysis, erythema multiforme, and fixed drug eruptions. Obviously the pathologist must recognize the clinical setting so that the appropriate diagnosis can be made. GVHD is one of the new illnesses associated with a skin rash and fever, and in this case the skin rash is a very early and extremely helpful finding (228).

Acute GVHD is commonly seen after solid organ or bone marrow transfusion and is rarely seen after nonirradiated blood product transfusions in immunocompromised hosts. The erythematous rash erupts first on the palms, soles, and ears, and then on the trunk, face, and extremities. The rash is pruritic and is often described as feeling like a sunburn. As it intensifies, the rash becomes bright and confluent. In severe reactions, bullous lesions, epidermal necrolysis, and a positive Nikolsky sign will be seen. The second most common organ involved is the liver and then the gastrointestinal tract. Fever usually precedes the rash, and the rash precedes the other organ system involvement. This is another example of a palms and soles erythematous skin rash. The erythroderma of the skin rash is quite striking. The prognosis of the patient correlates with the gradation and severity of the skin biopsy with grade 4 having a 95% to 100% mortality.

UNIQUE RECREATION AND OCCUPATION-ASSOCIATED RASH AND FEVER SYNDROMES

Many occupations and recreational activities bring the participant in close contact with animals, water, soil, or allergens, increasing the likelihood of the development of an AFR syndrome. Most infections involving the skin that develop as a result of these exposures present as a focal involvement without a subsequent diffuse skin presentation. Examples of these include sporotrichosis (gardener), *Mycobacterium marinum* (tropical fish enthusiast), cat scratch disease (veterinarian), plague (recreational exposure to southwestern United States), herpetic whitlow (respiratory therapist), and cutaneous anthrax (exposure to contaminated animal materials such as hides). Many of the other infections that might be acquired by these exposures and are associated with diffuse skin involvement, such as leptospirosis, cutaneous larva migrans, toxoplasmosis, and rickettsiae illnesses, have already been mentioned. We have chosen to highlight here several of the remaining syndromes that may present a confusing clinical picture.

"Hot tub" folliculitis is most commonly manifest by the development of a generalized pustular folliculitis usually developing 1 to 2 days after exposure to a contaminated hot tub or whirlpool. *P. aeruginosa* is the most commonly identified pathogen (229,230). The area covered by the bathing suit is most dramatically affected. Some infected bathers also report swollen breasts, sore throat, earache, and occasionally, abdominal cramps. About 10% of infected patients develop fever. The rash usually resolves within 7 days.

Herpes gladiatorum is a primary HSV infection (usually HSV-1) acquired from the close contact and trauma associated mainly with wrestling and rugby. Lesions may be on the head, extremities, or trunk. Headache, sore throat, and fever are common. Approximately 10% may have an associated conjunctivitis or blepharitis (231,232). The unusual distribution of lesions may prompt a consideration of varicella, zoster, or impetigo as an etiology unless this important exposure history is obtained. A pustular dermatitis due to infection with *Enterobacteriaceae* has also been described in association with mud wrestling (dermatitis palaestrae limosae) (233).

The increased use of latex gloves among health care workers has led to an increased recognition of allergic reactions (234). The most common reaction is a delayed hypersensitivity manifest by erythema and pain or pruritus of the hands beginning about 48 hours after exposure. A second, less common, reaction is an immediate urticarial contact dermatitis. This reaction, beginning on the hands, may become generalized and be associated with other symptoms of IgE-mediated illness such as wheezing, conjunctivitis, and anaphylaxis. Mild cases resolve in 1 to 2 hours without treatment. More severe cases should be treated as any other systemic allergic reaction.

REFERENCES

1 **Wenner HA.** Virus diseases associated with cutaneous eruptions. Progr Med Virol 1973;16:269–336.

2 **Cherry JD.** Cutaneous manifestations of systemic infections. In: Feigin RD, Cherry JD, eds. Textbook of Pediatric Infectious Diseases, 3rd ed, vol. 1. 1992;755–782.

3 **Powwell KR.** Filatow-Dukes' disease. Epidermolytic toxin-producing staphylo-

cocci as the etiologic agent of the fourth childhood exanthem. Am J Dis Child 1979;133:88–91.

4 Yamanishi K, Shiraki K, Kondo T, et al. Identification of human herpesvirus-6 as a causal agent for exanthem subitum. Lancet May 14, 1988:1065–1067.

5 Shapiro L. On the numbered exanthemata. Clin Pediatri 1967;6:611–612.

6 Cherry JD, Jhan CL. Exanthem and enanthem associated with mumps virus infection. Arch Environ Health 1966;12: 518–521.

7 Lerner AM, Cherry JD, Klein JO, Finland M. Infections with reoviruses. N Engl J Med 1962;267:947–952.

8 Ruzicka T, Rosendahl C, Braun-Falco O. A probable cause of rotavirus exanthem. Arch Dermatol 1985;121:253–254.

9 Timar L, Budai J, Gero A, Lakos A, Rapi K. Rare complications and unusual syndromes associated with Epstein-Barr virus. 1985;4:212–213. Letters.

10 Baumgarter JD, Glauser MP, Burgo-Black AL, Black RD, Pyndiah N, Chiolero R. Severe cytomegalovirus infection in multiply transfused, splenectomised, trauma patients. Lancet. July 10, 1982:63–66.

11 Coopman SA, Johnson RA, Platt R, Stern RS. Cutaneous disease and drug reactions in HIV infections. N Engl J Med 1993; 328:1670–1674.

12 Young EJ. Human brucellosis. Rev Infect Dis 1983;5:821–842.

13 Harrison DL. A case of human ornithosis presenting as an obscure febrile illness associated with macular rash. Gen Pract Forum 1962:245–246.

14 Spelman DW. Q-fever: A study of 111 consecutive cases. Med J Aust 1982;1:547–553.

15 Harris AA, Pattage JC, Kessler HA, Zeihen M, Levin S. Psittacosis bacteremia in a patient with sarcoidosis. Ann Intern Med 1984;101:502–503.

16 Suringa WR, Bank LJ, Ackerman AB. Role of measles virus in skin lesions and Koplik's spots. N Engl J Med 1970;283: 1139–1142.

17 Rauh LW, Schmidt R. Measles immunization with killed virus vaccine. Am J Child 1965;109:232–237.

18 Hall WJ, Hall CB. Atypical measles in adolescents; evaluation of clinical and pulmonary function. Ann Intern Med 1979;90:882–886.

19 Martin DB, Weiner LB, Nieburg PI, Blair DC. Atypical measles in adolescents and young adults. Ann Intern Med 1979;90: 877–881.

20 Edmonson MB, Addiss DG, McPherson JT, Berg JI, Circo SR, Davis JP. Mild measles and secondary vaccine failure during a sustained outbreak in a highly vaccinated population. JAMA 1990;253: 2467–2471.

21 Markowitz LE, Chandler FW, Roldan EO, et al. Fatal measles pneumonia without rash in a child with AIDS. J Infect Dis 1988;158:480.

22 Schiff GM. Titered lots of immune globulin. Efficacy in the prevention of rubella. Am J Dis Child 1969;118:322.

23 Johnson RE, Hall AB. Rubella arthritis. N Engl J Med 1958;258:743.

24 Tunnessen WW Jr. Erythema infectiosum, roseola, and enteroviral exanthems. Infectious Diseases. In: Gorback SL, Blacklow NR, eds. Philadelphia: WB Saunders, 19:1120–1125.

25 Chou S. Human herpesvirus 6 infection and associated disease. J Lab Clin Med 1993;121:368–393.

26 Carl M, Tibbs CW, Dobson ME, Papparello S, Dasch GA. Diagnosis of acute typhus infection using the polymerase chain reaction. J Infect Dis 1990; 161:791–793.

27 Zdrodovskii PF, Golinevich HM. Classical Typhus. In: Zdrodovskii PF, Golinevich HM, eds. The Rickettsial Diseases. Pergamon Press, 1960:217–236.

28 Zdrodovskii PF, Glonevich HM. In: Zdrodovskii PF, Glonevich HM, eds. The Rickettsial Diseases. Pergamon Press, 1960:236–246.

29 McDade JE, Shepard CC, Redus MA, et al. Evidence of *Rickettsia prowazekii* infections in the United States. Am J Trop Med Hyg 1980;29:277–284.

30 Dumler JS, Taylor JP, Walker DH. Clinical and laboratory features on murine typhus in south Texas, 1980 through 1987. JAMA 1991;266:1365–1370.

31 Slipapojakul K, Chayakul P, Krisanapan S, Slipopojakul K. Murine typhus in Thailand: clinical features, diagnosis and treatment. Q J Med 1993;86:43–47.

32 Raoult D, Brouqui P, Marchou B, Gastaut J-A. Acute and chronic Q-fever in patients with cancer. Clin Infect Dis 1992;14:127–130.

33 **DuPont HT, Raoult D, Brouqui P, et al.** Epidemiologic features and clinical presentation of acute Q-fever in hospitalized patients: 323 French cases. Am J Med 1992;93:427–431.

34 **Truck WPG, Howitt G, Turnberg A, et al.** Chronic Q-fever. Q J Med 1976;45:193–217.

35 **Goldman DP, Artenstein AW, Bolan CD.** Human ehrlichiosis: a newly recognized tick-borne disease. Am Fam Phy 1992;46:199–208.

36 **Dumler JS, Sutker WL, Walker DH.** Persistent infection with *Ehrlichia chaffeensis*. Clin Infect Dis 1993;17:903–905.

37 **Fichtenbaum CJ, Peterson LR, Weil GL.** Ehrlichiosis presenting as a life-threatening illness with features of the toxic shock syndrome. Am J Med 1993;95:351–356.

38 **Trape JF, Duplantier JM, Bougannali H, et al.** Tick-borne borreliosis in West Africa. Lancet 1991;337:473–475.

39 **Fihn S, Larson EB.** Tick-borne relapsing fever in the Pacific Northwest: an underdiagnosed illness? West J Med 1980;133:203–209.

40 **Spach DH, Liles WC, Campbell GL, Quick RE, Anderson DE, Fritsche TR.** Tick-borne diseases in the United States. N Engl J Med 1993;329:936–947.

41 **Horton JM, Blaser MJ.** The spectrum of relapsing fever in the Rocky Mountains. Arch Intern Med 1985;145:871–875.

42 **Schmidt DR, Winn RE, Keefe TJ.** Leptospirosis—epidemiology features of a sporadic case. Arch Intern Med 1989;149:1878–1880.

43 **Humphry T, Sanders S, Stadius M.** Leptospirosis mimicking MLNS. 1977;91:853–854. Letters.

44 **Ehrenkranz NJ, Ventura AK, Cuadrado RR, Pond WL, Porter JE.** Pandemic dengue in Caribbean countries and the southern United States—past, present and potential problems. N Engl J Med 1971;285:1460–1469.

45 **Malison MD, Waterman SH.** Dengue fever in the United States: a report of a cluster of imported cases and review of the clinical, epidemiologic and public health aspects of the disease. JAMA 1983;249:496–500.

46 **Schlesinger RW.** Dengue viruses. Virology Monographs vol 16. New York: Springer-Verlag, 1977:86–90.

47 **Monath TP.** Viral febrile illnesses. Strickland GT, ed. In: Hunter's tropical medicine 7th ed. Philadelphia: WB Saunders, 1991:200–219.

48 **Freier JE.** Eastern equine encephalomyelitis. Lancet 1993;342:1281–1285.

49 **Goodpasture HC, Poland JD, Francy DB, Bowen GS, Horn KA.** Colorado tick fever: clinical, epidemiologic, and laboratory aspects of 228 cases in Colorado in 1973–1974. Ann Intern Med 1978;88:303–310.

50 **Spruance SL, Bailey A.** Colorado tick fever: a review of 115 laboratory confirmed cases. Arch Intern Med 1973;131:288–293.

51 **Tesh RB.** Arthritides caused by mosquito-borne viruses. Ann Rev Med 1982;33:31–40.

52 **Niklasson B, Espmark A, LeDuc JW, et al.** Association of sindbis-like virus with Ockelbo disease in Sweden. Am J Trop Med Hyg 1984;1212–1217.

53 **Kennedy AC, Flemming J, Solomon L.** Chikungunya viral arthropathy: a clinical description. J Rheum 1980:7:231–236.

54 **Gilman RH, Terminel M, Levine MM, et al.** Relative efficacy of blood, urine, rectal scrub, bone marrow and rose spot cultures for recovery of *Salmonella typhi* in typhoid fever. Lancet 1975;1:1211–1213.

55 **Kaplowitz LG, Fisher JJ, Sparling PF.** Rocky Mountain spotted fever: a clinical dilemma. Curr Clin Topic Infect Dis 89–108.

56 **Kirk JL, Fine DP, Sexton DJ, Muchmore HG.** Rocky Mountain spotted fever—a clinical review based on 48 confirmed cases, 1943–1986. Medicine 1990;69:35–45.

57 **Griffith GL, Luce EA.** Massive skin necrosis in Rocky Mountain spotted fever. South Med J 1978;71:1337–1340.

58 **Kirkland KB, Marcom PK, Sexton DJ, Sumler JS, Walker DH.** Rocky Mountain spotted fever complicated by gangrene: report of six cases and review. Clin Infect Dis 1993;16:629–634.

59 **Salgo MP, Telzak EE, Currie B, et al.** A focus of Rocky Mountain spotted fever within New York City. N Engl J Med 1988;318:1345–1348.

60 **Westerman EL.** Rocky Mountain spotless fever. Arch Intern Med 1982;142:1106–1107.

61 **Woodward TE.** Rocky Mountain spotted fever: epidemiological and early clinical

signs are keys to treatment and reduced mortality. J Infect Dis 1984;150:465–468.

62 **Green WR, Walker DH, Cain BG.** Fatal viscerotropic Rocky Mountain spotted fever. Am J Med 1978;64:523–528.

63 **Walker DH, Lesesne HR, Varma VA, Thancker WC.** Rocky Mountain spotted fever mimicking acute cholecystitis. Arch Intern Med 1985;145:2194–2196.

64 **Turner RC, Chaplinski TJ, Adams HG.** Rocky Mountain spotted fever presenting as thrombocytopenic purpura. Am J Med 1986;81:153–157.

65 **Tzianabos T, Anderson BE, McDade JE.** Detection of *Rickettsia rickettsii* DNA in clinical specimens by using polymerase chain reaction technology. J Clin Microbiol 1989;27:2866–2868.

66 **Sexton DJ, Corey GR.** Rocky Mountain "spotless" and "almost spotless" fever: a wolf in sheep's clothing. Clin Infect Dis 1992;15:439–448.

67 **Chapel TA.** The signs and symptoms of secondary syphilis. Sex Transm Dis 1980; 7:161–170.

68 **Loveday C, Bingham JS.** Changes in circulating immune complexes during the Jarisch Herxheimer reaction in secondary syphilis. Eur J Clin Microbiol Infect Dis 1993;12:185–191.

69 **Huff JC, Weston WL.** Recurrent erythema multiforme. Medicine 1989;68:133–140.

70 **Cherry JD, Hurwitz WS, Welliver RC.** *Mycoplasma pneumoniae* infections and exanthems. J Peds 1975;87:369–373.

71 **Christenson B.** An outbreak of tularemia in the northern part of central Sweden. Scand J Infect Dis 1984;16:285–290.

72 **Levy M, Shear NH.** *Mycoplasma pseumoniae* infections and Stevens-Johnson syndrome. Clin Peds 1991;30:42–49.

73 **Chan LS, Soong HK, Foster CS, Hammerberg C, Cooper KD.** Ocular cicatrical pemphigoid occurring as a sequela of Stevens-Johnson syndrome. JAMA 1991;266:1543–1546.

74 **Hughes RD, Roberts C.** Hand, foot, mouth disease associated with coxsackie A9 virus. Lancet 1972;2:751.

75 **Raffin BJ, Freemark M.** Streptobacillary rat-bite fever: a pediatric problem. Pediatr 1979;64:214–217.

76 **Thyresson N.** Acrodermatitis enteropathica. Report of a case healed with zinc therapy. Acta Dermato Venerol (Stockholm) 1974;54:383–385.

77 **Neldner KH, Hagler L, Wise WR, Stifel FB, Lufkin EG, Herman RH.** Acrodermatitis enteropathica. Arch Dermatol 1974;110:711–721.

78 **McDonald JC, MacLean JD, McDade JE.** Imported rickettsial disease: clinical and epidemiologic features. Am J Med 1988; 85:799–805.

79 **Paterson PY, Taylor W.** Rickettsialpox. Bull NY Acad Med 1966;42:579–587.

80 **Brettman LR, Lewin S, Holzman RS, et al.** Rickettsialpox: report of an outbreak and a contemporary review. Medicine 1981;60:363–372.

81 **Silpapojakul K, Ukkachoke C, Krisanapan S, Siplapojakul K.** Rickettsial meningitis and encephalitis. Arch Intern Med 1991;151:1753–1757.

82 **Rapmund G.** Rickettsial diseases of the Far East: new perspectives. J Infect Dis 1984;149:330–338.

83 **Wang JG, Walker DH.** Identification of spotted fever groups rickettsiae from human and tick sources in the People's Republic of China. J Infect Dis 1987;156: 665–669.

84 **Sexton DJ, Dwyer B, Kemp R, Graves S.** Spotted fever group rickettsial infections in Australia. Rev Infect Dis 1991;13:876–886.

85 **Bitten, hot, and mostly spotty.** Lancet 1991;337:143–144. Editorial.

86 **Scrub typhus pneumonia.** Lancet November 5, 1988:1062.

87 **Okada T, Jange Y, Kobayashi Y.** Causative agent of spotted fever group rickettsiosis in Japan. Infect Immunol 1990;58:887–892.

88 **Moraga FA, Martinez-Riog A, Alonso JL, Boronat M, Domingo F.** Boutonneuse fever. Arch Dis Child 1982;57:149–151.

89 **Font-Creus B, Bella-Cueto F, Espejo-Arenas E, et al.** Mediterranean spotted fever: a cooperative study of 227 cases. Rev Infect Dis 1985;7:635–642.

90 **Hudson PJ, McPetrie R, Kitchener-Smith J, Eccles J.** Vesicular rash associated with infection due to *Rickettsia australis*. Clin Infect Dis 1994;18:118–119.

91 **Kemper CA, Spivack AF, Deresiniski SC.** Atypical papulovesicular rash due to infection with *Rickettsia conorii*. Clin Infect Dis 1992;15:591–594.

92 **Brouqui P, Dupont HT, Drancourt M, Bourgeade A, Raoult D.** Spotless Boutonneuse fever. Clin Infect Dis 1992; 14:114–116.

93   **Yagupsky P, Wolack B.** Fatal Israeli spotted fever in children. Clin Infect Dis 1993;17:850–853.

94   **Berger B.** Erythema chronicum migrans of Lyme disease. Arch Dermatol 1984; 120:1017–1021.

95   **Gear JHS, Miller GB.** The clinical manifestations of Rhodesian trypanosomiasis: an account of cases contracted in the Okavanago Swamps of Botswana. Am J Trop Med Hyg 1986;35:1146–1152.

96   **Mahmoud AAF, Warren KS.** Algorithms in the diagnosis and management of exotic diseases. XI. African Trypanosomiasis. J Infect Dis 1976;133:487–491.

97   **Bisno AL.** Group A streptococcal infections and acute rheumatic fever. N Engl J Med 1991;325:783–793.

98   **Miller RA, Brancato F, Holmes KK.** *Corynebacterium haemolyticum* as a cause of pharyngitis and scarlitinaform rash in young adults. Ann Intern Med 1986; 105:867–872.

99   **Tofte RW, Williams DN.** Toxic shock syndrome. Evidence of a broad clinical spectrum. JAMA 1981;246:2163–2167.

100   **Chesney PJ, Davis JP, Purdy WK, Wand PJ, Chesney RW.** Clinical manifestations of toxic shock syndrome. JAMA 1981; 246:741–748.

101   **Bergdoll MS, Reiser RF, Crass BA, Robbins BA, Davis JP.** A new staphylococcal enterotoxin F associated with toxic shock syndrome *Staphylococcus aureus* isolates. Lancet 1981:1018–1021.

102   **Bell DM, Morens DM, Holman RC, et al.** Kawasaki syndrome in the United States. Am J Dis Child 1983;137:211–214.

103   **Melish ME, Hicks RM, Larson EJ.** Mucocutaneous lymph node syndrome in the United States. Am J Dis Child 1976;130: 599–607.

104   **Newberger JW, Takahashi M, Burns JC, et al.** The treatment on Kawasaki syndrome with intravenous gamma globulin. N Engl J Med 1986;315:341–347.

105   **Morris JG, Black RE.** Cholera and other vibrios in the United States. N Engl J Med 1985;312:343–350.

106   **Chren MM, Lazarus HM, Bickers DR, Landefield CS.** Rashes in immunocompromised cancer patients. Arch Dermatol 1993;129:175–181.

107   **Balandran L, Rothschild H, Pugh N, Seabury J.** A cutaneous manifestation of systemic candidiasis. Ann Intern Med 1973;78:400–403.

108   **Kressel B, Szewczyk, Tuazon CU.** Early clinical recognition of disseminated candidiasis by muscle and skin biopsy. Arch Intern Med 1978;138:429–433.

109   **Jarowski CI, Fialk MA, Murray HW, et al.** Fever, rash, and muscle tenderness. Arch Intern Med 1978;138:544–546.

110   **Arena FP, Perlin M, Brahman H, Weiser B, Armstrong D.** Fever, rash and mylagias of disseminated candidiasis during antifungal therapy. Arch Intern Med 1981; 141:1233.

111   **Tashjian LS, Abramson JS, Peacock JE.** Focal hepatic candidiasis: a distinct clinical variant for candidiasis in immunocompromised patients. Rev Infect Dis 1984;6:689–702.

112   **Wingard JR, Merz WG, Saral R.** *Candida tropicalis*: a major pathogen in immunocompromised patients. Ann Intern Med 1979;91:539–543.

113   **Fine JD, Miller JA, Harrist TJ, Haynes HA.** Cutaneous lesions in disseminated candidiasis mimicking ecthyma gagrenosum. Am J Med 1981;70:1133–1135.

114   **Suster S, Rosen LB.** Intradermal bullous dermatitis due to candidiasis in an immunocompromised patient. JAMA 1987;258:2106–2107.

115   **Hitchcock CA, Pye GW, Troke PF, Johnson EM, Warnock DW.** Fluconazole resistance in *Candida glabrata*. Antimicrob Agent Chemother 1993;37:1962–1965.

116   **Wingard JR, Merz WG, Rinaldi MG, Miller CB, Karp JE, Saral R.** Association of *Torulopsis glabrata* infections with fluconazole prophylaxis in neutropenic bone marrow transplant patients. 1993;37: 1847–1849.

117   **McQuillen DP, Zingman BS, Meunier F, Levitz SM.** Invasive infections due to *Candida krusei*: report of ten cases of fungemia that include three cases of endophthalmitis. Clin Infect Dis 1992;14: 472–478.

118   **Dupont B, Drouhet E.** Cutaneous, ocular, and osteoarticular candidiasis in heroin addicts: new clinical and therapeutic aspects in 38 patients. J Infect Dis 1985;152: 577–590.

119   **Bardwell A, Hill DW, Runyon BA, Koster FT.** Disseminated macronodular cutaneous candidiasis in chronic alcoholism. Arch Intern Med 1986;146:385–386.

120 Bisbe J, Miro JM, Latorre X, et al. Disseminated candidiasis in addicts who use brown heroin: report of 83 cases and review. Clin Infect Dis 1992;15:910–923.

121 Eidbo J, Sanchez RL, Tschen JA, Ellner KM. Cutaneous manifestations of histoplasmosis in the acquired immune difficiency syndrome. Am J Surg Path 1993;17:110–116.

122 Wallace RJ, Tanner D, Brennan PJ, Brown BA. Clinical trial of clarithromycin for cutaneous (disseminated) infection due to Mycobacterium chelonae. Ann Intern Med 1993;119:482–486.

123 Straus WL, Ostroff SM, Jernigan DB, et al. Clinical and epidemiologic characteristics of Mycobacterium haemophilum, an emerging pathogen in immunocompromised patients. Ann Intern Med 1994; 120:118–125.

124 Gamis AS, Gudnason T, Giebink GS, Ramsay NKC. Disseminated infection with fusarium in recipients of bone marrow transplant. Rev Infect Dis 1991; 13:1077–1088.

125 Blazar BR, Hurd DD, Snover DC, Alexander JW, McGlave PB. Invasive fusarium infections in bone marrow transplant recipients. Am J Med 1984;77:645–650.

126 Chaulk CP, Smith PW, Feagler JR, Verdirame J, Commers JR. Fungemia due to fusarium solani in an immunocompromised child. Ped Infect Dis 1986;5: 363–366.

127 Richardson SE, Bannatyne RM, Summerbell RC, Miliken J, Gold R, Weitzman SS. Disseminated fusarial infection in the immunocompromised host. Rev Infect Dis 1988;10:1171–1180.

128 Moorjani H, Kapila R. Factitious dermatoses: an enigma for the infectious disease consultant. Infect Med 1994;11:81–82.

129 Forstrom L, Winklemann RK. Factitial panniculitis. Arch Dermatol 1974;110:747–750.

130 Wykoff. Delusions of parasitosis: a review. Rev Infect Dis 1987;9:433–436.

131 Hannuksela M, Ahvonen P. Skin manifestations in human yersinosis. Ann Clin Res 1975;7:368–373.

132 Turner TW, Wilkinson DS. Pasteurella pseudotuberculosis as a cause of Erythema nodosum. Br J Dermatol 1969;81:8236.

133 Luzar MJ, Caldwell JH, Mekkjian H, Thomas FB. Yersinia enterocolitica infection presenting as chronic enteropathic arthritis. Arth Rheum 1983;26:1163–1168.

134 Taylor PR, Weinstein WM, Bryner JH. Campylobacter fetus infection in human subjects: association with raw milk. Am J Med 1979;66:779–782.

135 West BC, Todd JR, Lary CH, Blake LA, Fowler MER, King JW. Leprosy in six isolated residents of northern Louisiana. Arch Intern Med 1988;148:1987–1991.

136 Beall GN. Urticaria: a review of laboratory and clinical observations. 131–151.

137 Patamasucon P, Schaad B, Nelson JD. Melioidosis. J Pediatr 1982;100:175–182.

138 Pollowitz JA. Acute urticaria associated with shigellosis: a case report. Ann Allergy 1980;45:302–303.

139 Daye S, McHenry JA, Roscelli JD. Pruritic rash associated with cat scratch disease. Pediatrics 1988;81:559–561.

140 Parish LC, Schwartzman RM. Zoonoses of dermatological interest. Semin Dermatol 1993;12:57–64.

141 Ingber A, Trattner A, Cleper R, Sandbacnk M. Morbidity of brown recluse spider bites. Acta Derm Venereol (Stockholm) 1991;71:337–340.

142 Orkin M, Maiback H. Current concepts in parasitology. This scabies pandemic. N Engl J Med 1978;298:496–498.

143 Charlesworth EN, Johnson JL. An epidemic of canine scabies in man. Arch Dermatol 1974;110:572–574.

144 Taplin D, Porcelain SL, Mainking TL, et al. Community control of scabies: a model based on use of permethrin cream. Lancet 1991;337:1016–1018.

145 Paterson WB, Allen BR, Beveridge GW. Norwegian scabies during immunosuppressive therapy. Br Med J 1973;4:211–212.

146 Regan AM, Metersky ML, Craven DE. Nosocomial dermatitis and pruritus caused by pigeon mite infestation. Arch Intern Med 1987;147:2185–2187.

147 Dienstag JL, Rhodes AR, Bhan AK, Dvorak AM, Mihm MC, Wands JR. Urticaria associated with acute viral hepatitis type B. Studies of pathogenesis. Ann Intern Med 1978;89:34–40.

148 Castellano A, Schweitzer R, Tong MH, Omata M. Papular acrodermatitis of childhood and hepatitis B infection. Arch Dermatol 1978;114:1530–1532.

149 Taieb A, Plantin P, Pasquier PDU, Guillet G, Maleville J. Br J Dermatol 1986;115:49–59.

150 Schneider JA, Poley JR, Millunchick EW, Orcutt MA, deTriquet JM. Papular acrodermatitis (Gianotti-Crosti syndrome) in a child with anicteric hepatitis B, virus subtype Adw. J Pediatr 1982; 101:219–222.

151 Cherry JD, Lerner AM, Klein JO, et al. Coxsackie A-9 infection with exanthems with particular reference to urticaria. Pediatrics 1963;31:819–823.

152 Clark WD, Cox PM, Ratner LH, Correa-Coronas R. Acute Schistosomiasis mansoni in 10 boys. Ann Intern Med 1970;73: 379–385.

153 From the Centers of Disease Control. JAMA 1992;267:2581–2586.

154 Leighton PM, MacSween HM. Strongyloides stercoralis. The cause of an urticarial-like eruption of 65 years' duration. Arch Intern Med 1990;150:1747–1748.

155 Harris RA, Musher DM, Fainstein V, Young EJ, Clarridge J. Disseminated strongyloidiasis. Diagnosis made by sputum examination. JAMA 1980;244:65–66.

156 Milder JE, Walzer PD, Kilgore G, Rutherford I, Klein M. Clinical features of Strongyloides stercoralis infection in an endemic area of the United States. Gastroenterology 1981;80:1481–1498.

157 Nutman TB, Reese W, Poindexter RW, Ottesen EA. Immunologic correlates of the hyperresponsive syndrome of loiasis. J Infect Dis 1988;157:544–550.

158 Nutman TB, Miller KD, Mulligan M, Ottensen EA. Loa loa infection in temporary residents of endemic regions: recognition of a hyperresponsiveness syndrome with characteristic clinical manifestations. J Infect Dis 1986;154:10–18.

159 Rakita RM, White AC Jr, Kielhofner MA. Loa loa infection as a cause of migratory angioedema: report of three cases from the Texas Medical Center. Clin Infect Dis 1993;17:691–694.

160 VanDellen RG, Ottensen EA, Gocke TM, Neafie RC. Loa loa—an unusual case of chronic urticaria and angioedema in the United States. JAMA 1985;253:1924–1925.

161 Sacks HN, Williams DN, Eifrig DE. Loiasis. Report of a case and review of the literature. Arch Intern Med 1976;136:914–915.

162 MacLean JD, Poirier L, Gyorkos TW, et al. Epidemiologic and serologic definition of primary and secondary trichinosis in the Arctic. J Infect Dis 1992;165:908–912.

163 Frayha RA. Trichinosis-related polyarteritis nodosa. Am J Med 1981;71:307–312.

164 Duke BOL. Onchocerciasis. Br Med J 1981;283:961–962.

165 Jacobs RF, Hsi S, Wilson CB, Benjamin D, Smith AL, Morrow R. Apparent meningococcemia: clinical features of disease due to Haemophilus influenzae and Neisseria meningitidis. Pediatrics 1983;72: 469–472.

166 Strong WB. Petechiae and streptococcal pharyngitis. Am J Dis Child 1969;117:156–169.

167 Benoid FL. Chronic meningococcemia. Case report and review of the literature. Am J Med 1963;35:103–112.

168 Frothingham TE. Echovirus type 9 associated with three cases simulating menigococcemia. N Engl J Med 1958;259: 484–486.

169 Gear JHS. Clinical aspects of African viral hemorrhagic fevers. Rev Infect Dis 1989; 11(S4):S777–S782.

170 LeDuc JW. Epidemiology of hemorrhagic fever viruses. Rev Infect Dis 1983;11(S4): S730–S735.

171 Monath TP. Yellow fever: a medically neglected disease. Report on a seminar. Rev Infect Dis 1987;9:165–174.

172 Bruno P, Hassel LH, Brown J, Tanner W, Lau A. The protean manifestations of hemorrhagic fever with renal syndrome. Ann Intern Med 1990;113:385–391.

173 Kenyon RH, Peters CJ. Actions of complement of Junin virus. Rev Infect Dis 1989;11(S4):S771–S776.

174 Chapman LE, Wilson ML, Hall DB, et al. Risk factors for Crimean-Congo hemorrhagic fever in rural northern Senegal. J Infect Dis 1991;164:686–692.

175 Settergren B, Juto P, Trollfors B, Wadell G, Norrby SR. Clinical characteristics of nephropathia epidemica in Sweden: prospective study of 74 cases. Rev Infect Dis 1989;11:921–926.

176 Yao ZQ, Yang WS, Zhang WB, Bai XF. The distribution and duration of Hantaan virus in the body fluids of patients with hemorrhagic fever with renal syndrome. J Infect Dis 1989;160:218–224.

177 Huggins JW. Prospects for treatment of viral hemorrhagic fevers with ribavirin, a broad-spectrum antiviral drug. Rev Infect Dis 1989;11(S4):S750–S762.

178 **McCromick JB, King IJ, Webb PA, et al.** Lassa fever. Effective therapy with ribavirin. N Engl J Med 1986;314:20–26.

179 **Huggins JW, Hsiang CM, Cosgriff TM, et al.** Prospective, double-blind, concurrent, placebo-controlled clinical trial of intravenous ribavirin therapy of hemorrhagic fever with renal syndrome. J Infect Dis 1991;164:1119–1127.

180 **Bohan A, Peter BR, Bowman RL, Pearson CM.** A computer-assisted analysis of 153 patients with polymyositis and dermatomyositis. Medicine 1977;56:255–286.

181 **Plotkin GR, Patel BR, Shas VN.** Behcet's syndrome complicated by cutaneous leukocytoclastic vasculitis. Arch Intern Med 1985;145:1913–1915.

182 **Jorizzo JL, Schmalsteig FC, Solomon AR, et al.** Thalidomide effects in Behcet's syndrome and pustular vasculitis. Arch Intern Med 1986;146:878–881.

183 **Fauci AS, Haynes BR, Katz P.** The spectrum of vasculitis. Clinical, pathologic, immunologic, and therapeutic considerations. Ann Intern Med 1978;89:660–676.

184 **deShazo RD, Levinson AI, Lawless OJ, Weisbaum G.** Systemic vasculitis with coexistent large and small vessel involvement. JAMA 1977;238:1940–1942.

185 **Mason AMS, Gumpel JM, Golding PL.** Sjogren's syndrome—a clinical review. Semin Arthritis 1973;2:301–303.

186 **McAdam LP, O'Hanlan MA, Bluestone R, Pearson CM.** Relapsing polychondritis: prospective study of 23 patients and a review of the literature. Medicine 1976; 55:193–215.

187 **Wong KF, Chan JKC.** Am J Med 1992; 93:177–180.

188 **Hertzman PA, Blevins WL, Mayer J, Greenfield B, Ting M, Gleich GJ.** Association of the eosinophilia-myalgia syndrome with the ingestion of tryptophan. N Engl J Med 1990;322:869–873.

189 **Culpepper RC, Williams RG, Mease PJ, Koepsell TD, Kobayashi JM.** Natural history of the eosinophilia-myalgia syndrome. Ann Intern Med 1991;115:437–442.

190 **Alonso-Ruiz A, Calabozo M, Perez-Ruiz F, Mancebo L.** Toxic oil syndrome. A long-term follow-up of a cohort of 332 patients. Medicine 1993;72:285–294.

191 **Fernandez-Herlihy L.** Eosinophilic fasciitis: report of a 22-year follow up study. Arthritis Rheum 1981;24:97–98.

192 **Pouchot J, Sampalis JS, Beaudet F, et al.** Adult Still's disease: manifestations, disease course, and outcome in 462 patients. Medicine 1991;70:118–136.

193 **Landry M, Muller SA.** Generalized pustular psoriasis. Arch Dermatol 1972; 105:711–716.

194 **Stewart AF, Battaglini-Sabetta J, Millstone L.** Hypocalcemia-induced pustular psoriasis of von Zumbusch. Ann Intern Med 1984;100:677–680.

195 **Karvonen S-L.** Acne fulminans: report of clinical findings and treatment of twenty-four patients. J Am Acad Dermatol 1993; 28:572–579.

196 **Goldstein B, Chalker DH, Lesher JL.** Acne fulminans. South Med J 1990;83: 705–708.

197 **Roujeau J-C, Bioulac-Sage P, Bourseau C, et al.** Acute generalized exanthemous pustulosis. Arch Dermatol 1991;127:1333–1338.

198 **Ross MG, Tucker DC, Hayashi RH.** Impetigo herpetiformis as a cause of postpartum fever. Obstet Gynecol 1984; 64(suppl):49S–51S.

199 **Kanel KT, Kroboth FJ, Swartz WM.** Pyoderma gangrenosum with myelofibrosis. Am J Med 1987;82:1031–1034.

200 **Castillo LE, Winslow DL, Pankey GA.** Wound infection and septic shock due to *Vibrio vulnificus*. Am J Trop Med Hyg 1981;30:844–848.

201 **Klontz KC, Lieb S, Schreiber M, Janowski HT, Baldy LM, Gunn RA.** Syndromes of Vibrio vulnificus infections. Clinical and epidemiologic features in Florida cases, 1981–1987. Ann Intern Med 1988;114:343–348.

202 **Mitchell LA, Tingle AJ, Shukin R, Sangeorzan JA, McCune J, Braun DK.** Chronic rubella vaccine-associated arthropathy. Arch Intern Med 1993;153:2268–2274.

203 **Ware R.** Human parovirus infection. J Pediatr 1989;114:343–348.

204 **Cockerell CJ.** Human immunodeficiency virus infection and the skin. A crucial interface. Arch Intern Med 1991;151:1295–1303.

205 **Goodman DS, Tepliz ED, Wishner A, et al.** Prevalence of cutaneous disease in patients with acquired immunodeficiency syndrome (AIDS) or AIDS-related complex. J Am Acad Dermatol 1987;17:210–220.

206 **Kaplan MH, Sadick N, McNutt NS, et al.** Dermatologic findings and manifestations

of acquired immunodeficiency syndrome (AIDS). J Am Acad Dermatol 1987;16:485–506.

207 **Laurence J.** Dermatological manifestations of HIV infection. Infect Med 1987; 241–246.

208 **Buchness MR, Lim HW, Hatcher VA, Sanchez M, Soter NA.** Eosinophilic pustular folliculitis in the acquired immunodeficiency syndrome. Treatment with ultraviolet B phototherapy. N Engl J Med 1988;318:1183–1186.

209 **Cone LA, Woodward DR, Byrd RG, Schultz K, Kopp SM, Schilevert PM.** A recalcitrant desquamating disorder associated with toxin-producing staphylococci in patients with AIDS. J Infect Dis 1992;165:638–643.

210 **Patterson JW, Kitces EN, Neafie RC.** Cutaneous botrymycosis in a patient with acquired immunodeficiency syndrome. J Am Acad Dermatol 1987;16:238–242.

211 **Hulbert TV, Larson RA.** Hyperkeratotic (Norwegian) scabies with gram-negative bacteremia as the initial presentation of AIDS. CID 1992;14:1164–1165.

212 **Hicks CB, Benson PM, Lupton GP, Tramont EC.** Seronegative secondary syphilis in a patient infected with the human immunodeficiency virus (HIV) and Kaposi's sarcoma. Ann Intern Med 1987; 107:492–495.

213 **Spence MR.** Syphilis and infection with the human immunodeficiency virus. Ann Intern Med 1987;107:587.

214 **Shulkin D, Tripoli L, Abell E.** Lues maligna in a patient with human immunodeficiency virus infection. Am J Med 1988;85:425–427.

215 **Safrin S, Kemmerly S, Plotkin B, et al.** Foscarnet-resistant herpes simplex virus infection in patients with AIDS. J Infect Dis 1994;169:193–196.

216 **Norris SA, Kessler HA, Fife KH.** Severe progressive herpetic whitlow caused by an acyclovir resistant virus in a patient with AIDS. J Infect Dis 1988;157:209–210.

217 **Quale J, Teplitz E, Augenbraun M.** Atypical presentation of chancroid in a patient infected with the human immunodeficiency virus. Am J Med 1990;88: 543N–544N.

218 **Dever LL, Martin JW, Seaworth B, Jorgenson JH.** Varied presentation and responses to treatment of infections caused by *Mycobatecteria haemophilum* in

patients with AIDS. CID 1992;14:1195–1200.

219 **Wheat LJ, Slama TG, Zeckel ML.** Histoplasmosis in the acquired immunodeficiency syndrome. Am J Med 1985; 78:203–210.

220 **Bonner JR, Alexander WJ, Dismukes WE, et al.** Disseminated histoplasmosis in patients with the acquired immunodeficiency syndrome. Arch Intern Med 1984:144:2178–2181.

221 **Concus AP, Helfand RF, Imber MJ, Lerner ES, Sharpe RJ.** Cutaneous cryptococcus mimicking molluscum contagiosum in a patient with AIDS. J Invest Dermatol 1988;158:897–898.

222 **Koehler JE, Quinn FD, Berger TG, Leboit PE, Tappero JW.** Isolation of Rochalimaea species from cutaneous and osseous lesions of bacillary angiomatosis. N Engl J Med 1992;327:1625–1631.

223 **Koehler JE, LeBoit PE, Egbert BM, Berger TG.** Cutaneous vascular lesions and disseminated cat-scratch disease in patients with the acquired immunodeficiency syndrome (AIDS) and AIDS-related complex. 1988;109:449–455.

224 **Litwin MA, Williams CM.** Cutaneous *Pneumocystis carnii* infection mimicking Kaposi's sarcoma. Ann Intern Med 1992;117:48–49.

225 **Wiley CA, Safrin RE, Davis CE, et al.** Acanthambe meningoencephalitis in a patient with AIDS. J Invest Dermatol 1987;155:130–133.

226 **Routledge PA, Scolding NJ.** Disseminated-to-skin Kala-azar and the acquired immunodeficiency syndrome. Ann Intern Med 1988;108:490–491.

227 **Svec F.** Porphyria cutanea tarda as initial presentation of the acquired immunodeficiency syndrome in two patients. J Invest Dermatol 1990;161:1032–1033.

228 **Vogelsang GB, et al.** Acute graft versus host disease: clinical characteristics in the cyclosporine era. Medicine 1988;67:163.

229 **McCausland WJ, Cox PJ.** Pseudomonas infection traced to a motel whirlpool. JEH 1975;35:455–459.

230 **Washburn J, Jacobson JJ, Marston E, Thorsen B.** Pseudomonas aeruginosa rash associated with a whirlpool. JAMA 1976; 235:2205–2207.

231 **Goodman RA, Thacker SB, Solomon SL, Osterholm MT, Hughes JM.** Infectious diseases in competitive sports. JAMA 1994;271:862–867.

232 **Belongia EA, Goodman JL, Holland EJ, et al.** An outbreak of herpes gladiatorum at a high-school wrestling camp. N Engl J Med 1991;325:906–910.

233 **Alder AL, Altman J.** An outbreak of mud-wrestling-induced pustular derma-titis in college students. JAMA 1993;269: 502–504.

234 **Berkley MZ, Luciano J, James WB.** Latex glove allergy. A survey of the US Army dental corps. JAMA 1992;268:2695–2697.

Prophylaxis in Bowel Surgery

RONALD LEE NICHOLS
JAMES WILLIAM C. HOLMES

The dramatic decrease in postoperative wound infection rates reported in the United States after elective colon resection during the last decade compared with earlier authoritative studies appears to be due primarily to the improvements in the approaches of preoperative intestinal antisepsis (1,2). These decreased infection rates after colon resection are not apparent in the recently reported European Danop trial where rates of infection exceed 20% (3).

We collectively reviewed many of the important historical aspects of preoperative bowel preparation over 20 years ago (4). It was apparent at that time that surgeons knew that the colon contained a luxuriant aerobic bacterial flora, which was excluded from the rest of the body by the normal mucous membrane barrier. If this barrier were disturbed by disease or trauma or if the colon were opened to the peritoneal cavity, bacteria escaped and invaded adjacent tissues, often producing serious infection. Because the colonic lumen must be opened during many operations and because such operations are associated with some infectious morbidity, a reliable method of sterilizing colonic content has been the objective of surgeons throughout this century. During the last 20 years great advances have been made in preoperative intestinal antisepsis due primarily to the fact that the bacteriologic techniques developed allowed for the isolation of the predominant anaerobic microflora, including *Bacteroides fragilis*. This in turn resulted in major modifications of our approaches to preoperative colon preparation and a much improved reduction of postoperative infections.

HISTORICAL ASPECTS

Primitive attempts at intestinal antisepsis made use of charcoal, chlorine, naphthalene, iodoform, and salicylates (5). These agents did not reduce the incidence of infection and were often responsible for toxic complications. The introduction of sulfonamides in the late 1930s, however, offered hope for effective preoperative intestinal antisepsis. Garlock and Seley (6) published a preliminary report in which only one wound infection occurred among 21 patients given oral sulfanilamide before elective operations of the colon. The authors concluded that preoperative administration of sulfanilamide resulted in reduced postoperative morbidity. Unfortunately, a definitive study on this subject was never published by the authors.

During the ensuing three decades, numerous clinical studies of various oral antibiotic preparations used for intestinal antisepsis were reported. Most of these studies were retrospective in nature and inadequately controlled. All of the antibiotic regimens studied were chosen to be effective against the aerobic colonic microflora thought at the time to be the major cause of postoperative infections. These reports fueled a debate regarding the value of various schemes of preoperative antibiotic preparation but failed to reach any clear conclusions about the ideal antibiotic regimen or whether the chosen antibiotics were better than mechanical preparation alone (7).

This chapter reviews some of the major studies on mechanical cleansing, oral antibiotics, and complications of the various colon preparations that resulted in the confusion, which existed until the mid-1970s.

EARLY ATTEMPTS OF PREOPERATIVE ORAL ANTIBIOTIC PREPARATION

Most early studies of nonabsorbable oral antibiotics also used some form of mechanical cleansing. Antibiotics alone had been noted to have a minimal effect on suppressing the colonic aerobes unless the bulk of fecal material had also been removed. Poth (8) was the first to characterize the ideal oral antiseptic for the intestine as having the properties of broad bacterial spectrum, low toxicity, stability in the presence of digestive enzymes, capacity to prevent development or overgrowth of resistant bacteria, and rapidity of action. Other important characteristics mentioned were limited absorption, activity in the presence of food, thereby permitting continued dietary intake in the preoperative period, capacity to aid in mechanical cleansing of the intestine without inducing dehydration, lack of tendency to irritate the gastrointestinal mucosa, and lack of interference with normal tissue growth and repair. Qualities such as low dosage requirement, solubility in water, palatability, inhibition of excessive fungal growth, and administration restricted to use only as an intestinal antiseptic were also included.

Cohn later indicated that it would be difficult for any single agent to fulfill these formidable characteristics (9). He stressed that the three major requirements for an effective intestinal antiseptic were rapid, highly bactericidal activity against pathogenic organisms and low local as well as systemic toxicity, together with limited absorption from the intestine. He also reported on the efficacy of 48 different intestinal antiseptic regimens, given usually for 72 hours, on suppressing the human aerobic and anaerobic colonic microfloras. Once again it should be noted that before the acceptance in the mid-1970s of *B. fragilis* as the predominant fecal constituent and frequent cause of postoperative infection after colon surgery, the antibiotic agents chosen as intestinal antiseptics were primarily effective against the aerobic colonic flora. These oral agents included the sulfonamides, tetracyclines, and aminoglycosides. A review of these early studies and the complications associated with these approaches has been published and will not be addressed in this chapter (4).

BACTERIOLOGY OF THE GASTROINTESTINAL TRACT

The human gastrointestinal tract in utero is sterile (5). Within a few hours of birth, the oral and anal orifices are colonized, and organisms can be cultured from the rectum. The intestinal flora at this time is variable and is derived from the environment of the infant. A few days after birth a more stable gastrointestinal flora begins to establish itself. The bacteria that colonize the colon at this time depend on whether the newborn infant is formula fed or breast fed. The stool of the breast-fed infant is characterized by large concentrations of gram-positive organisms, predominantly *Lactobacillus bifidus*. The stool flora of formula-fed infants is more complex with a predominance of gram-negative aerobic and anaerobic organisms and resembles that of children eating a mixed diet.

Smith and Crabb (10) studied the stool flora of a variety of newborn animals and human infants. During the early weeks of life, the flora was similar in all species but as the animals grew older, differences developed. Bacteroides and lactobacilli were the most common organisms found in the stool of human infants, and clostridia, coliforms, or streptococci predominated in the feces of lower animals. *Staphylococcus aureus* was never isolated from animals and appeared only in human stool. Because of such differences in fecal flora of animals and man, the results of studies of antibiotic preparation of the colon in lower animals must be applied with considerable caution to human beings.

During the last 20 years, many thoughtfully designed and scientifically accurate studies have outlined the gastrointestinal flora in both healthy and diseased colons (11). These reports have demonstrated that anaerobic, non-sporulating, gram-negative rods, predominantly *Bacteroides* species, are the most prevalent bacteria in the colon. These anaerobic microorganisms are 1000 to 100,000 times more numerous than aerobic coliforms. Stool specimens usually contain 10^{10} to 10^{11} anaerobic *Bacteroides* species per gram, and aerobic coliforms number 10^6 to 10^8 organisms per gram. Other major fecal organisms are aerobic lactobacilli, anaerobic lactobacilli or bifidobacilli, and streptococci. The minor bacterial constituents of human stool include proteus, pseudomonas, clostridia, and staphylococci.

Most recently emphasis has been placed on studying both the luminal- and mucosal-associated colonic flora (12,13). These qualitatively and quantitatively different populations of colonic bacteria appear to have varying degrees of importance concerning bacterial translocation, anastomotic healing, and development of wound and intra-abdominal infections.

RISK FOR INFECTION IN COLON SURGERY

Many clinical studies of risk factors for infection in specific operative procedures were published during the 1980s. Knowledge of the presence or absence of these risk factors in the perioperative period may allow for alterations of infection control techniques in the studies conducted during the 1990s (14).

Kaiser and colleagues (15) in a study of elective colon resection and different approaches to preoperative antibiotic prophylaxis have shown a direct correlation between the duration of the operation and the postoperative infection rate. In operations lasting less than 3 hours, no infections were identified when the antibiotic prophylaxis was with a parenteral agent alone or a combination of oral and parenteral agents. However, in operations lasting more than 4 hours, a significant reduction in infection was observed in patients who received the combination prophylactic regimen. Coppa and Eng (16) in a similar study of elective colon resection have stressed that postoperative wound infections are associated with the duration of operation and location of the colonic resection (intraperitoneal colon resection versus rectal resection). These authors showed that the wound infection rate in high-risk patients with long operations (over 215 minutes) and rectal resection could significantly benefit from the use of a combination of oral and parenteral prophylactic antibiotics. Other studies confirmed that abdominal-perineal resections and operations lasting more than 3.5 hours are associated with higher postoperative infection rates (17).

Whether primarily to repair the injured colon or to do a colostomy has been the subject of a recent prospective study of colonic injuries after penetrating abdominal trauma (18). The authors, using logistic regression analysis, have identified that transfusion with 4 units or more, more than two associated injuries, significant intraperitoneal contamination, and increasing colon injury severity scores correlate significantly with postoperative wound and intra-abdominal infections. They concluded that nearly all penetrating colon wounds can be repaired primarily regardless of risk factors. It should, however, be noted that the finding of a colonic perforation and the performance of a colostomy during exploration for penetrating abdominal trauma have been identified to be the prime risk factors for postoperative infections (19,20).

MECHANICAL PREPARATION BEFORE COLON SURGERY

Historically, mechanical preparation by means of purgation, enemas, and dietary restriction was used in nearly all patients undergoing elective operations of the colon. Clinical experience long ago demonstrated that mechanical removal of gross feces from the colon was associated with decreased morbidity and mortality rates in patients undergoing operations of the colon.

Although there was no universally accepted regimen for mechanical preparation of the colon, in most schemes preparations in hospitalized patients with a nonobstructed colon were carried out during a 48- to 72-hour period and included a low-residue diet for one or two days and, often, a clear liquid diet on the day immediately preceding operation. Daily use of cathartics and enemas in various combinations were common components. Saline enemas were preferred by some surgeons to reduce the electrolyte loss that accompanies repeated enemas.

Did thorough mechanical preparation influence the numbers and composition of the colonic flora? Gliedman and his associates (21) studied the effect of saline irrigation on closed loops of canine colon. Saline irrigation resulted in a progressive reduction of total bacterial count, which was related linearly to the volume of saline irrigation. Tyson and Spaulding (22) showed that mechanical preparation of the colon decreased the fecal bacterial population from 10^8 or 10^9 to 10^6 or 10^7 organisms per gram of stool. This decrease was shown to persist for 12 to 18 hours after completion of the mechanical preparation. Bornside and Cohn (23), on the other hand, found that 72 hours of mechanical preparation did not result in any decrease in numbers of fecal microorganisms. Our study of 12 patients undergoing a vigorous 72-hour mechanical bowel preparation with dietary restriction, cathartics, and enemas showed only a significant reduction in the mean concentration of coliforms within various segments of the colonic lumen and stool (24). Obligate anaerobes, the major constituents of the colonic microflora, and other aerobic and microaerophilic bacteria were not significantly altered. Our conclusion was that vigorous mechanical cleansing reduces total fecal mass, but the residual bowel contents harbor microflora, a potential source of wound infection following colonic resections.

The modern approaches to mechanical cleansing still vary considerably (25). In comparison to 1979, when a survey of surgeons' preferences for preoperative colon preparation indicated that 5 to 16% of surgeons relied solely on mechanical cleansing (26), a 1990 survey of 500 active board-certified colorectal surgeons revealed that all who answered the survey (72%) used antibiotics in addition to mechanical cleansing (27).

Mechanical Preparation Approaches in Elective Operation

Modern approaches in the nonobstructive elective procedure fall into two general categories: 1) whole gut lavage with either an electrolyte solution, 10% mannitol or polyethylene glycol on the day before operation and 2) standard mechanical cleansing that uses dietary restriction, cathartics, and enemas for a 2-day period. In most patients the majority of the preparation is accomplished on an outpatient basis. Our approach to the two alternative

Table 3.1.   Suggested Approach to Preoperative Preparation for Elective Colon Resection

Two Days before Surgery (at home)	The Day Before Surgery (at home or in hospital if necessary)	Day of Surgery
Dietary restriction: low residue or liquid diet	Admit in moring (if necessary)	Operation at 8 AM
Magnesium sulfate, 30 mL of 50% solution (15 g) PO at 10 AM, 2 PM, and 6 PM	Clear liquid diet, IV fluids as needes	A single dose of antibiotic with broad spectrum aerobic/anaerobic activity given IV by anesthesia personnel in operating room just before incision. Repeat dosage if operation lasts over 2 h
Fleet® enemas until diarrhea efluent clear in the evening	Magnesium sulfate, in dosage given above at 10 AM and 2 PM	
	OR	
	Whole gut lavage with Golytely® (1 L/h for 2–3 h until diarrhea effluent clear) beofre administration of oral antibiotic, starting at 9 AM and ending at the latest at noon	
	No enemas	
	All patients receive neomycin and erythromycin base, 1 g each PO at 1 PM, 2 PM, and 11 PM	

techniques of mechanical cleansing as well as antibiotic coverage is offered in Table 3.1.

The choice of mechanical cleansing technique depends primarily on the surgeon's preference. Traditional bowel preparation including dietary restriction, cathartics, and enemas, if carried out for an unnecessarily long period of time (3 to 5 days), will be associated with less patient acceptability, greater patient fatigue, and other related complications than other cleansing techniques. Similarly, whole gut irrigation techniques previously recommended that use large amounts of fluid (10 to 15L) should be discouraged. Mannitol in varying concentrations has been recommended by some for use in lavage solutions (28). Other studies (29,30) have warned about the possibility of developing clinical dehydration when 15% mannitol is used and also of colonic explosions with the use of electrocautery when mannitol was used without oral antibiotics. The use of polyethylene glycol-electrolyte lavage solutions appears today to be the preferred cleansing method before elective colorectal surgery (30–32). It is advisable in these cost-conscious days to perform the preoperative bowel preparation, when possible, on an outpatient basis, thereby saving hundreds of dollars per admission (33,34).

Mechanical Preparation in the Partially Obstructed Patient

In patients presenting with partially obstructing lesions of the large bowel, surgery is more often urgent than elective. These individuals often will not tolerate a rapid mechanical preoperative bowel preparation as shown in Table 3.1 due to the potential of impacting stool proximal to the obstructing lesion and thereby converting a partial to a complete obstruction. Fortunately, these patients will most often tolerate decelerated mechanical bowel preparation. Such a partially obstructed patient who is stable and in good clinical condition is admitted to the hospital while undergoing preoperative bowel preparation. Resuscitation with parenteral fluids and their continuation at a maintenance rate is usually necessary although many patients will tolerate clear liquids by mouth. Fleets® phosphosoda is also given orally in 10-cc aliquots at hourly intervals for six doses on day 2 preoperatively and is repeated starting at 6 AM on preoperative day one. If the patient develops worsening abdominal distention or signs of complete obstruction, the oral mechanical bowel preparation is stopped and the patient is prepared for urgent surgery using an appropriate perioperative parenteral antimicrobial agent or agents. In the patient who tolerates the decelerated mechanical bowel preparation, oral preoperative antibiotic prophylaxis is given and surgery is done the following morning using an additional dose of perioperative parenteral antibiotic (Table 3.2).

Mechanical Approach in Emergent Colon Operation

Emergency situations often require immediate surgical intervention precluding preoperative mechanical and oral antibiotic bowel preparation. In selected patients with limited intra-abdominal disease and without peritonitis or free pus, resection of the diseased segment of large bowel with primary anastomosis is possible. This is routinely done without the benefit of preoperative mechanical bowel preparation in patients with lesions of the right colon. Under identical clinical settings, emergency surgery for distal colonic lesions presents a greater challenge. Intraoperative antegrade colonic lavage following resection of the diseased distal segment of colon or rectum will facilitate primary anastomosis in many cases. Although this technique has a place in the surgeon's armamentarium, it is not recommended if the surgeon is operating alone. It is most often useful when adequate assistance is available that allows a group effort to prevent loss of control of either the proximal or distal ends of the lavage circuit, which would result in gross fecal contamination of the abdominal cavity with disastrous results in the postoperative course of the patient (35,36). Perioperative coverage with parenteral antibiotic agents with aerobic and anaerobic activity is indicated in these emergency procedures (see Table 3.2).

It should be emphasized that all prospective clinical studies using appropriate oral or parenterally administered antibiotics have shown a benefit over mechanical cleansing, whereas the use of inappropriate antibiotics most often

Table 3.2. Selected Single and Combination Parenterally Administered Antibiotic Agents That Cover Facultative/Anaerobic Colonic Microflora

Facultative Coverage (to be combined with a drug having anaerobic activity)	Anaerobic Coverage (to be combined with a drug having facultative activity)	Facultative—Anaerobic Coverage—Single Agents
Amikacin	Chloramphenicol	Ampicillin-sulbactam
Aztreonam	Clindamycin	Cefotetan
Cefotaxime	Metronidazole	Cefoxitin
Ceftriaxone		Ceftizoxime
Ciprofloxacin		Imipenem-cilastatin
Gentamicin		Piperacillin-tazobactam
Tobramycin		Ticarcillin-clavulanic acid

does not show advantages over mechanical preparation above (Table 3.3) (37–49). The use of placebo control studies in clinical trials of antibiotic prophylaxis in colon surgery have been abandoned since the early 1980s (50).

CURRENTLY USED APPROACHES TO ANTIBIOTIC PREPARATION BEFORE COLON SURGERY

The use of antibiotics in addition to mechanical cleansing is currently the standard of care before colon surgery (25,27,34). A recent survey of 352 board-certified, active colon and rectal surgeons has shown that all use this combined approach before operations on the colon (27). It is also generally agreed that the antibiotics chosen should be able to suppress both the colonic aerobes and anaerobes. However, some disagreement continues concerning which route of administration is preferred. Advocates of oral administration typically emphasize the importance of reducing the number of microorganisms in the colonic lumen before opening the colon, whereas those who advocate parenteral administration emphasize the importance of adequate tissue levels of antibiotics. It appears today that the great majority of surgeons prefer to use a combination of both oral and parenteral antibiotic agents before elective colon resection.

Oral Antibiotics Alone

Early studies did not consider significant the predominant role of the obligate anaerobes in the human colonic microflora or their frequent isolation from postoperative infections when appropriate anaerobic collection and culturing were exercised. The fact that many anaerobes were resistant to antimicrobial agents commonly used for bowel preparation made it likely that regimens previously recommended had been pharmacologically inadequate (51). There-

Table 3.3.   Prospective Clinical Trials Conducted during the 1970s Comparing the Use of Mechanical Cleansing Alone with Mechanical Cleansing and Antibiotics in Elective Colon Resection

Year (Reference)	Patients (No.)	Antibiotic	Route	Infection Rate (%)	
				Mechanical Cleansing Alone	Mechanical Cleansing and Antibiotics
1973 (37)	87	Cephaloridine	Parenteral	44	34*
1978 (38)	20	Neomycin-erythromycin	Oral	30	0*
1974 (39)	196	Neomycin	Oral	43	41*
		Neomycin-tetracycline	Oral	43	5†
1975 (40)	80	Gentamicin	Parenteral	31	34*
1975 (41)	50	Kanamycin-metronidazole	Oral	44	8†
1976 (42)	67	Cephalothin	Parenteral	27	24*
1977 (43)	87	Cephalothin	Parenteral	59	17†
1977 (44)	75	Cephalothin	Parenteral	21	19*
1977 (45)	116	Neomycin-erythromycin	Oral	43	9†
1978 (46)	118	Doxycycline	Parenteral	42	9†
1978 (47)	71	Kanamycin-metronidazole	Oral	46	12†
1978 (48)	110	Neomycin-metronidazole	Oral	42	18†
1979 (49)	83	Metronidazole	Parenteral	77	34†

* Not significant.
† Significant at $P < .05$.

fore, it became apparent that use of effective antimicrobial agents for oral bowel preparation required the knowledge of the normal bowel flora, the capacity of various fecal bacteria to produce infections, the frequency with which each species of microorganisms is involved in infection, and the patterns of antimicrobial sensitivity of these pathogens. On the basis of these questions we organized a series of prospective, randomized clinical trials. The combination of neomycin and erythromycin base was chosen for trial because these drugs were likely to be effective in controlling both aerobic and anaerobic fecal pathogens and at that time were not generally used for treatment of infections. In addition, these antibiotic agents were well tolerated by patients and were relatively inexpensive.

The objective of our first study was to determine the effectiveness of the neomycin-erythromycin base as compared with antibiotic regimens recommended for bowel preparation by other recognized experts. The results of this study indicated that although most of the recommended antibiotic regimens reduced the concentration of aerobes in the colon, the preparation with neomycin-erythromycin base was most effective in reducing the numbers of both aerobic and anaerobic fecal pathogens (51).

We next turned to a prospective, randomized, clinical trial of the effectiveness of preparation with neomycin-erythromycin base in controlling wound infections in patients with disease of the colon (38). By the time 20 patients had been entered in this trial, the rate of septic complications among patients who did not receive antibiotics was 30%. No septic complications had occurred among 10 antibiotic-treated patients, but three serious wound infections and one death had occurred among 10 control patients. Clinically, the difference seemed quite clear to our surgical residents, and the study was stopped. Unfortunately, because of the small numbers involved, the difference was not statistically significant.

Over the next five years, data were collected from two Veterans Administration cooperative studies. These prospective, randomized, and double-blind studies were conducted with patients undergoing elective colonic resection (26,45). In the first study, the effectiveness of short-term, low-dose, preoperative, oral neomycin and erythromycin base combined with vigorous purgation compared with placebo and the same mechanical preparation was proved (45). The overall rate of directly related septic complications was 43% in the group given a placebo and 9% in the group given neomycin and erythromycin base.

The second Veterans Administration cooperative study was designed to compare the commonly advocated parenteral use of cephalothin with oral neomycin and erythromycin base as preoperative preparation before elective colonic resection (26). In this prospective, randomized, double-blind study, groups receiving the following regimens were compared: intravenous cephalothin and oral neomycin-erythromycin base. All groups received the same mechanical preparation. The addition of patients to the group given intravenous cephalothin was stopped after 10 months because sequential analysis of the data indicated that this method of prophylaxis resulted in significantly higher numbers of septic complications. The incidence of wound infections was 30%, and the overall incidence of septic complications was 39% in patients receiving only intravenous cephalothin combined with mechanical cleansing. The incidence of septic complications was only 6% in the groups receiving the oral neomycin and erythromycin base.

Other oral antibiotic combinations, which usually included combinations of neomycin or kanamycin with either metronidazole or tetracycline, have been used successfully compared to either mechanical preparation alone (see Table 3.3) or to parenteral antibiotic agents (Table 3.4) (52–80).

The three oral regimens now most frequently used are: an aminoglycoside with erythromycin base, an aminoglycoside with metronidazole, and an aminoglycoside with tetracycline. The regimen most often chosen in the United States is neomycin-erythromycin base, which was introduced in 1972 (51). In

Table 3.4. Prospective Studies of Oral and Parenteral Antibiotics Regimens in Patients Receiving Mechanical Cleansing

Year (Reference)	Patients (No.)	Neomycin and Erythromycin Base Given to All Patients	Antibiotic	Route	Infection Rate (%)
1976 (52)	144	Yes	Cefazolin	Parenteral	6
			Placebo		16*
1978 (53)	79	No	Neomycin-erythromycin	Oral	12
			Cephaloridine	Parenteral	13[†]
1978 (54)	79	No	Neomycin-erythromycin	Oral	25
			Neomycin-metronidazole	Oral	5*
1979 (55)	93	No	Metronidazole-kanamycin	Oral	32
			Metronidazole-kanamycin	Parenteral	7*
1979 (26)	193	No	Neomycin-erythromycin	Oral	6
			Cephalothin	Parenteral	30*
1979 (56)	77	No	Kanamycin	Oral	46
			Kanamycin-erythromycin	Oral	13*
1979 (57)	126	No	Thalazole	Oral	49
			Metronidazole-thalazole	Oral	13*
1979 (58)	59	Yes	Placebo	Parenteral	4
			Clindamycin-gentamicin	Parenteral	7[†]
1979 (59)	34	No	Cephalothin	Parenteral	31
			Cefamandole	Parenteral	33[†]
1982 (60)	92	Yes	Cefazolin	Parenteral	13
			Ceftizoxime	Parenteral	7[†]
			Cefoxitin	Parenteral	3[†]
1982 (61)	102	No	Doxycycline	Parenteral	13
			Cefoxitin	Parenteral	18[†]
1982 (62)	74	No	Cephalothin	Parenteral	25
			Cefoxitin	Parenteral	4[†]
			Metronidazole	Parenteral	4[†]
1983 (63)	123	No	Neomycin-erythromycin	Oral	2
			Cephaloridine	Parenteral	12*

Table 3.4. *Continued*

Year (Reference)	Patients (No.)	Neomycin and Erythromycin Base Given to All Patients	Antibiotic	Route	Infection Rate (%)
1983 (64)	104	Yes	Placebo	Parenteral	35
			Cefazolin	Parenteral	7*
			Ticarcillin	Parenteral	5*
1983 (15)	119	No	Neomycin-erythromycin	Oral	
			plus cefazolin	Parenteral	3
			Cefoxitin	Parenteral	12[†]
1983 (65)	241	Yes	No additional antibiotics		18
			Cefoxitin	Parenteral	7*
1983 (66)	100	No	Cefoxitin	Parenteral	12
			Metronidazole-gentamicin	Parenteral	12[†]
1983 (67)	1082	Yes	Placebo	Parenteral	8
			Cephalothin	Parenteral	6[†]
1984 (68)	57	Yes	Cefonicid	Parenteral	6
			Cefoxitin	Parenteral	10[†]
1984 (69)	93	No	Neomycin-erythromycin	Oral	9
			Metronidazole-gentamicin	Parenteral	27*
1985 (70)	267	No	Tinidazole-doxycycline	Parenteral	3
			Tinidazole	Parenteral	10*
1986 (71)	86	No	Moxalactam	Parenteral	12
			Metronidazole-gentamicin	Parenteral	13[†]
1986 (72)	60	No	Neomycin-erythromycin	Oral	41
			Metronidazole-ceftriaxone	Parenteral	10*
1987 (73)	100	Yes	Cefazolin	Parenteral	3[†]
			Cefoxitin	Parenteral	3[†]
			Cefotaxime	Parenteral	14
1987 (74)	167	No	Ticarcillin-clavilanic acid	Parenteral	2
			Tinidazole	Oral	14*
1988 (75)	239	Variable	Cefotetan	Parenteral	12
			Cefoxitin	Parenteral	8[†]

Table 3.4. *Continued*

Year (Reference)	Patients (No.)	Neomycin and Erythromycin Base Given to All Patients	Antibiotic	Route	Infection Rate (%)
1988 (76)	119	No	Neomycin-metronidazole plus metronidazole	Oral Parenteral	14
			Metronidazole	Parenteral	28*
1988 (16)	310	No	Neomycin-erythromycin plus cefoxitin	Oral Parenteral	5
			Cefoxitin	Parenteral	18*
1989 (77)	102	No	Neomycin-erythromycin plus cefazolin	Oral Parenteral	11
			Metronidazole	Parenteral	32*
1989 (78)	403	No	Cefoxitin	Parenteral	11
			Cefotetan	Parenteral	9†
1989 (79)	54	No	Neomycin-erythromycin	Oral	4
			Metronidazole-ceftriaxone	Parenteral	7†
1993 (80)	196	No	Ceftriaxone	Parenteral	6
			Metronidazole-gentamicin	Parenteral	17*

* Significant at $P < .05$.
† Not significant.

Europe and Australia, physicians often prefer kanamycin-metronidazole or neomycin-metronidazole.

The timing of the administration of these oral agents appears to be critical (81,82). It is recommended that 1 g each of neomycin and erythromycin base be given at 1:00 PM, 2:00 PM, and 11:00 PM on the day before surgery (6 g total) (see Table 3.1). Surgery should then be scheduled for about 8:00 AM the next day. If the operation must be scheduled for later in the day, the times at which the oral agents are administered should be changed accordingly to preserve the 19 hours of preparation time. Giving more than three doses of oral antibiotics as prophylaxis is unwarranted and may induce the emergence of resistant flora (83). Authoritative reviews of antibiotic prophylaxis in colon surgery confirm the value of the oral neomycin-erythromycin base preparation in preventing infection after elective colon resection (84). The pharmacokinetics of the oral neomycin-erythromycin base preparation have been studied in healthy volunteers (81) and in patients undergoing elective colon resection (82). The findings suggest that when adequate mechanical preparation is also carried out, significant intraluminal (local) and serum (systemic) levels of erythromycin and significant local levels of neomycin are present and that both techniques may help prevent infection after colon operation.

Parenteral Antibiotic Alone

In 1969, the first prospective, randomized, double-blind study published on parenteral antibiotic prophylaxis in elective colon resection used cephaloridine administered intramuscularly during the perioperative period (85). This study revealed a significant reduction of postoperative infections (30% to 7%) in the group of patients receiving antibiotics and mechanical preparation when compared to patients who received mechanical preparation alone. Other clinical studies using the same or similar first-generation cephalosporins for prophylaxis failed, however, to show efficacy of this approach when compared to placebo (mechanical preparation alone) (37) or to oral neomycin and erythromycin base (26,63). However, Kaiser et al. (15) did not observe differences in postoperative infectious complications in operations of less than 4 hours when parenteral first-generation cefazolin (1.8-hour half-life) was compared to oral neomycin and erythromycin and parenteral cefazolin. Other clinical studies comparing parenteral cephalosporin alone in this setting showed lack of efficacy unless the antibiotic agent possessed aerobic and anaerobic activity (see Table 3.4). Parenteral agents in this setting that have shown efficacy alone or in combination with an aminoglycoside include cefoxitin, cefotetan, metronidazole, and doxycycline. Most investigators recommend the perioperative use of one to five doses of parenteral agents during the 24-hour period shortly before and after operation. A recent multicenter study showed that a single dose of cefotetan was equal in efficacy to multiple-dose cefoxitin in preventing infection after colon resection (75). Many of the clinical studies designed to test various parenteral antibiotic agents have given all or some of the patients oral neomycin-erythromycin, which, in our minds, discredits the value of the parenteral regimens in preventing infections (see Table 3.4).

The worst result ever published using neomycin and erythromycin base reported a 41% infection rate compared to a 10% rate with parenteral metronidazole and ceftriaxone (72). To add to the confusion and to further cast a cloud of doubt on these results, the other center in this two-center trial has recently reported a 3.7% infection rate with the oral agents compared to 7.4% rate with the parenteral agents (79). We leave it to responsible surgeons to read these two very different studies and reach their own conclusions.

Parenteral antibiotics are currently used alone for preoperative colon preparation by fewer than 10% of actively involved colon and rectal surgeons who were surveyed in 1990 (27).

Combination Oral and Parenteral Antibiotics

Most surgeons presently use both oral and parenteral antibiotic agents in addition to mechanical cleansing as preoperative preparation before elective colon resection in hopes of further reducing the postoperative infection rate (25,27). In a survey of more than 500 surgeons reported in 1979 only 8% used systemic antibiotics alone, 37% used oral antibiotics alone, and 49% used oral plus systemic antibiotics before colon surgery (26). Recently, a survey of over 360 colon and rectal surgeons revealed that more than 88% used both oral and systemic antibiotic agents before elective colon resection (27). The most commonly used agents were neomycin and erythromycin and a parenterally administered second-generation cephalosporin that has aerobic and anaerobic activity.

Condon et al. (67) reported the results of a 5-year cooperative Veterans Administration study of more than 1000 patients undergoing elective colon surgery, comparing oral neomycin-erythromycin base with and without parenteral perioperative cephalothin. In this study the infection rate was not significantly different and was below 9% in both groups.

Studies using oral neomycin and erythromycin base in combination with newer systemic agents with both aerobic and anaerobic coverage such as cefoxitin, cefotetan, or ceftizoxime have shown a low incidence of infections (60). It appears at this time, with somewhat conflicting evidence, that the addition of one dose of parenteral cephalosporin with aerobic and anaerobic activity given intravenously within 30 minutes of incision may be beneficial when added to mechanical and oral antibiotic bowel preparation. The use of the parenteral antibiotic may provide a fail-safe mechanism in cases when the oral agents have been administered in inappropriate time sequences or in cases when the time of operation has been delayed.

Topical Prophylaxis

Another possible approach to the prevention of wound infection in colon surgery is the use of topically administered antibiotics such as ampicillin, which was first shown to be effective in 1967 (86). Although the results of that study are difficult to evaluate because other routes of antibiotic administration were used and some patients undergoing emergency colon procedures without mechanical bowel preparation were included, it should be pointed out that only one of 36 patients (3%) who received topical ampicillin experienced infectious complications. However, the concomitant use of additional parenteral antibiotic agents in most of the patients has confused the strength of the message. In recent studies, no advantage was gained by adding topical ampicillin where adequate oral or parenteral regimens were used (87,88). The use of so-called instant preparation of the colon, in which povidone-iodine solutions are instilled or injected into the colonic lumen, has been studied experimentally and clinically, but has not been generally adopted (89).

INTRAOPERATIVE COLONIC LAVAGE

One-stage resection and anastomosis is currently an accepted technique in emergency surgery of the right side of the colon in a patient given appropriate parenteral antibiotics. For lesions of the left side of the colon requiring rapid or immediate surgical intervention, intraoperative lavage is a useful supplement to a surgeon's armamentarium. We have performed the lavage successfully in many patients in the following manner. A ring-type plastic wound protector is inserted at the time of laparotomy in all patients. The obstructed segment is resected and removed from the operative field. The splenic and hepatic flexures are mobilized allowing easy mechanical manipulation of the large bowel.

The abdominal cavity is then protected from the proximal colon with laparotomy pads, towels, and plastic barrier drapes. Following mobilization of hepatic and splenic flexures, laparotomy pads are used to isolate the distal ileum and colon from other abdominal contents and the operating field. The distal colonic segment is brought over the field through a sterile, sticky, small aperture plastic drape. A Steridrape irrigation pouch is placed over the small aperture drape to contain the distal stapled end of the colon. A purse-string suture is placed in the antimesenteric border of the ileum approximately 5 cm proximal to the ileocecal valve. A no. 18 Foley catheter with a 5-mL balloon is inserted through an ileotomy in the center of the purse-string suture. The Foley catheter is passed through the ileocecal valve so that the inflated balloon lies snugly within the cecum on the valve. The purse-string suture is then tightened and tied with a bow onto the shaft of the catheter. An alternative method is to perform an appendectomy and introduce the catheter through the stump, which is ducked as the purse-string suture is tied when the catheter is withdrawn at the end of the irrigation. The distal stapled end of the colon is held off the field over a sterile receptacle as the staple line is resected, thus opening the bowel. We do not use a sterile conduit tube for outflow but rely on direct manual control of the open end. The cecum is held by the surgeon and an assistant holds the transected distal colonic end securely and inspissated stool is manually expressed while small amounts of saline solution are instilled proximally to soften it if necessary. The stool present in patients with chronic obstruction has often undergone liquefaction, resulting in a pasty to fluid consistency that is easier to remove with lavage. The irrigation is performed with warm saline solution. Once gross evacuation of stool is complete, the warmed irrigation fluid is administered as rapidly as possible while the colon is manually agitated. It is more efficient to administer the saline solution from bags each containing 3000 mL. A circulator is assigned to control the inflow of saline solution. Colonic lavage is continued until the effluent is clear, which usually requires 6 to 9 L warm saline solution. The distal contaminated colon is then excised with a linear stapling device and handed off field. The Foley ligature is untied, the balloon is deflated, and the catheter is withdrawn as the purse-string suture is tied. A sterile laparotomy pad is held around the catheter as it is withdrawn to minimize fecal contamination. The ileotomy site is closed transversely with Lembert sutures. The rectal stump is washed out from below with sterile saline solution. Gloves and instruments are changed before performing a primary anastomosis. The distal rectal washout device can be saved to test the anastomosis for leakage (water or airtight) following its completion. An intraoperative lavage takes approximately 30 minutes; therefore, only low-risk, stable patients should be selected for this procedure. The intraoperative lavage requires a group effort and is therefore not recommended for use by a solitary surgeon. The use of antimicrobial or antiseptic solutions for lavage or peritoneal irrigation is not recommended because they are frequently absorbed with the possible end point of increased toxicity and they lack definite evidence of improved efficacy.

SUMMARY

The busy colon and rectal surgeon deals daily with a sea of bacteria. Using good surgical judgment as well as time-honored techniques and innovative equipment the postoperative results are generally good. The role that appropriately administered efficacious antibiotics play in this scenario should not be underestimated and can only be realized when historical controls are evaluated.

The results of these studies of antibiotic bowel preparation suggest that many different approaches may be equally effective in reducing infection after elective colonic resection. Certain features, however, appear to be common to most of the studies:

1   Oral antibiotic regimens with both aerobic and anaerobic activity (e.g., neomycin/erythromycin base) were used.

2   The oral agents were given in limited doses the day before operation.

3   Addition of systemic antibiotic agents without broad-spectrum coverage to the oral regimen generally did not improve the results.

4   Use of broad-spectrum parenteral antibiotic agents alone was associated with a lower infection rate than the use of systemic agents having only limited coverage.

5   Addition of a broad-spectrum parenteral antibiotic to the oral antibiotics may further reduce the postoperative infection rate.

6   Parenteral or oral antibiotics should be administered only for short periods of time during the perioperative period.

Since the general acceptance of the approach outlined above, infection rates have decreased and the number of clinical studies reported has drastically decreased. The authors do feel, however, that there is a need for further study to outline possible benefits of other appropriate regimens (34).

REFERENCES

1 **Ad Hoc Committee of the Committee on Trauma, Division of Medical Sciences, National Academy of Sciences—National Research Council.** Factors influencing the incidence of wound infection. Ann Surg 1964;160(suppl):32–81.

2 **Haley RW, Culver DH, Morgan WM, et al.** Identifying patients at high risk of surgical wound infection. Am J Epidemiol 1985; 121:206–215.

3 **Surgical Wound Infection Study.** In: Paine L, ed. Hospital management international (Yearbook). 1990:274–278.

4 **Nichols RL, Condon RE.** Preoperative preparation of the colon. Surg Gynecol Obstet 1971;132:323–337.

5 **Riddell MI.** A review of the literature on preoperative prophylaxis of the bowel with antibacterial agents. Am J Med Sci 1952; 223:301–315.

6 **Garlock JH, Seley GP.** The use of sulfanilamide in surgery of the colon and rectum; preliminary report. Surgery 1939;5:787–790.

7 **Tyson RR, Spaulding EH.** Antibiotic preparation of the bowel—a chimera. In: Finland M, Ingelfinger FJ, Relman AS, eds. Controversy in Internal Medicine. Philadelphia: WB Saunders, 1966:615–621.

8 **Poth EJ.** Intestinal antisepsis in surgery. JAMA 1953;153:1516–1521.

9 **Cohn I Jr.** Intestinal Antisepsis. Springfield: Charles C. Thomas, 1968:1–245.

10 **Smith WH, Crabb WE.** The fecal-bacterial flora of animals and man; its development in the young. J Pathol Bacteriol 1961;82:53–66.

11 **Nichols RL.** Prophylaxis for surgical infections. In: Gorbach SL, Bartlett JG, Blacklow NR, eds. Infectious Diseases. Philadelphia: WB Saunders, 1992:393–403.

12 **Lindsey JT, Smith JW, MCluggage SG Jr, et al.** Effects of commonly used bowel preparations on the large bowel mucosal-associated and luminal microflora in the rate model. Dis Colon Rectum 1990;33:554–560.

13 **Smith MB, Goradia VK, Holmes JW, et al.** Suppression of the human mucosal-related colonic microflora with prophylactic parenteral and/or oral antibiotics. World J Surg 1990;14:636–641.

14 **Nichols RL.** Surgical wound infection. Am J Med 1991;91(S3B):54s–64s.

15 **Kaiser AB, Herrington JL Jr, Jacobs JK, et al.** Cefoxitin versus erythromycin, neomycin, and cefazolin in colorectal operations. Ann Surg 1983;198:525–530.

16 **Coppa GF, Eng K.** Factors involved in antibiotic selection in elective colon and rectal surgery. Surgery 1988;104:853–858.

17 **Tartter PI.** Determinants of postoperative stay in patients with colorectal cancer: implications for diagnostic-related groups. Dis Colon Rectum 1988;31:694–698.

18 **George SM Jr, Fabian TC, Voeller GR, et al.** Primary repair of colon wounds: a prospective trial in nonselected patients. Ann Surg 1989;209:728–734.

19 **Nichols RL, Smith JW, Klein DB, et al.** Risk of infection after penetrating abdominal trauma. N Engl J Med 1984;311:1065–1070.

20 **Nichols RL, Smith JW, Robertson GD, et al.** Prospective alterations in therapy for penetrating abdominal trauma. Arch Surg 1993;128:55–64.

21 **Gliedman ML, Grant RN, Vestal BL, et al.** Impromptu bowel cleansing and sterilization. Surgery 1958;43:282–287.

22 **Tyson RR, Spaulding EH.** Should antibiotics be used in large bowel preparations? Surg Gynecol Obstet 1959;108:623–626.

23 **Bornside GH, Cohn I Jr.** Intestinal antisepsis; stability of fecal flora during mechanical cleansing. Gastroenterology 1969;57:569–573.

24 **Nichols RL, Gorbach SL, Condon RE.** Alteration of intestinal microflora following preoperative mechanical preparation of the colon. Dis Colon Rectum 1971;14:123–127.

25 **Nichols RL.** Bowel preparation. In: Meakins JL, ed. Surgical Infections. Diagnosis and Treatment. III Prevention of Infections. New York: Scientific American Medicine, 1994:151–159.

26 **Condon RE, Bartlett JG, Nichols RL, et al.** Preoperative prophylactic cephalothin fails to control septic complications of colorectal operations. Results of controlled clinical trial. A Veterans Administration Cooperative Study. Am J Surg 1979;137:68–74.

27 **Solla JA, Rothenberger DA.** Preoperative bowel preparation. A survey of colon and rectal surgeons. Dis Colon Rectum 1990; 33:154–159.

28 Jagelman DG, Fazio VW, Lavery IC, et al. A prospective, randomized, double-blind study of 10% mannitol mechanical bowel preparation combined with oral neomycin and short-term, perioperative intravenous Flagyl as prophylaxis in elective colorectal resections. Surgery 1985;98:861–865.

29 Beck DE, Harford FJ, DiPalma JA. Comparison of cleansing method in preparation for colonic surgery. Dis Colon Rectum 1985;28:491–495.

30 Beck DE, Harford FJ, DiPalma JA, et al. Bowel cleansing with polyethylene glycol-electrolyte lavage solution. South Med J 1985;78:1414–1416.

31 Fleites RA, Marshall JB, Eckhauser ML, et al. The efficacy of polyethylene glycol-electrolyte lavage solution versus traditional mechanical bowel preparation for elective colonic surgery: a randomized prospective, blinded clinical trial. Surgery 1985;98:708–716.

32 Wolff BG, Beart RW Jr, Dozois RR, et al. A new bowel preparation for elective colon and rectal surgery: a prospective randomized trial. Arch Surg 1988;123:895–899.

33 Frazee RC, Roberts J, Symmonds R, et al. Prospective randomized trial of inpatient vs. outpatient bowel preparation for elective colorectal surgery. Dis Colon Rectum 1992;35:223–226.

34 Gorbach SL, Condon RE, Conte JE Jr, et al. General guidelines for the evaluations of new anti-infective drugs for prophylaxis of surgical infections—evaluations of new anti-infective drugs for surgical prophylaxis. Clin Infect Dis 1992;15(suppl 1):S313–S338.

35 Muir EG. Safety in colonic resection. Proc Royal Soc Med 1968;61:401–408.

36 Murray JJ, Schoetz DJ Jr, Coller JA, et al. Intraoperative colonic lavage and primary anastomosis in nonelective colon resection. Dis Colon Rectum 1991;34:527–531.

37 Evans C, Pollack AV. The reduction of surgical wound infection by prophylactic parenteral cephaloridine: a controlled clinical trial. Br J Surg 1973;60:434–437.

38 Nichols RL, Broido P, Condon RE, et al. Effect of preoperative neomycin-erythromycin intestinal preparation on the incidence of infectious complications following colon surgery. Ann Surg 1973;178:453–462.

39 Washington JA II, Dearing WH, Judd ES, et al. Effect of preoperative antibiotic regimen on development of infection after intestinal surgery: prospective, randomized, double-blind study. Ann Surg 1974;108:567–572.

40 Burton BC, Hughes ESR, Cuthbertson AM. Prophylactic use of gentamicin in colonic and rectal surgery. Med J Aust 1975;2:846–850.

41 Goldring J, McNaught W, Scott A, et al. Prophylactic oral antimicrobial agents in elective colon surgery: a controlled trial. Lancet 1975;2:997–999.

42 Brote I, Gillquist J, Hojer H. Prophylactic cephalothin in gastrointestinal surgery. Acta Chir Scand 1976;142:238–245.

43 Kjellgren K, Sellstrom H. Effect of prophylactic systemic administration of cephalothin in colorectal surgery. Acta Chir Scand 1977;143:473–477.

44 Burdon JGW, Morris IJ, Hunt P, et al. A trial of cephalothin sodium in colon surgery to prevent wound infection. Arch Surg 1977;112:1169–1173.

45 Clarke JS, Condon RE, Bartlett JG, et al. Preoperative oral antibiotics reduce septic complications of colon operations: results of a prospective, randomized, double-blind clinical study. Ann Surg 1977; 186:251–259.

46 Hojer H, Wetterfors J. Systemic prophylaxis with doxycycline in surgery of the colon and rectum. Ann Surg 1978;187:362–368.

47 Gillespie G, McNaught W. Prophylactic oral metronidazole in intestinal surgery. J Antimicrob Chemother 1978;4(suppl):29–32.

48 Matheson DM, Arabi Y, Baxter-Smith D, et al. Randomized multicentre trial of oral bowel preparation and antimicrobials for elective colorectal operations. Br J Surg 1978;65:597–600.

49 Eykyn SJ, Jackson BT, Lockhart-Mummery HE, et al. Prophylactic perioperative intravenous metronidazole in elective colorectal surgery. Lancet 1979;2:761–764.

50 Baum ML, Anish DS, Chalmers TC, et al. A survey of clinical trials of antibiotic prophylaxis in colon surgery: evidence against further use of no-treatment controls. N Engl J Med 1981;305:795–799.

51 Nichols RL, Condon RE, Gorbach SL, et al. Efficacy of preoperative antimicrobial preparation of the bowel. Ann Surg 1972; 176:227–232.

52 Stone HH, Hooper CA, Kolb LD, et al. Antibiotic prophylaxis in gastric, biliary

and colonic surgery. Ann Surg 1976; 184:443–452.

53 Lewis RT, Allan CM, Goodall RG, et al. Antibiotics in surgery of the colon. Can J Surg 1978;21:339–341.

54 Brass C, Richards GK, Ruedy J, et al. The effect of metronidazole on the incidence of postoperative wound infection in elective colon surgery. Am J Surg 1978;135:91–96.

55 Keighley MRB, Arabi Y, Alexander-Williams J. Comparison between systemic and oral antimicrobial prophylaxis in colorectal surgery. Lancet 1979;1:894–897.

56 Wapnick S, Guinto R, Reizis I, et al. Reduction of postoperative infection in elective colon surgery with preoperative administration of kanamycin and erythromycin. Surgery 1979;85:317–321.

57 Taylor SA, Cawdery HW, Smith J. The use of metronidazole in the preparation of bowel for surgery. Br J Surg 1979;66:191–192.

58 Barber MS, Hirschberg BC, Rice CL, et al. Parenteral antibiotics in elective colon surgery? A prospective, controlled clinical study. Surgery 1979;86:23–29.

59 Slama TG, Carey LC, Fass RJ. Comparative efficacy of prophylactic cephalothin and cefamandole for elective colon surgery: results of a prospective, randomized, double-blind study. Am J Surg 1979;137: 593–596.

60 Maki DG, Aughey DR. Comparative study of cefazolin, cefoxitin and ceftizoxime for surgical prophylaxis in colorectal surgery. J Antimicrob Chemother 1982;10(suppl C):281–287.

61 Ivarsson L, Darle N, Kewenter JG, et al. Short-term systemic prophylaxis with cefoxitin and doxycycline in colorectal surgery—a prospective, randomized study. Am J Surg 1982;144:257–261.

62 Panichi G, Pantosti A, Giunchi G, et al. Cephalothin, cefoxitin or metronidazole in elective colon surgery? A single blind randomized trial. Dis Colon Rectum 1982; 25:783–786.

63 Edmondson HT, Rissing JP. Prophylactic antibiotics in colon surgery. Arch Surg 1983;118:227–231.

64 Portnoy J, Kagan E, Gordon PH, et al. Prophylactic antibiotics in elective colorectal surgery. Dis Colon Rectum 1983; 26:310–313.

65 Coppa GE, Eng K, Gouge TH, et al. Parenteral and oral antibiotics in elective colon and rectal surgery: a prospective and randomized trial. Am J Surg 1983;145:62–65.

66 McDonald PJ, Karran SJ. A comparison of intravenous cefoxitin and a combination of gentamicin and metronidazole as prophylaxis in colorectal surgery. Dis Colon Rectum 1983;26:661–664.

67 Condon RE, Bartlett JG, Greenlee H, et al. Efficacy of oral and systemic antibiotic prophylaxis in colorectal operations. Arch Surg 1983;118:496–502.

68 Fabian TC, Mangiante EC, Boldreghini SJ. Prophylactic antibiotics for elective colorectal surgery or operation for obstruction of the small bowel: a comparison of cefonicid and cefoxitin. Rev Infect Dis 1984;6(suppl 4):S896–S900.

69 Figueras-Felip J, Basilio-Bonet E, Lara-Eisman F, et al. Oral is superior to systemic antibiotic prophylaxis in operations upon the colon and rectum. Surg Gynecol Obstet 1984;158:359–362.

70 Norwegian Study Group for Colorectal Surgery. Should antimicrobial prophylaxis in colorectal surgery include agents effective against both anaerobic and aerobic microorganisms? A double-blind, multicenter study. Surgery 1985;97:402–407.

71 McCulloch PG, Blamey SL, Finlay IG, et al. A prospective comparison of gentamicin and metronidazole and moxalactam in the prevention of septic complications associated with elective operations of the colon and rectum. Surg Gynecol Obstet 1986;162:521–524.

72 Weaver M, Burdon DW, Youngs DJ, et al. Oral neomycin and erythromycin compared with single-dose systemic metronidazole and ceftriaxone prophylaxis in elective colorectal surgery. Am J Surg 1986;151:437–442.

73 Jones RN, Wojeski W, Bakke J, et al. Antibiotic prophylaxis of 1036 patients undergoing elective surgical procedures. Am J Surg 1987;153:341–346.

74 University of Melbourne Colorectal Group: Systemic Timentin® is superior to oral tinidazole for antibiotic prophylaxis in elective colorectal surgery. Dis Colon Rectum 1987;30:786–789.

75 Jagelman DG, Fabian TC, Nichols RL, et al. Single dose cefotetan versus multiple dose cefoxitin as prophylaxis in colorectal surgery. Am J Surg 1988;155(suppl 5A):71–76.

76 Playforth MJ, Smith GMR, Evans M, et al. Antimicrobial bowel preparation—oral, parenteral or both? Dis Colon Rectum 1988;31:90–93.

77 Khubchandani IT, Karamchandani MC, Sheets JA, et al. Metronidazole vs. erythromycin, neomycin and cefazolin in prophylaxis for colon surgery. Dis Colon Rectum 1989;32:17–20.

78 Periti P, Mazzei T, Tonelli F, et al. Single dose cefotetan versus multiple dose cefoxitin—antimicrobial prophylaxis in colorectal surgery. Dis Colon Rectum 1989; 32:121–127.

79 Kling PA, Dahlgren S. Oral prophylaxis with neomycin and erythromycin in colorectal surgery—more proof for efficacy than failure. Arch Surg 1989;124: 705–707.

80 Morris WT. Ceftriaxone is more effective than gentamicin/metronidazole prophylaxis in reducing wound and urinary tract infections after bowel operations: results of a controlled, randomized, blind clinical trial. Dis Colon Rectum 1993;36:826–833.

81 Nichols RL, Condon RE, DiSanto AR. Preoperative bowel preparation: erythromycin base serum and fecal levels following oral administration. Arch Surg 1977; 112:1493–1496.

82 DiPiro JT, Patrias JM, Townsend RJ, et al. Oral neomycin sulfate and erythromycin base before colon surgery: a comparison of serum and tissue concentrations. Pharmacotherapy 1985;5:91–94.

83 Kaiser AB. Antimicrobial prophylaxis in surgery. N Engl J Med 1986;315:1129–1138.

84 Antimicrobial prophylaxis in surgery. Med Lett Drugs Ther 1993;35:91–94.

85 Polk HC Jr, Lopez-Mayor JF. Postoperative wound infections. A prospective study of determinant factors and prevention. Surgery 1969;66:97–103.

86 Nash AG, Hugh TB. Topical ampicillin and wound infection in colon surgery. Br Med J 1967;1:471–472.

87 Juul P, Merrild U, Kronborg O. Topical ampicillin in addition to a systemic antibiotic prophylaxis in elective colorectal surgery: a prospective randomized study. Dis Colon Rectum 1985;28:804–806.

88 Salvati EP, Rubin J, Eisenstat TE, et al. Value of subcutaneous and intraperitoneal antibiotics in reducing infection in clean contaminated operations of the colon. Surg Gynecol Obstet 1988;167:315–318.

89 Jones FE, DeCosse JJ, Condon RE. Evaluation of "instant" preparation of the colon with povidone-iodine. Ann Surg 1976; 184:74–79.

Update on Diagnosis of *Clostridium difficile*-Associated Diarrhea

JAMES DEMAIO
JOHN G. BARTLETT

Clostridium difficile was originally described as an enteric pathogen in animals in 1977 and in patients in 1978 (1–3). The early work indicated that it produced a potent cytopathic toxin and the initial assumption was that this toxin was responsible for clinical expression with diarrhea and colitis. From 1978 through 1980, most of the current data concerning *C. difficile* were established. The cytotoxin assay, as described in the initial report, remained the only diagnostic test of choice for several years. The latex agglutination assay was introduced in the mid-1980s, but it had a fundamental flaw. It was intended to detect toxin A, but actually detected another protein product that had no apparent biologic importance. Thus, the cytotoxin assay remained the standard diagnostic test until the early 1990s. During the past three to four years, there has been an avalanche of new diagnostic tests designed to detect toxin A, toxin B, or the organism. These tests vary in sensitivity and specificity, and many are relatively early in development. Most laboratories are now using these alternative tests, but few clinicians are aware of which tests are being used, their relative merits, or how decisions to select tests by laboratory directors are made. This chapter reviews the state of the art with regard to detection of *C. difficile*-associated diarrhea and colitis.

CLINICAL FEATURES

Clostridium difficile-associated enteric disease should be suspected in any patient who develops diarrhea during antibiotic use or within two weeks following discontinuation of antibiotics. *C. difficile*-associated disease is only rarely found in the absence of antibiotic exposure. However, cancer chemotherapy (4) and antivirals (5) have been infrequently implicated as inciting factors. Pseudomembranous colitis without antecedent antibiotic exposure is another setting in which *C. difficile* toxin has been detected (6,7).

The spectrum of gastrointestinal disease associated with C. *difficile* is broad. Patients may present with "nuisance" diarrhea, nonspecific colitis, or pseudomembranous colitis (PMC). Asymptomatic carriage may also occur in both healthy and hospitalized individuals. The frequency with which C. *difficile* is detected is directly dependent on the severity of illness. The most accurate studies measuring frequency were probably done between 1977 and 1980 when the full spectrum of disease was commonly seen. More recent work has generally involved patients with early stage disease or has lacked endoscopy. According to the earlier work, C. *difficile* toxin is found in 2 to 10% of asymptomatic patients receiving clindamycin, ampicillin, and cephalosporins; 10 to 20% of patients with antibiotic-associated diarrhea; 50 to 70% of patients with antibiotic-associated colitis and 90 to 100% of patients with antibiotic-associated PMC (8,9). The prevalence of C. *difficile* within a particular subpopulation of patients will affect the positive predictive value of the diagnostic methods used.

Eighty to 90% of patients with antibiotic-associated diarrhea have negative toxin assays for C. *difficile*. Most toxin-negative cases have no alternative explanation. Clinical features that distinguish positive and negative C. *difficile* cases have not been well studied. However, it appears that toxin-negative cases of antibiotic-related diarrhea are more likely to be dose related and less likely to be associated with evidence of inflammation (cramps, fecal leukocytes, or fever). Symptoms typically respond when the antimicrobial agent is simply discontinued or reduced in dose. In contrast, C. *difficile*-associated enteric complications are not dose related, often persist following discontinuation of the implicated antimicrobial agent, or show evidence of colonic inflammation. The essential differences between antibiotic-associated diarrhea due to C. *difficile* and antibiotic-associated diarrhea with no clear etiology are summarized in Table 4.1.

EPIDEMIOLOGY

Clostridium difficile is by far the most common enteric pathogen causing nosocomial diarrhea and has been implicated in major epidemics in hospitals and nursing homes (10–12). Because C. *difficile* is a spore-forming organism, it can readily persist and spread throughout the hospital environment. Although the organism can be isolated from stool from only 0 to 2% of healthy adults, intestinal carriage rates may be as high as 20% in hospitalized patients. Detection of C. *difficile* is important both for treatment of the individual and also for the purpose of infection control. Strain typing schemes (which require stool culture rather than toxin assays) may be valuable in expanding our knowledge of C. *difficile* epidemiology and in assisting with control measures for epidemics.

Table 4.1. Comparison of Antibiotic-Associated Diarrhea due to *Clostridium difficile* and Enigmatic Cases

Variable	Antibiotic-Associated Diarrhea/Colitis	
	Due to C. difficile	*Enigmatic Cases*
Most common implicated drugs	Clindamycin, ampicillin, cephalosporins	Clindamycin, tetracycline, ampicillin, some cephalosporins
Relationship of illness to dose	Not dose related	Dose related
Response to drug withdrawal	Symptoms often persist	Symptoms usually resolve
Clinical Features		
Intestinal	Watery diarrhea, cramps	Watery diarrhea
Constitutional	Fever and leukocytosis common	Usually none
History	Noncontributory	History of diarrhea with same or other antibiotics
Complications	Toxic megacolon, ileus, leukemoid reaction, hypoalbuminemia, high fever, arthritis (rare)	Rarely serious
Evidence of colitis	Cramps, WBCs in feces; colitis or PMC evident by endoscopy or CT scan	Colitis uncommon
Epidemiology	Epidemic or endemic in hospitals and nursing homes	Sporadic
Treatment	Discontinue implicated drug; administer vancomycin or metronidazole	Discontinue antibiotic or reduce dose

CT = computerized tomography; PMC = pseudomembranous colitis; WBCs = white blood cells.

PATHOPHYSIOLOGY

Clostridium difficile-associated enteric disease is mediated by two toxins, toxin A and toxin B. Both toxins are large molecular weight proteins of about 300,000 daltons. Toxin A was originally called the "enterotoxin" because it appears to be responsible for clinical expression of diarrhea and colonic inflammation. Toxin B was originally called the "cytotoxin" because it is responsible for characteristic actinomorphic changes in tissue culture cells. Although there is a case report of a strain that produces toxin B to the exclusion of toxin A (13), virtually all isolated, toxigenic strains produce both toxins simultaneously. The implication is that the detection of toxin B is nearly always accompanied by toxin A. The precise sequence of events leading to diarrhea or colitis are currently unknown. The most widely accepted hypothesis is that the normal flora of the intestinal tract and becomes permissive to the replication of vegetative forms of *C. difficile* with concomitant toxin production. The severity of disease is probably modulated by a complex interaction between the quantity of toxin A present (which depends on the toxigenic potential of the strain and the rate of replication), humoral or secretory antibodies, colonic proteolytic enzymes, the competitive flora, and possibly the presence of toxin B.

GENERAL PRINCIPLES OF *Clostridium difficile* DIAGNOSIS

The diagnosis of *C. difficile*-associated diseases has focused on three approaches. The first approach is the detection of specific anatomic changes in the patient's colonic mucosa. *C. difficile* toxin A causes a severe inflammatory reaction with bloody fluid accumulation in small bowel and colon loop assays in all rodent models (14,15). The disease encountered in the hamster model largely involves the cecum and, to a lesser extent, the colon (16,17). In clinical practice, *C. difficile*-induced inflammatory changes are restricted to the colon with the small bowel remaining unaffected. A rare exception is in patients with an ileostomy who may have disease in the distal ileum. The inflammatory changes in the colonic mucosa may allow a diagnosis to be made by colonoscopic or radiologic methods.

The second approach to diagnosis has focused on detection of the organism itself. Investigators have used Gram stain, culture methods, and the polymerase chain reaction (PCR) to identify *C. difficile* in stool specimens. There have also been extensive efforts to develop typing schemes to better understand the organism's epidemiology.

Finally, most clinicians rely on tests designed to detect *C. difficile* toxin as a marker of disease. These include cytotoxin assays, enzyme-linked immunosorbent assays (ELISA), latex agglutination, and dot-immunobinding assays to detect the toxin A or B in stool samples. The following sections of this chapter examine each diagnostic method in detail. Table 4.2 summarizes the performance times, sensitivities, and specificities of currently available tests.

Colonoscopy

Direct visualization of the intestinal mucosa was one of the earliest techniques used to diagnose *C. difficile*-associated colitis. The presence of pseudomembranes is nearly pathognomonic for this condition. Pseudomembranes appear as raised yellow-green plaques that may be attached by thin stalks to a friable mucosa. Histologically, they are composed of mucin, fibrin, poly-

Table 4.2. Diagnostic Tests for *Clostridium difficile*

	Tissue Culture Assay	Latex Particle Agglutination	Enzyme Immunoassay	Dot Immunoblot	Polymerase Chain Reaction	Culture
References	45, 89, 92–94	106–121	90, 92–94, 132, 133	134	85, 135–137	28–32, 45
Source	Commercial microtiter well system available	Commercially available	Five brands commercially available	Commercially available	Experimental, not yet commercially available	Variety of media are commercially available
Product Detected	Toxin B	Glutamate dehydrogenase	Toxin A or toxin A plus toxin B	Toxin A	Toxin A gene, toxin B gene, or both	Organism
Time Required	18–48 h	30 min	2–4 h	30 min	2–4 h	28–72 h
Clinical Correlations	Best sensitivity with proper dilutions; excellent specificity	Least sensitive and specific; + results require confirmation	Good sensitivity; excellent specificity	Initial studies promising	Excellent sensitivity; good specificity	Excellent sensitivity but poor specificity

morphonuclear leukocytes, and sloughed colonic mucosal cells. Endoscopic visualization of the plaques may be more sensitive than biopsy. The pseudomembranes are relatively fragile, and at least one study has shown that they do not consistently survive processing in pathology (18).

Up to 91% of patients with pseudomembranes will have lesions less than 60 cm from the anal verge (19,20). Most patients, therefore, require only flexible sigmoidoscopy to make the diagnosis. The presence of pseudomembranes, however, varies considerably with the severity of illness. Talbot and colleagues were able to show that 71% of patients with severe colitis had pseudomembranes, whereas pseudomembranes were only present in 23% of those with mild disease (21). Mild cases may show only a nonspecific colitis with friable, edematous colonic mucosa.

The increased awareness of C. difficile-associated disease and the increasing availability of toxin assays has led to recognition at an earlier stage of illness. Concerns about cost, fear of perforation during endoscopic examination in severe cases, and the relative ease of cytotoxin assays have removed sigmoidoscopy and colonoscopy from the forefront of diagnosis. However, a role for endoscopic visualization may still exist in cases requiring rapid diagnosis if laboratory results will be delayed. Colonoscopy may also be used to monitor response in patients who are initially refractory to therapy.

Radiologic Techniques

Although radiologic procedures are not the primary means of diagnosing C. difficile-associated colitis, severe PMC may be suggested by findings on plain abdominal films, barium enema studies, abdominal computerized tomography (CT), or abdominal ultrasound. Plain films may reveal giant "thumbprinting" or wide bands of thickened bowel wall (22,23). Barium enemas are relatively contraindicated in the presence of PMC due to the risk of perforation during air insufflation. However, when such studies have been performed, raised plaques, oval filling defects, and a shaggy luminal contour have sometimes been noted (22,24). Fishman and colleagues reviewed the abdominal CT findings in 26 patients with documented PMC (25). Irregular mucosal thickening with an average depth of 14.7 mm and wide haustral folds were suggestive of the diagnosis. These findings are restricted to the colon and ascitic fluid is often present as well. The finding on ultrasound of thickened mucosal folds and intramural lucencies has occasionally confirmed the diagnosis (26).

It must be emphasized that none of these radiologic findings is pathognomonic for C. difficile-associated disease. Most mild to moderate cases of colitis will present with normal or near-normal radiologic studies. Although severe PMC may be suggested by radiologic studies in the appropriate clinical setting, final diagnosis requires endoscopic visualization of PMC or toxin assay. Radiologic procedures are not a definitive method for diagnosing C. difficile-associated gastrointestinal disease, but they may call attention to this possibility when done for other indications.

Detection of *Clostridium difficile*

Gram Stain   The Gram stain of fecal specimens plays no role in the diagnosis of *C. difficile*-associated diarrhea. Because fecal concentrations of *C. difficile* are generally 10^5 to 10^7/g stool, this organism accounts for less than 1% of the colonic flora. Furthermore, other species of Clostridia that appear identical on Gram stain are frequent normal inhabitants of the gastrointestinal tract. These factors lead to the extremely low sensitivity and specificity of Gram-stained specimens (27). Fecal leukocytes may be present in 30 to 50% of patients with *C. difficile* diarrhea; this finding supports the diagnosis but is also nonspecific.

Culture   *Clostridium difficile* was given its species name because of early difficulties in successfully culturing the organism. Nonselective media are not satisfactory for culture because of the rapid overgrowth of other fecal bacteria. A major advance was the development of a selective medium, cycloserine cefoxitin-fructose agar (CCFA) by George et al. in 1978 (28). *C. difficile* produces flat, yellow-green, ground–glass-appearing colonies on CCFA. Colonies may fluoresce yellow after prolonged incubation.

Since the introduction of CCFA media, numerous modifications have been tried to further increase the sensitivity of cultures. Lower concentrations of cycloserine (250 μg/mL) and cefoxitin (8 μg/mL) have been recommended as less inhibitory to *C. difficile* growth while still retaining selectivity (29). Other media such as cycloserine mannitol agar (CMA) and cycloserine-mannitol blood agar (CMBA) have also been developed. The relative effectiveness of these media is debated. Although some studies show CMBA to be more effective than CMA or CCFA (30,31), at least one study contradicts this finding (32).

The addition of p-cresol or its metabolic precursor p-hydroxy phenyl acetic acid increases the selectivity of both broth and solid media culture systems (28,33–35). p-Cresol is a unique metabolic product of *C. difficile*, which is highly inhibitory to most other bacterial species. Unfortunately, it may also be relatively inhibitory to *C. difficile* with a subsequent loss of sensitivity at high concentrations (28). Taurocholate has been used to increase spore germination and, therefore, increase sensitivity (36–38). Although 0.1% taurocholate appears to increase the yield of positive cultures when only a small number of spores are present, such as during environmental sampling, it provides little advantage in testing fecal specimens (38).

Because *C. difficile* is a spore-forming organism, both alcohol shock and heat shock have been used to suppress other fecal bacteria. The results of studies have been contradictory. Some studies have shown alcohol shock (30,31,39) or heat shock (40) to increase sensitivity, whereas others have demonstrated the reverse (41,42). Again, alcohol shock and heat shock probably increase the sensitivity in situations where small numbers of spores are present, such as in asymptomatic carriers (40), due to the suppression of bacterial overgrowth. However, these techniques may decrease sensitivity in symptomatic infection where a relatively large number of vegetative forms of *C. difficile* are present.

Although solid media have generally been preferred, several selective broth media have been developed. Cycloserine-cefoxitin-fructose broth (43) and cycloserine cefoxitin gentamicin (44) broth offer excellent sensitivity in growing *C. difficile*. However, because colonial morphology and fluorescence are apparent only on solid media, broth culture offers no advantage.

Current culture techniques have a relatively high sensitivity. Sensitivity of culture approaches 100% in specimens that are positive in the cytotoxin assay. An excellent study by Walker and associates showed a sensitivity of 89% when culture was compared to clinical assessment (45). Unfortunately, the benefit of high sensitivity is negated by a low specificity (74%). Symptomatic disease is secondary to toxin A and possibly toxin B. Culture cannot distinguish toxin-positive strains, toxin-negative strains, and asymptomatic carriage. Stool cultures show that as many as 20% of inpatients are asymptomatic carriers (46). Unlike most enteric bacterial infections, culture plays only a secondary role in *C. difficile*-associated disease.

Cultures may be desired in the context of evaluating some nosocomial outbreaks because culture is required to identify carriers as potential sources of epidemiologic spread or to use strain typing to track epidemic strains. It is also conceivable that isolated strains would be useful for antimicrobial sensitivity testing, especially in the setting of treatment failures or relapses. However, most studies show that isolated strains are always susceptible to levels of vancomycin and metronidazole that are achieved in the colon. To our knowledge, in vitro resistance has never been an explanation for either drug failure or relapses.

Typing Schemes

Over the last decade, various typing schemes have been proposed to facilitate epidemiologic studies of *C. difficile*. Delmee and colleagues have identified specific serogroups (A, B, C, D, F, G, H, I, K, and X) on the basis of slide agglutination and, more recently, ELISA (47–50). Serogroup A is further divided into types A1 to A12 on the basis of sodium dodecyl sulfate-polyacryl amide gel electrophoresis (SDS-PAGE) patterns (51). This system has been successfully used to study the epidemiology of a *C. difficile* outbreak on an orthopedic unit (52). Although the investigators have tried to draw correlations between serogroups and various patient populations, these correlations do not appear to remain constant between studies.

Chromosomal restriction endonuclease analysis (REA) has also been evaluated as a typing system (53–55). This technique produces numerous reproducible strain profiles that can be correlated with antibiograms (53) and other typing schemes (54). REA has been used successfully to study both relapses (56) and a nursing home outbreak (57).

The SDS-PAGE technique has been used alone by a number of investigators to separate strains. Tabaqchali and colleagues have proposed one such typing scheme based on SDS-PAGE of 35S-methionine-labeled proteins from *C. difficile* (58–60). Strain patterns are divided into groups A to E and W to Z. Other PAGE typing systems have produced an even greater number of strain patterns (61–63).

Pyrolysis mass spectrometry has been used by two groups to investigate *C. difficile* outbreaks in England (64,65). Plasmid fingerprinting (61), antibiograms (64), bacteriophage systems (66), restriction fragment length polymorphism (RFLP) (62), and immunoblotting (61,62,67) have also been tried.

The relative merits of these techniques are unknown because only a few studies have compared different schemes simultaneously. Wolfhagen and colleagues compared RFLP, REA, PAGE, and immunoblotting (62). They concluded that results from REA and PAGE were difficult to interpret secondary to the excessive number of bands produced. RFLP and immunoblotting were felt to be the superior techniques. Mulligan and colleagues compared plasmid fingerprinting, PAGE, serotyping, and immunoblotting (61). They also found PAGE results to be excessively complex and difficult to interpret. The effectiveness of plasmid fingerprinting was limited by the lack of plasmids in some *C. difficile* isolates. Immunoblotting was again felt to give the most reproducible and useful results.

At the present time there is no consensus on the relative merits of the typing schemes reviewed. The indications for using these techniques are vague and most regard them as research tools that are not offered by clinical laboratories.

Cytotoxin Assay   The presence of *C. difficile* toxin B will cause highly characteristic actinomorphic changes in fibroblast cell lines and cytopathic changes in virtually all cell lines. This effect is neutralized by *Clostridium sordellii* antitoxin and by *C. difficile* toxin B antitoxin. The demonstration of this cytotoxicity and its neutralization by *C. sordellii* antitoxin was an initial early breakthrough in detection of the putative agent of PMC (1,68–71). At present, many feel that the tissue culture cytotoxin assay (CTA) remains the "gold standard" in diagnosing *C. difficile*-associated diarrhea (72,73).

Stools are usually tested directly, although broth cultures of isolated strains may be tested to facilitate identification and to determine toxigenic potential. Some strains of *C. sordellii* will produce a cytopathic toxin that is neutralized by *C. sordellii* antitoxin, but the changes in fibroblast cell lines are not the characteristic actinomorphic changes noted with *C. difficile*. Other species of Clostridia do not produce cytopathic toxins.

Methods of specimen handling are variable and critical. Liquid stool should be filtered and tested undiluted. Semisolid stool is diluted 1:4 in buffered saline. Some laboratories routinely dilute specimens at 1:10 or 1:40, but these higher dilutions will increase the false negative rate by 10 to 15% (69,74). To avoid breakdown of the toxin, stool samples should be stored at 4°C if a delay before testing is anticipated. Toxin degradation has been directly correlated to increasing temperature (69) and is presumably due to proteolytic enzymes in stool.

A variety of cell lines including Chinese hamster ovary, rat hepatoma, Y1 adrenal cells, HeLa cells, and human epithelium (HEp-2) have been used for cell culture (75–78). These appear equally sensitive in detecting *C. difficile* toxin B. Cells can be grown in shell vials or microtiter plates (79). Results may be read in only 4 hours if there is a high toxin titer. However, the standard method for most laboratories is an initial reading at 18 to 24 hours and a final reading at 48 hours. Neutralization with antitoxin may be done sequentially after demonstrating cytopathic effects. This step delays results by an additional 24 hours. The alternative is to test filtered stool with and without antitoxin simultaneously.

Many laboratories perform serial dilutions and report titers of *C. difficile* cytotoxin. There is a near perfect correlation between toxin titers and severity of disease in the hamster model (80). However, toxin titers have never proven to be a useful clinical tool and do not correlate well with the severity of illness in human beings (67).

A major concern has been that the CTA usually detects only toxin B, whereas it is toxin A that causes the major physiologic changes responsible for disease. Fortunately, one toxin is not normally present without the other. Although a toxin A-positive, toxin B-negative strain has been described (81), such strains are rare. The genes for toxin A and toxin B are separated by only 1.2 kb on the *C. difficile* chromosome (82–84). PCR studies imply that nontoxigenic strains of *C. difficile* lack both the toxin A and toxin B gene completely (85–87). In vitro studies also show that toxin A and toxin B are expressed under identical culture conditions. Thus, the great majority of specimens will show either both toxins or neither.

Another concern with the CTA has been the lack of tissue culture facilities at most hospitals. This problem has been alleviated by the development of commercially available microtiter plates. The Toxi-titer system (Bartels Immunodiagnostic Supplies, Inc., Bellevue, WA) uses microtiter wells pre-seeded with human fibroblasts (88). The wells are sealed with plastic covers to prevent drying and have a shelf life of 2 weeks. The Cytotoxi Test (Advanced Clinical Diagnostics, Toledo, OH) uses a mammalian epithelial cell line in a similar system (89). Both tests have been shown to have sensitivities and specificities approximating traditional CTA systems (87,88,90,91).

Because CTA is commonly considered the "gold standard" test, it is difficult to accurately determine its sensitivity and specificity. However, studies that have carefully defined true positive and true negative results based on clinical assessment, culture, and other laboratory tests, such as electroimmunoassay (EIA), yield sensitivities of 78 to 100% and specificities of 95 to 99.8% (45,89,92–94). This sensitivity compares favorably with other antigen assays because of the extraordinary potency of toxin B (95,96).

Counterimmunoelectrophoresis Although CTA is highly sensitive and specific, final results may not be available for 24 to 48 hours. The need for a rapid diagnostic test led to the development of various immunodiagnostic assays during the early 1980s. Although initial reports with counterimmunoelectrophoresis (CIE) were encouraging (97,98), further studies revealed this technique to have a low positive predictive value (17 to 54%) (99,100). The antitoxins used in CIE cross-reacted with *C. difficile* antigens other than toxin A and toxin B, as well as with antigens present on other bacterial species (101). Attempts have been made to remove cross-reacting antitoxin by absorption to whole *C. difficile* cells (102), but CIE is currently felt not to be a useful technique due to its poor sensitivity and specificity (72,103–105).

Latex Agglutination A latex agglutination test, Culturette Brand Rapid Latex Test (Marion Scientific, Kansas City, MO), was originally designed to detect toxin A. This test has been shown, however, not to specifically detect either toxin A or toxin B (106–109). Rather, the test-reactive protein is actually glutamate dehydrogenase (110,111). Cross-reactivity with various bacterial species has been clearly documented (107,112). Although the test has been shown to have a high negative predictive value (91 to 99%), it has a very low positive predictive value. It may be reasonable to use the latex agglutination test as a rapid screen and eliminate from further study those samples testing negative. However, all positive samples should be confirmed by CTA to avoid overdiagnosis (91,113–121).

Gas-Liquid Chromatography High-pressure gas-liquid chromatography (GLC) has been used to screen for the metabolic byproducts of *C. difficile* in both enrichment broth (33,122,123) and also directly in stool specimens (124–126). The presence of isocaproic acid (33,91) and p-cresol (33,34,121) peaks have been the most consistent indicators of *C. difficile*. However, the results of GLC testing have been highly variable. Some investigators have found a high sensitivity and specificity (118,121). However, Levett found a low sensitivity for both metabolic byproducts (126). Pepersack and colleagues found a high negative predictive value, but a low positive predictive value (125). Although GLC may play a role in epidemiologic studies (43), its inconsistent results and low positive predictive value make it unsatisfactory for clinical diagnosis.

Enzyme-Linked Immunosorbent Assay Enzyme-linked immunosorbent assay technology has been developed to detect *C. difficile* toxins with the potential advantages of rapid results, technical ease of performance, and use of commercially available reagents. Systems based on either polyclonal (74,127–129) or monoclonal (127,130,131) antibodies have been used to capture toxin A (45,74,127,128) or toxin B (45,74,128). Tests using noncommercial reagents have shown sensitivities of 61 to 80% and specificities of 96 to 100% when compared to CTA (45,74). Because the ELISA and CTA detect toxin in the nanogram and picogram ranges, respectively, the lower sensitivities noted in the ELISA tests are expected.

Currently, reagents for ELISA tests are available from at least five commercial sources. The Cytoclone A+B EIA (Cambridge Biotech Corporation) detects both toxin A and toxin B. The Premier *C. difficile* Toxin A EIA (Meridian Diagnostics), the Techlab *C. difficile* Tox-A Test EIA (Techlab), the Bartels Prima System *C. difficile* Toxin A EIA, and the Vidas *C. difficile* Toxin A immunoassay (Vitek Systems Inc.) detect only toxin A. All commercial systems use monoclonal antibodies.

Table 4.3 displays the published sensitivities, specificities, and predictive values of commercial EIAs when compared to CTA and clinical correlations (90,92–94,132,133). Although ELISA testing has a lower sensitivity than CTA, it may still play a role in the diagnostic laboratory. However, both the test's limitations and also its clinical correlation must be considered to avoid underdiagnosis.

Dot-Immunobinding Assay   A dot-immunobinding assay, C. diff-CUBE (Difco Laboratories, Detroit, MI), has been developed for the rapid detection of toxin A (120,134). In this test, the filtered supernatant from diluted stool specimens is allowed to contact a membrane that will bind toxin A. Mouse monoclonal antibody directed against toxin A is added. The presence of the membrane-bound toxin A–monoclonal antibody complex is demonstrated using antimouse IgG-horse radish peroxidase and a chromogenic substrate. Positive samples show a blue-green color change in 3 minutes. The initial clinical trial demonstrated a sensitivity of 67% and a specificity of 84% when compared to the CTA (134). Due to the low positive predictive value (36%) and

Table 4.3.   The Calculated Sensitivities, Specificities, Positive Predictive Values and Negative Predictive Values of Commercially Available ELISA Tests Compared to the Cytotoxin Assay and Clinical Correlation

Test (Reference)	Sensitivity (%)	Specificity (%)	PPV (%)	NPV (%)
Premier Toxin A (90)	69.0	100	NC	NC
Cytoclone Toxin A+B (90)	84.5	100	NC	NC
Premier Toxin A (92)	85.0	98.0	87	98
Premier Toxin A (132)	65.0	99.6	NC	NC
Cytoclone Toxin A+B (132)	75.5	97.8	NC	NC
Vidas Toxin A (132)	65.4	100	NC	NC
Vidas Toxin A (94)	63.0	75.0	50	99
Premier Toxin A (93)	86.6	99.0	94.7	97.4
Premier Toxin A (133)	87	98	77	99
Cytoclone Toxin A+B (133)	89	99	90	99
Prima Toxin A (133)	87	96	65	99
Techlab Toxin A (133)	87	95	60	99

PPV, positive predictive value; NPV, negative predictive value; NC, not calculated.

high negative predictive value (95%), this test will probably be effective only as an initial screen. If these predictive values are correct, all positive tests will need to be confirmed by CTA.

Polymerase Chain Reaction A number of different PCR assays have been developed for the detection of *C. difficile*, but none is commercially available at present. Gumerlock and colleagues developed a PCR assay based on the amplification of a unique 270 bp fragment of the *C. difficile* 16S RNA (135). Although this technique can detect the presence of *C. difficile* in stool specimens with a very high sensitivity, it cannot discriminate between toxigenic and nontoxigenic strains. Other investigators have amplified gene fragments that encode for either toxin A (86,136–138) or toxin B (137,139). McMillin and colleagues have successfully developed a multiplex PCR assay that can amplify and detect toxin A and toxin B gene fragments simultaneously (86). None of these techniques has been tested in a large clinical trial, but preliminary nonclinical (85,136) and clinical (135,137) testing suggests a very high sensitivity and specificity.

Unprocessed stool filtrates contain substances that are inhibitory to the PCR reaction (135) necessitating use of relatively complex neutralization and extraction procedures. Widespread use of PCR will depend on simplification of laboratory procedures and concerns for specificity.

CONCLUSION

Clostridium difficile is widely recognized as the major identifiable cause of antibiotic-associated diarrhea and colitis. It is so dominant as a nosocomial enteric pathogen that some authorities propose that screening for *C. difficile* be done as a contingency for any further microbial studies of stool in patients with hospital-acquired diarrhea. It is relatively easy to identify indications for the test. It is much more difficult to design guidelines for selection of the test to be done, the need for confirmatory tests, and the need for sequential tests as a method to follow response to therapy. Many laboratories rely on the tissue culture assay because it is considered the "gold standard" and appears to have the highest sensitivity and specificity providing it is done with stool dilutions that do not exceed 1:4. Alternative antigen detection methods have the advantage of earlier results and easier technical accommodation in the laboratory routine. Probably, the most popular at present is EIA with commercially available reagents from various suppliers. Due to lower sensitivity, negative tests in difficult cases may require repeat testing or testing with an alternative technique. The latex agglutination assay appears to have relatively good sensitivity, but poor specificity so that positive assays should probably be confirmed with alternative tests. Culture is sensitive if done properly, but it is technically demanding and relatively nonspecific and results are always delayed. The dot-blot immunoassay for toxin and PCR for detection of toxigenic strains are newly introduced techniques. Unfortunately, most clinicians are not aware of the relative merits of the various tests.

REFERENCES

1 **Bartlett JG, et al.** Antibiotic-associated pseudomembranous colitis due to toxin producing clostridia. N Engl J Med 1978; 298:531.

2 **George RH, et al.** Identification of *Clostridium difficile* as a cause of pseudomembranous colitis. Br Med J 1978; 1:695.

3 **George WL, et al.** Aetiology of antimicrobial-agent-associated colitis. Lancet 1978; i:802.

4 **Silva J, et al.** Inciting and etiologic agents of colitis. Rev Inf Dis 1984;6(suppl 1):S214.

5 **Colarian J.** *Clostridium difficile* colitis following antiviral therapy in the acquired immunodeficiency syndrome. Am J Med 1988;84:1081.

6 **Wald A, et al.** Nonantibiotic-associated pseudomembranous colitis due to toxin-producing Clostridia. Ann Intern Med 1980;92:798.

7 **Peikin S, et al.** Role of *Clostridium difficile* in non–antibiotic-associated pseudomembranous colitis. Gastroenterology 1980; 79:948.

8 **Bartlett JG, et al.** Clinical and laboratory observations in *Clostridium difficile* colitis. Am J Clin Nutr 1980;33:2521.

9 **Viscidi R, et al.** Isolation rates and toxigenic potential of *Clostridium difficile* isolates from various patient populations. Gastroenterology 1981;81:5.

10 **Bentley DW.** *Clostridium difficile*-associated disease in long-term care facilities. Infect Control Hosp Epidemiol 1990;11: 434.

11 **Yee J, et al.** *Clostridium difficile* disease in a department of surgery. Arch Surg 1991; 126:241.

12 **Cartmill TD, et al.** Nosocomial diarrhoea due to a single strain of *Clostridium difficile*: a prolonged outbreak in elderly patients. Age Ageing 1992;21:245.

13 **Lyerly DM, et al.** Characterization of toxin A-negative, toxin B-positive strain of *Clostridium difficile*. Infect Immun 1992; 60:4633.

14 **Czuprynski CJ, et al.** Pseudomembranous colitis in *Clostridium difficile*-monoassociated rats. Infect Immun 1983; 39:1368.

15 **Lyerly DM, et al.** Effects of *Clostridium difficile* toxins given intragastrically to animals. Infect Immun 1985;47:349.

16 **Bartlett JG, et al.** Clindamycin-associated colitis due to a toxin producing species of Clostridium in hamsters. J Infect Dis 1977;136:701.

17 **Lusk RH, et al.** Clindamycin induced enterocolitis in hamsters. J Infect Dis 1978;137:464.

18 **Sumner HW, et al.** Rectal biopsy in clindamycin-associated colitis. Arch Pathol 1975;99:237.

19 **Tedesco FJ.** Antibiotic associated pseudomembranous colitis with negative proctosigmoidoscopy examination. Gastroenterology 1979;77:295.

20 **Tedesco FJ, et al.** Rectal sparing in antibiotic-associated pseudomembranous colitis: a prospective study. Gastroenterology 1982;83:1259.

21 **Talbot RW, et al.** Changing epidemiology, diagnosis and treatment of *Clostridium difficile* toxin-associated colitis. Br J Surg 1986;73:457.

22 **Stanley RJ, et al.** The spectrum of radiographic findings in antibiotic-related pseudomembranous colitis. Radiology 1974;111:519.

23 **Stanley RJ, et al.** Plain-film findings in pseudomembranous colitis. Radiology 1976;118:7.

24 **Rubesin SE, et al.** Pseudomembranous colitis with rectosigmoid sparing on barium studies. Radiology 1989;170: 811.

25 **Fishman EK, et al.** Pseudomembranous colitis: CT evaluation of 26 cases. Radiology 1991;180:57.

26 **Oei TK, et al.** Pseudomembranous colitis: an ultrasound diagnosis. Eur J Radiol 1992;15:154.

27 **Shanholtzer CJ, et al.** Prospective study of gram-stained stool smears in diagnosis of *Clostridium difficile* colitis. J Clin Microbiol 1983;17:906.

28 **George WL, et al.** Selective and differential medium for isolation of *Clostridium difficile*. J Clin Microbiol 1979;9:214.

29 **Levett PN.** Effect of antibiotic concentration in a selective medium on the isolation of *Clostridium difficile* from faecal specimens. J Clin Pathol 1985;38:233.

30 **Marler LM, et al.** Comparison of five cultural procedures for isolation of *Clostridium difficile* from stools. J Clin Microbiol 1992;30:514.

31 **Bartley SL, et al.** Comparison of media for the isolation of *Clostridium difficile* from fecal specimens. Lab Med 1991;22:335.

32 **Iwen PC, et al.** Comparison of media for screening of diarrheic stools for the recovery of *Clostridium difficile*. J Clin Microbiol 1989;27:2105.

33 **Levett PN, et al.** Gas chromatographic identification of *Clostridium difficile* and detection of cytotoxin from a modified selective medium. J Clin Pathol 1985;38:82.

34 **Phillips KD, et al.** Rapid detection and presumptive identification of *Clostridium difficile* by p-cresol production on a selective medium. J Clin Pathol 1981;34:642.

35 **Hafiz S, et al.** *Clostridium difficile*: isolation and characteristics. J Med Microbiol 1976; 9:129.

36 **Wilson KH, et al.** Use of sodium taurocholate to enhance spore recovery on a medium selective for *Clostridium difficile*. J Clin Microbiol 1982;15:443.

37 **Wilson KH.** Efficiency of various bile salt preparations for stimulation of *Clostridium difficile* spore germination. J Clin Microbiol 1983;18:1017.

38 **O'Farrell, et al.** A selective enrichment broth for the isolation of *Clostridium difficile*. J Clin Pathol 1984;37:98.

39 **Clabots CR, et al.** Detection of asymptomatic *Clostridium difficile* carriage by an alcohol shock procedure. J Clin Microbiol 1989;27:2386.

40 **Hanff PA, et al.** Use of heat shock for culturing *Clostridium difficile* from rectal swabs. Clin Infect Dis 1993;16(suppl 4): S245.

41 **Borriello SP, et al.** Simplified procedure for the routine isolation of *Clostridium difficile* from faeces. J Clin Pathol 1981; 34:1124.

42 **Riley TV, et al.** Comparison of alcohol shock enrichment and selective enrichment for the isolation of *Clostridium difficile*. Epidemiol Infect 1987;99:355.

43 **Buchanan AG.** Selective enrichment broth culture for detection of *Clostridium difficile* and associated cytotoxin. J Clin Microbiol 1984;20:74.

44 **Carroll SM, et al.** A selective broth for *Clostridium difficile*. Pathology 1983;15:165.

45 **Walker RC, et al.** Comparison of culture, cytotoxicity assays, and enzyme-linked immunosorbent assay for toxin A and toxin B in the diagnosis of *Clostridium difficile*-related enteric disease. Diagn Microbiol Infect Dis 1986;5:61.

46 **McFarland LV, et al.** Nosocomial acquisition of *Clostridium difficile* infection. N Engl J Med 1989;320:204.

47 **Delmee M, et al.** Use of an enzyme-linked immunoassay for *Clostridium difficile* serogrouping. J Clin Microbiol 1993;31: 2526.

48 **Delmee M, et al.** Serogrouping of *Clostridium difficile* strains by slide agglutination. J Clin Microbiol 1985;21:323.

49 **Toma S, et al.** Serotyping of *Clostridium difficile*. J Clin Microbiol 1988;26:426.

50 **Delmee M, et al.** Characterization of flagella of *Clostridium difficile* and their role in serogrouping reactions. J Clin Microbiol 1990;28:2210.

51 **Delmee M, et al.** Comparison of serogrouping and polyacrylamide gel electrophoresis for typing *Clostridium difficile*. J Clin Microbiol 1986;24:991.

52 **Delmee M, et al.** Application of a technique for serogrouping *Clostridium difficile* in an outbreak of antibiotic-associated diarrhoea. J Infect 1986;13:5.

53 **Peerbooms PG, et al.** Application of chromosomal restriction endonuclease digest analysis for use as a typing method for *Clostridium difficile*. J Clin Pathol 1987; 40:771.

54 **Clabots CR, et al.** Development of a rapid and efficient restriction endonuclease analysis typing system for *Clostridium difficile* and correlation with other typing systems. J Clin Microbiol 1993;31:1870.

55 **Pear SM, et al.** Decrease in nosocomial *Clostridium difficile*-associated diarrhea by restricting clindamycin use. Ann Intern Med 1994;120:272.

56 **O'Neill GL, et al.** Relapse versus reinfection with *Clostridium difficile*. Epidemiol Infect 1991;107:627.

57 **Simor AE, et al.** Infection due to *Clostridium difficile* among elderly residents of a long-term-care facility. Clin Infect Dis 1993;17:672.

58 **Tabaqchali S, et al.** Method for the typing of *Clostridium difficile* based on polyacrylamide gel electrophoresis of 35-S methionine labeled proteins. J Clin Microbiol 1986; 23:197.

59 **Heard SR, et al.** Immunoblotting to demonstrate antigenic and immunogenic differences among nine standard strains of *Clostridium difficile*. J Clin Microbiol 1986; 24:384.

60 **Tabaqchali S, et al.** Typing scheme for *Clostridium difficile*: Its application in clinical and epidemiological studies. Lancet 1984;1(8383):935.

61 **Mulligan ME, et al.** Immunoblots and plasmid fingerprints compared with serotyping and polyacrylamide gel electrophoresis for typing *Clostridium difficile*. J Clin Microbiol 1988;26:41.

62 **Wolfhagen MJ, et al.** Comparison of typing methods for *Clostridium difficile* isolates. J Clin Microbiol 1993;31:2208.

63 **Wexler H, et al.** Polyacrylamide gel electrophoresis patterns produced by *Clostridium difficile*. Rev Infect Dis 1984; 6(suppl 1): S229.

64 **Magee JT, et al.** An investigation of a nosocomial outbreak of *Clostridium difficile* by pyrolysis mass spectrometry. J Med Microbiol 1993;39:345.

65 **Cartmill TD, et al.** Nosocomial infection with *Clostridium difficile* investigated by pyrolysis mass spectrometry. J Med Microbiol 1992;37:352.

66 **Sell TL, et al.** Bacteriophage and bacteriocin typing scheme for *Clostridium difficile*. J Clin Microbiol 1983;17:1148.

67 **McFarland LV, et al.** Correlation of immunoblot type, enterotoxin production, and cytotoxin production with clinical manifestations of *Clostridium difficile* infection in a cohort of hospitalized patients. Infect Immun 1991;59:2456.

68 **Willey SH, et al.** Cultures for *Clostridium difficile* in stools containing a cytotoxin neutralized by *Clostridium sordellii* antitoxin. J Clin Microbiol 1979;10:880.

69 **Chang T, et al.** Cytotoxicity assay in antibiotic-associated colitis. J Infect Dis 1979; 140:765.

70 **Chang T.** Neutralization of *Clostridium difficile* toxin by *Clostridium sordellii* antitoxins. Infect Immun 1978;22:418.

71 **Rifkin GD, et al.** Neutralization by *Clostridium sordellii* antitoxin of toxins implicated in clindamycin-induced cecitis in the hamster. Gastroenterology 1978;75: 422.

72 **Bartlett JG.** Antibiotic-associated diarrhea. Clin Infect Dis 1992;15:573.

73 **Pothoulakis C, et al.** Diagnostic tests for *Clostridium difficile* diarrhoea and colitis: past, present and future. J Gastroenterol Hepatol 1993;8:311.

74 **Laughon BE, et al.** Enzyme immunoassays for detection of *Clostridium difficile* toxins A and B in fecal specimens. J Infect Dis 1984;149:781.

75 **Donta ST, et al.** Effects of *Clostridium difficile* toxin on tissue cultured cells. J Infect Dis 1980;141:218.

76 **Maniar AC, et al.** Detection of *Clostridium difficile* toxin with McCoy cell monolayers and cell suspensions and comparison with HeLa cell assay. J Clin Microbiol 1984;19:294.

77 **Murray PR, et al.** Detection of *Clostridium difficile* cytotoxin in HEp-2 and CHO cell lines. Diagn Microbiol Infect Dis 1983;1: 331.

78 **Donta ST, et al.** Differential effects of *Clostridium difficile* toxins on tissue-cultured cells. J Clin Microbiol 1982;15:1157.

79 **George RH.** A micro-method for detecting toxins in pseudomembranous colitis. J Clin Pathol 1979;32:303.

80 **Bartlett JG, et al.** Antibiotic-induced lethal enterocolitis in hamsters: studies with eleven agents and evidence to support the pathogenic role of toxin-producing Clostridia. Am J Vet Res 1978;39:1525.

81 **Borriello SP, et al.** Molecular, immunological, and biological characterization of a toxin A-negative, toxin B-positive strain of *Clostridium difficile*. Infect Immun 1992;60:4192.

82 **Phelps CJ, et al.** Construction and expression of the complete *Clostridium difficile* toxin A gene in *Escherichia coli*. Infect Immun 1991;59:150.

83 **Dove CH, et al.** Molecular characterization of the *Clostridium difficile* toxin A gene. Infect Immun 1990;58:480.

84 **Johnson JL, et al.** Cloning and expression of the toxin B gene of *Clostridium difficile*. Curr Microbiol 1990;20:397.

85 **Kuhl SJ, et al.** Diagnosis and monitoring of *Clostridium difficile* infections with the polymerase chain reaction. Clin Infect Dis 1993;16(suppl 4):S234.

86 **Kato N, et al.** Identification of toxigenic *Clostridium difficile* by the polymerase chain reaction. J Clin Microbiol 1991; 29:343.

87 **Milligan DE, et al.** Simultaneous detection of toxin A and toxin B genetic deter-

minants of *Clostridium difficile* using the multiplex polymerase chain reaction. Can J Microbiol 1992;38:81.

88 **Wu TC, et al.** Evaluation of a commercial kit for the routine detection of *Clostridium difficile* cytotoxin by tissue culture. J Clin Microbiol 1986;23:792.

89 **Walpita P, et al.** Mammalian epithelial cell line kit for detection of *Clostridium difficile* toxin. J Clin Microbiol 1993;31:315.

90 **Doern GV, et al.** Laboratory diagnosis of *Clostridium difficile*-associated gastrointestinal disease: comparison of a monoclonal antibody enzyme immunoassay for toxins A and B with a monoclonal antibody enzyme immunoassay for toxin A only and two cytotoxicity assays. J Clin Microbiol 1992;30:2042.

91 **Nachamkin I, et al.** Evaluation of a commercial cytotoxicity assay for detection of *Clostridium difficile* toxin. J Clin Microbiol 1986;23:954.

92 **DiPersio JR, et al.** Development of a rapid enzyme immunoassay for *Clostridium difficile* toxin A and its use in the diagnosis of *C. difficile*-associated disease. J Clin Microbiol 1991;29:2724.

93 **DeGirolami PC, et al.** Multicenter evaluation of a new enzyme immunoassay for detection of *Clostridium difficile* enterotoxin A. J Clin Microbiol 1992;30:1085.

94 **Shanholtzer CJ, et al.** Comparison of the VIDAS *Clostridium difficile* toxin A immunoassay with *C. difficile* culture and cytotoxin and latex tests. J Clin Microbiol 1992;30:1837.

95 **Sullivan NM, et al.** Purification and characterization of toxins A and B of *Clostridium difficile*. Infect Immun 1982;35:1032.

96 **Tucker KD, et al.** Toxin A of *Clostridium difficile* is a potent cytotoxin. J Clin Microbiol 1990;28:869.

97 **Welch DF, et al.** Identification of toxigenic *Clostridium difficile* by counterimmunoelectrophoresis. J Clin Microbiol 1980;11:470.

98 **Ryan RW, et al.** Rapid detection of *Clostridium difficile* toxin in human feces. J Clin Microbiol 1980;12:776.

99 **Wu TC, et al.** Evaluation of the usefulness of counterimmunoelectrophoresis for diagnosis of *Clostridium difficile*-associated colitis in clinical specimens. J Clin Microbiol 1983;17:610.

100 **Kurzynski TA, et al.** The use of CIE for the detection of *Clostridium difficile* toxin in stool filtrates: laboratory and

clinical correlation. Am J Clin Pathol 1983;79:370.

101 **West SE, et al.** Problems associated with counterimmunoelectrophoresis assays for detecting *Clostridium difficile* toxin. J Clin Microbiol 1982;15:347.

102 **Ryan RW, et al.** Improved immunologic detection of *Clostridium difficile* antigen by counterimmunoelectrophoresis. Diagn Microbiol Infect Dis 1983;1:59.

103 **Tilton RC, et al.** Varying results of counterimmunoelectrophoresis for the detection of *Clostridium difficile* toxins. J Infect Dis 1982;146:449.

104 **Levine HG, et al.** Counterimmunoelectrophoresis vs. cytotoxicity assay for the detection of *Clostridium difficile* toxin. J Infect Dis 1982;145:398.

105 **Jarvis W, et al.** Comparison of bacterial isolation, cytotoxicity assay, and counterimmunoelectrophoresis for the detection of *Clostridium difficile* and its toxin. J Infect Dis 1983;147:778.

106 **Lyerly DM, et al.** Characterization of cross-reactive proteins detected by Culturette Brand Rapid Latex Test for *Clostridium difficile*. J Clin Microbiol 1988;26:397.

107 **Lyerly DM, et al.** Commercial latex text for *Clostridium difficile* toxin A does not detect toxin A. J Clin Microbiol 1986;23:622.

108 **Borriello SP, et al.** Analysis of latex agglutination test for *Clostridium difficile* toxin A (D-1) and differentiation between *C. difficile* toxins A and B and latex reactive protein. J Clin Pathol 1987;40:573.

109 **Kamiya S, et al.** Evaluation of commercially available latex immunoagglutination test kit for detection of *Clostridium difficile* D-1 toxin. Microbiol Immunol 1986;30:177.

110 **Lyerly DM, et al.** Identification of the latex test-reactive protein of *Clostridium difficile* as glutamate dehydrogenase. J Clin Microbiol 1991;29:2639.

111 **Willis DH, et al.** Confirmation that the latex-reactive protein of *Clostridium difficile* is a glutamate dehydrogenase. J Clin Microbiol 1992;30:1363.

112 **Miles BL, et al.** Evaluation of a commercial latex test for *Clostridium difficile* for reactivity with *C. difficile* and cross-reactions with other bacteria. J Clin Microbiol 1988;26:2452.

113 **Shahrabadi MS, et al.** Latex agglutination test for detection of *Clostridium difficile* toxin in stool samples. J Clin Microbiol 1984;20:339.

114   **Patel N, et al.** Comparison of cell culture cytotoxicity, latex agglutination and enzyme immunoassays for the detection of *C. difficile*-associated disease. 92nd General Meeting of the American Society for Microbiology, New Orleans, Louisiana, May 30, 1992. Abstract.

115   **Kurzynski TA, et al.** Evaluation of C. diff.-CUBE test for detection of *Clostridium difficile*-associated diarrhea. Diagn Microbiol Infect Dis 1992;15:493.

116   **Bennett RG, et al.** Evaluation of a latex agglutination test for *Clostridium difficile* in two nursing home outbreaks. J Clin Microbiol 1989;27:889.

117   **Woods GL, et al.** Clinical comparison of latex agglutination and cytotoxin assay for detection of *Clostridium difficile* toxin in feces. Lab Med 1988;19:649.

118   **Sherman ME, et al.** Evaluation of a latex agglutination test for diagnosis of *Clostridium difficile*-associated colitis. Am J Clin Pathol 1988;89:228.

119   **Bowman RA, et al.** Latex particle agglutination for detecting and identifying *Clostridium difficile*. J Clin Pathol 1986;39: 212.

120   **Woods GL, et al.** Comparison of a dot immunobinding assay, latex agglutination, and cytotoxin assay for laboratory diagnosis of *Clostridium difficile*-associated diarrhea. J Clin Microbiol 1990;28:855.

121   **Kelly MT, et al.** Commercial latex agglutination test for detection of *Clostridium difficile*-associated diarrhea. J Clin Microbiol 1987;25:1244.

122   **Johnson LL, et al.** Identification of *Clostridium difficile* in stool specimens by culture-enhanced gas-liquid chromatography. J Clin Microbiol 1989;27:2218.

123   **Nunez-Montiel OL, et al.** Norleucine-tyrosine broth for rapid identification of *Clostridium difficile* by gas-liquid chromatography. J Clin Microbiol 1983;17:382.

124   **Brooks JB, et al.** Studies of stools for pseudomembranous colitis, rotaviral, and other diarrheal syndromes by frequency-pulsed electron capture gas-liquid chromatography. J Clin Microbiol 1984;20:549.

125   **Pepersack F, et al.** Use of gas-liquid chromatography as a screening test for toxigenic *Clostridium difficile* in diarrhoeal stools. J Clin Pathol 1983;36:1233.

126   **Levett PN.** Detection of *Clostridium difficile* in faeces by direct gas liquid chromatography. J Clin Pathol 1984;37:117.

127   **Lyerly DM, et al.** Monoclonal and specific polyclonal antibodies for immunoassay of *Clostridium difficile* toxin A. J Clin Microbiol 1985;21:12.

128   **Aronsson B, et al.** Enzyme immunoassay for detection of *Clostridium difficile* toxins A and B in patients with antibiotic-associated diarrhoea and colitis. Eur J Clin Microbiol 1985;4:102.

129   **Krishnan C.** Detection of *Clostridium difficile* toxins by enzyme immunoassay. J Hyg Camb 1986;96:5.

130   **Muller F, et al.** Monoclonal antibodies specific for *Clostridium difficile* toxin B and their use in immunoassays. J Clin Microbiol 1992;30:1544.

131   **Depitre C, et al.** Detection of *Clostridium difficile* toxins in stools. Gastroenterol Clin Biol 1993;17:283.

132   **Barbut F, et al.** Comparison of three enzyme immunoassays, a cytotoxicity assay, and toxigenic culture for diagnosis of *Clostridium difficile*-associated diarrhea. J Clin Microbiol 1993;31:963.

133   **Merz CS, et al.** Comparison of four commercially available rapid enzyme immunoassays with cytotoxin assay for detection of *Clostridium difficile* toxin(s) from stool specimens. J Clin Microbiol 1994;32:1142.

134   **Kurzynski TA, et al.** Evaluation of C. diff-CUBE test for detection of *Clostridium difficile*-associated diarrhea. Diagn Microbiol Infect Dis 1992;15:493.

135   **Gumerlock PH, et al.** Use of the polymerase chain reaction for the specific and direct detection of *Clostridium difficile* in human feces. Rev Infect Dis 1991;13:1053.

136   **Kato N, et al.** Detection of toxigenic *Clostridium difficile* in stool specimens by the polymerase chain reaction. J Infect Dis 1993;167:455.

137   **Wren BW, et al.** Identification of toxigenic *Clostridium difficile* strains by using a toxin A gene-specific probe. J Clin Microbiol 1990;28:1808.

138   **Knudsen JD, et al.** Demonstration of toxin A and B by polymerase chain reaction and McCoy cell assay in clinical isolates of *Clostridium difficile* from Denmark. APMIS 1993;101:18.

139   **Gumerlock PH, et al.** Specific detection of toxigenic strains of *Clostridium difficile* in stool specimens. J Clin Microbiol 1993; 31:507.

Brucellosis: Current Epidemiology, Diagnosis, and Management

EDWARD J. YOUNG

Brucellosis is largely a disease of domestic animals. The causative agent is known, as are the routes of transmission from animals to man. Techniques for bacteriologic and serologic diagnosis are readily available but underused. A variety of antimicrobial agents active against brucellae are known, yet the most effective treatments for complications of human brucellosis are elusive. Elimination of brucellosis as a human pathogen can be accomplished by eradicating the disease in animals. The methods to accomplish this goal are also known. What is lacking throughout much of the world are the resources and the commitment.

EPIDEMIOLOGY

Brucellosis exists worldwide but is especially prevalent in the Mediterranean basin, the Arabian peninsula, the Indian subcontinent, and in parts of Mexico and Central and South America. In many countries, the status of brucellosis remains unknown owing to insufficient facilities for diagnosis and reporting. In brucellosis-free areas, the unregulated importation of animals for breeding purposes can have an impact on the incidence of the disease in animals and man.

Brucella abortus

In the United States, largely as a result of the Cooperative State-Federal Brucellosis Eradication Program begun in 1934, bovine brucellosis has been eradicated in all but a few southern states. Coincident with the enforcement of this program, which involves serologic testing of cattle, quarantine and slaughter of infected animals, and calfhood immunization with *B. abortus* strain 19 vaccine, the incidence of human brucellosis declined after World War II from more than 6000 to fewer than 100 cases per year. As effective as this program has been, it is estimated that less than half of all cases of human brucellosis diagnosed are reported (1).

Brucella melitensis

In contrast to B. abortus, the situation with regard to B. melitensis is less encouraging. In recent years the incidence of disease caused by B. melitensis has reached epidemic proportions in several areas, notably in the Middle East. In some instances, this apparent increase represented better surveillance and case identification. In Jordan, for example, brucellosis was not reportable until 1981. In 1985, when the disease was recognized to be a problem, the number of reported cases increased from fewer than 10 to more than 400 per year over the next 3 years (2). In Kuwait, the infection rate increased from 5.1 in 1982, to a high of 68.9/100,000 population in 1985 (3). Although steps were taken to combat this epidemic, the affects of the war with Iran on this effort remain to be determined.

The major source of human infection with B. melitensis is dairy products prepared from the milk of infected goats and sheep. In some countries camels are also believed to be a reservoir for brucellosis (4). In Peru, epidemics of human brucellosis have occurred periodically, coincident with epizootics of the disease in goats (5). The source is goat's milk cheese, which is consumed fresh to preserve its preferred flavor and aroma. Although boiling and pasteurizing are effective means to eliminate brucellae from milk, attempts to introduce such practices are met with great resistance; nothing is more difficult to change than traditional methods of preparing food.

Although B. melitensis has been eradicated from native goats in the United States, the importation of contaminated goat cheese from Mexico has resulted in outbreaks of human brucellosis in border states (6,7) and elsewhere (8). In Texas, the epidemiology of brucellosis has changed dramatically in recent years. Between 1977 and 1981, the majority of cases occurred in Caucasian men who had documented exposure to cattle or swine. In contrast, between 1982 and 1986, the preponderance of cases occurred in Hispanics of both sexes, and the source of infection was goat's milk products (9). Brucellosis is also a risk for travellers to countries where the disease is enzootic. Ingestion of local foods can result in infection that may not become symptomatic until the victim returns home (10). Unless a history of foreign travel is elicited, brucellosis may not be considered and the diagnosis will be delayed.

Brucella melitensis strain Rev-1 is an effective vaccine for caprine and ovine brucellosis. Widespread immunization of susceptible animals can significantly reduce the spread of brucellosis to human beings in areas where the milk supply is not safeguarded and where animal husbandry practices are substandard.

Brucella suis

Human infection with B. suis is most commonly associated with the slaughter of swine (11), and studies within abattoirs have documented the risk of aerosols as a mode of transmission (12). At the end of 1990 there were 65 domestic swine herds under quarantine in the southeastern United States (13). A recent outbreak of human brucellosis cases at a swine processing plant in North Carolina is believed to have resulted from the slaughter of swine purchased from unregulated suppliers.

In recent years, feral swine (domesticated pigs that have returned to the wild) have become an increasing source of brucellosis. Feral swine are widely distributed throughout the continental United States and Hawaii, where they have become a popular game animal (14). In Florida, it is estimated that about 50,000 feral swine are hunted annually (15), and the shipment of animals from Florida to a game preserve in Iowa resulted in transmission of the disease to a domestic herd (13). A similar situation has been reported in Australia, where an effective eradication program resulted in the elimination of bovine brucellosis in 1989. The incidence of human brucellosis fell concomitantly until 1986, when an increasing number of cases caused by B. suis were reported in Queensland. This change in epidemiology appears to be related to the growing demand for wild boar meat for export to France and Germany (16). Hunters of feral swine and wild boars are often unaware of the risk of brucellosis in these animals, and are exposed to brucellae during the process of butchering and dressing the carcasses. In addition, feral swine transported to swine brucellosis-free states for hunting purposes pose a risk to domestic swine and cattle with which they may commingle. The primary hosts of B. suis biovar 4 are reindeer and caribou of the Arctic and sub-Arctic areas of Alaska, Canada, and Siberia. Although cooking, curing, or smoking meat effectively kills brucellae, the tradition of ingesting raw meat or bone marrow, prevalent among Eskimo and Inuits, places them at risk of contracting brucellosis in this manner (17). Currently, there is no satisfactory method to immunize swine against B. suis, despite reports from China regarding strain-2 vaccine, which is alleged to induce immunity after oral administration (18).

Brucella canis

B. canis was identified by Carmichael in 1966 as the cause of abortions and whelping failures among kennel-bred beagles (19). The disease occurs worldwide in many breeds of dogs, including those of mixed ancestry, and possibly in other canine species as well. Since it was first shown to be a human pathogen in 1972, only a handful of cases have been reported, primarily among laboratory workers and owners of infected dogs (20,21). Unless organisms are recovered from blood or other tissues, the diagnosis of B. canis infection is difficult. Because it is a naturally rough species, antibodies to B. canis are not detected by standard brucellosis serologic tests, which use cell wall polysaccharide as the principal antigen. A *B. canis* whole cell microagglutination test has been devised to detect species-specific antibodies (22). However, it is not widely available. Most laboratories depend on a veterinary slide agglutination test to make a presumptive diagnosis, with a titer of 1:100 or greater after pretreatment of the serum with 2-mercaptoethanol (2ME) generally considered to be "significant" (23).

Occupational Hazards

Except for brucellosis linked to food, the vast majority of cases of human brucellosis can be traced to direct contact with animals, their carcasses, or their secretions. Hence, ranchers, veterinarians, abattoir workers, and laboratory personnel are at increased risk of contracting the disease. Veterinarians and animal health technicians have the added risk of exposure to live brucella vaccines. *B. abortus* strain 19 was isolated in 1923 by Buck from the milk of a Jersey heifer named Lady Victor's Matilda (24). After remaining at room temperature for more than a year, the isolate was found to have reduced virulence for cattle, and in 1940 it was approved by the U.S. Bureau of Animal Industry as a suitable vaccine against bovine brucellosis. Strain 19 was once used in the Soviet Union to immunize human beings. However, in the United States, the risk of adverse reactions was considered to be too high to justify its use. Moreover, a number of well documented cases of human brucellosis have been linked to accidental inoculation with strain 19 vaccine (25). With an estimated 10 million doses of strain 19 vaccine administered to cattle in the United States annually, it is surprising that more cases of strain 19 disease in human beings do not occur. In addition, studies with *B. melitensis* Rev-1 vaccine in volunteers showed that the margin between an innocuous dose and one leading to infection was too narrow to recommend its use in human beings.

Factors that appear to influence the outcome of brucella vaccine accidents include the route of exposure, the dose of vaccine inoculated, and the prior immune status of the victim. Spraying vaccine into the eyes carries a higher risk for infection than needle stick injuries, perhaps owing to the volume of vaccine inoculated. If the subject has preexisting antibodies to brucella at the time of injury, the outcome is generally a transient, self-limited local reaction, sometimes accompanied by systemic symptoms, such as fever and chills. This is believed to be an allergic response, although the nature of the reaction remains undefined. In the absence of preexisting antibodies, there is a risk of developing acute brucellosis, although this risk appears to be small (26). Management of brucella vaccine accidents includes a baseline serologic test for brucella antibodies, local wound care, and, when the eyes are involved, a course of antibiotics. Because tetracycline given as prophylaxis following a significant exposure may only delay the onset of infection, it is prudent to continue antibiotics for a full six-week course.

The brucellae are class 3 pathogens, requiring biologic safety cabinets and other containment equipment. The risk to laboratory personnel has been recognized since 1897, when the researchers MacFadyen in London and Carbone in Italy died as the result of accidental infection with *B. melitensis* (27). Over a 25-year period at the National Animal Disease Center, *Brucella* species were the most frequent class 3 organisms causing laboratory-associated infections (28). Aerosol contamination is often the route of transmission in laboratories, as was the case at a brucella vaccine production facility in Spain where a faulty air extraction system exposed employees to contaminated air (29). The failure to take appropriate precautions when handling clinical specimens is not only a risk in countries where brucellosis is endemic (30,31), but also in countries where the disease is rare and often unsuspected (32,33).

Abortion and Human-to-Human Transmission

The relationship of brucellosis to human abortion and the potential for human-to-human transmission are frequent questions. In animals, brucellae localize in the reproductive organs of both sexes, and spontaneous abortion is a frequent outcome of infection. It is postulated that erythritol, a polyhydric alcohol found in the placentae of certain animals, stimulates the growth of brucellae leading to abortion. Because erythritol is not found in the human placenta, it is theorized that this provides relative resistance to the acute placental form of brucellosis (34). Nevertheless, pregnant women who contract brucellosis can abort (35), and brucellae have been recovered from placentae, amniotic fluid, and fetal tissues (36). Spink summarized the data in his classic monograph, concluding that abortion can occur with the bacteremic phase of many bacteremic infections and that brucellosis is no exception (37).

Rare cases of brucellosis transmitted by blood transfusions (38) or bone marrow transplantation (39) have been reported; otherwise, the disease is not readily transmitted between human beings. Nevertheless, brucellae have been isolated from human spermatozoa (40), and in several cases, venereal transmission has been suspected (41,42). Although the evidence is circumstantial, it may be prudent to advise individuals with brucellosis to refrain from unprotected sexual activity until the infection is resolved.

Clinical Features: Common and Uncommon

The clinical manifestations of brucellosis are more protean even than those of syphilis and tuberculosis. Attempts have been made to categorize the disease into acute, subacute, and chronic according to the length and severity of symptoms, but such distinctions are purely arbitrary, because the onset is insidious in more than half the cases (43). Symptoms are nonspecific—notably, fever, anorexia, weight loss, malaise, profound fatigue, body and joint aches, mental inattention and depression. Sweating, often profuse, is characteristic and may have a peculiar odor. In contrast to the multitude of somatic complaints, there are often a paucity of abnormal physical findings other than fever. In cases caused by *B. melitensis*, periods of fever may be interspersed with periods of normal temperature, leading to the term *undulant fever*.

Brucellosis is a systemic illness in which any organ or system of the body can be involved. Because the brucellae are facultative intracellular pathogens, they localize within organs of the reticuloendothelial system, such as lymph nodes, liver, spleen, and bone marrow. Localized involvement of one or more organs is often termed a complication (44). The more common complications of brucellosis have been reviewed recently and will not be detailed here. These include osteoarticular (45), nervous system (46), cardiovascular (47), genitourinary (48), pulmonary (49), gastrointestinal (50), and dermatologic (51) manifestations.

Less common complications include deep tissue abscesses, which are more often caused by *B. suis* than other *Brucella* species (52,53). In addition, a variety of eye lesions have been described in association with brucellosis, most notably uveitis (54). Many of the ocular lesions in brucellosis are thought to represent a postinfectious immune reaction (55).

DIAGNOSIS

The diagnosis of brucellosis requires a high index of suspicion and careful attention to a history of contact with animals, foreign travel, or ingestion of "exotic" foods. A definitive diagnosis is made by recovering brucellae from blood, bone marrow, or other tissues. Routine laboratory tests are generally unremarkable, except that the white blood cell count is usually normal or low (56). Anemia, thrombocytopenia, and pancytopenia have been reported, and examination of the bone marrow may reveal hemophagocytosis (57).

Bacteriologic Diagnosis

Brucella species grow slowly in vitro, and the rate of isolation is low. When the disease is suspected, the laboratory should be alerted to maintain routine cultures for at least 30 days. Most clinical laboratories now use automated blood culture systems such as the Bactec, but the recovery times are still prolonged (58). Preliminary studies with the BACT/ALERT system using blood culture bottles seeded with *B. melitensis* indicated a shortening of the recovery time to several days (59). However, additional experience is needed. The lysis concentration technique has also been reported to improve the rate of isolation (60), but this technique is not routine in most laboratories.

Once a *Brucella* species is recovered, identification of the organism is best reserved for reference laboratories with appropriate biohazard equipment. However, many clinical laboratories now use commercial rapid identification systems. Caution is advised when using such systems because the biochemical profiles of the brucellae are not included in all computerized data bases. In several instances, *B. melitensis* has been incorrectly identified as *Moraxella* species by such systems (61,62). The application of polymerase chain reaction technology to the identification of *Brucella* species is underway but is not yet widely available (63).

Serologic Diagnosis

In the absence of bacteriologic confirmation, the diagnosis of brucellosis can be made by demonstrating high or rising titers of specific antibodies in the serum. A variety of serologic methods have been used, but the serum agglutination test (SAT) remains the standard against which others are compared (64). In 1965, Reddin and colleagues showed that the immune response in brucellosis is characterized by an initial rise in IgM antibodies within the first week of infection (65). Agglutination by this class of immunoglobulin can be destroyed by reacting it with disulfide reducing agents, such as 2ME or dithiothreitol (DTT) (66,67). Within the second week of infection, IgG antibodies (which are resistant to inactivation by 2ME or DTT) appear, after which both antibody isotypes continue to rise. After treatment with antibiotics, the titers decline slowly and generally disappear within two years. In some cases, however, low levels of IgM agglutinins can remain in the serum for months to years without evidence of continued infection. Because the SAT measures the total quantity of agglutinating antibodies (IgM + IgG), it is necessary to perform *both* the SAT and 2ME (or DTT) tests to determine the relative contributions of IgM and IgG in the reaction. This is important because the presence of a high titer of 2ME-resistant (IgG) antibodies correlates best with active disease (68). After treatment it is important to follow the decline in titers because a failure of the IgG titer to fall is often predictive of relapse or chronic infection (69–72).

Some authors contend that agglutination tests are too insensitive and favor instead an enzyme-linked immunosorbent assay (ELISA). Unfortunately, at present there is no standardized brucella antigen for ELISA, making it difficult to compare the results from different laboratories.

Regardless of the serologic method used, it is important to understand the limitations of the test. For example, in the SAT, many sera with high titers of antibody to *Brucella* fail to agglutinate at low dilutions owing to a prozone phenomenon. False negative results can be avoided by routinely diluting sera beyond 1:640 because the prozone will disappear at higher dilutions. In addition, false positive results have been reported owing to shared epitopes between *Brucella* species and other gram-negative bacteria, such as *Vibrio cholerae*, *Francisella tularensis*, and *Yersinia enterocolitica*. This is rarely a problem in diagnosis because cross-reacting antibodies are present in low titer and are destroyed by 2ME treatment.

The SAT has good interlaboratory reproducibility but there is still controversy among investigators as to what titer is "diagnostic." By convention, the end-point determination is considered to be the highest dilution of serum yielding a 2+ (50% agglutination) reaction. Some laboratories consider a titer of

1:80 or above to be significant, whereas others recommend a titer of 1:160 or above. In our experience, no single titer is always diagnostic, and serologic test results must be interpreted in light of historical, epidemiologic, and clinical data (64). Nevertheless, the majority of patients with active brucellosis have titers of 1:80 or above after treatment of the serum with 2ME (68). Studies in areas where brucellosis is enzootic show a high prevalence of IgM antibodies among asymptomatic individuals, suggesting either prior infection or subclinical disease (73).

Although humoral antibodies provide a means of establishing a diagnosis and may play some role in resistance, studies have shown that cell-mediated immunity predominates in recovery from brucellosis in animals and human beings (74). Coincident with the acquisition of cellular resistance is the development of delayed-type hypersensitivity to antigens of *Brucella* species. Although this can be demonstrated using a variety of skin test preparations, they are not standardized and are of no use in diagnosis.

MANAGEMENT

Hall reviewed the treatment of brucellosis, concluding that the most effective and least toxic chemotherapy is still undecided (75). There is little question that antimicrobial therapy improves symptoms, shortens the course of illness, and aids the body's natural defenses in eliminating the pathogen. However, Spink postulated that the intracellular milieu might protect brucellae against both drugs and humoral antibodies. In addition, he likened brucellosis to tuberculosis, in which the persistence of organisms is associated with the acquisition of hypersensitivity, which also contributes to some of the symptoms (37).

Although a variety of antimicrobial drugs are active in vitro against *Brucella* species, some have a wide range of minimal inhibitory concentrations (MICs) and clinical efficacy varies accordingly. Moreover, the results of standard in vitro susceptibility tests do not always predict clinical efficacy. For example, whereas Lang et al. reported low MICs for cefatriaxone against *B. melitensis*, patients treated with this drug failed to be cured (76). Overall, the wide variability in MICs of β-lactam antibiotics makes them less useful than other classes of drugs for treating brucellosis.

The tetracyclines have been the most effective class of antibiotics against the brucellae despite their bacteriostatic mode of action. Nevertheless, short courses of oxytetracycline were associated with relapse rates in excess of 70%. Consequently prolonged administration of tetracycline or combinations of drugs, such as oxytetracycline and streptomycin, were used in an attempt to reduce this unacceptably high rate of treatment failures (75). The combination of tetracycline given for four to six weeks plus streptomycin given for the initial one to two weeks became the standard therapy, and relapse rates declined to less than 10%. Although some studies reported that this combination of drugs was synergistic and bacteriocidal (77), others failed to demonstrate synergy depending on the *Brucella* species and the methods used (78). Rubinstein et al. recently obtained a better correlation between in vitro and clinical results using a method to measure the rates of killing of *B. melitensis* by various antibiotics alone and in combination (79). Although they could not demonstrate synergy using routine in vitro techniques, *B. melitensis* was sequentially killed more rapidly when streptomycin was used in combination with minocycline, ciprofloxacin, or rifampin than when any of these agents were used alone. Doxycycline, which has a longer half-life and is more lipophilic than tetracycline hydrochloride, has become the analogue of choice. Numerous studies have shown the superiority of the combination of oral doxycycline (200 mg/d) continued for 4 to 6 weeks plus intramuscular streptomycin (1 g/d) administered for the initial 2 to 3 weeks (80–83). When streptomycin was used alone in treating brucellosis, the results were disappointing (75). Therefore, many authorities prefer gentamicin in place of streptomycin owing to fewer side effects. Recommended doses range from 2 to 5 mg/kg/d in divided doses for the initial 5 to 10 days in combination with doxycycline.

Among other drugs with in vitro activity against *Brucella* species, rifampin, trimethoprim/sulfamethoxazole (TMP/SMZ), and the fluoroquinolones have been the most promising (75). Rifampin has a low MIC (0.05 to 4.0 µg/mL), is lipophilic, and achieves good levels in cerebrospinal fluid. Unfortunately, when used alone in doses of 10 to 20 mg/kg/d, the rate of relapse was unacceptably high. Nevertheless, the combination of doxycycline plus rifampin administered for 45 days is nearly comparable to doxycycline plus streptomycin (80,81,83).

Trimethoprim/sulfamethoxazole has found its principal use for treating brucellosis in children less than 8 years of age and in pregnancy, where the tetracyclines are contraindicated. To avoid relapse, four tablets of TMP/SMZ (standard formulation of 800 mg TMP/400 mg SMZ) are given daily for 4 to 6 weeks in combination with gentamicin for the initial 5 days (84). When used alone, the fluoroquinolones have a higher failure rate than other drugs with similar MICs (85). Consequently, currently available quinolone preparations should be reserved for combination therapy with other drugs, such as doxycycline.

Complications

Potentially life-threatening complications, such as meningitis and endocarditis, are rare, and insufficient numbers of patients have been studied to determine the most effective therapy. Nevertheless, most authorities agree that combinations of drugs are essential, and treatment should continue for a longer time than with uncomplicated brucellosis. Doxycycline plus streptomycin or gentamicin remain the principal drugs for both uncomplicated and localized disease. When the central nervous system is involved, treatment is generally continued for 6 to 9 months, and an agent with good penetration of the blood/brain barrier, such as rifampin, is often added (46,86). A similar approach is taken to brucella endocarditis, except that in addition to antibiotics, valve replacement surgery is often required (47,87).

Relapse

Relapse is confirmed by isolating brucellae from blood or other tissues of a patient with recurring symptoms some time after a course of treatment. Relapse generally occurs within weeks to months of stopping therapy, and with very few exceptions, is not caused by the emergence of antibiotic-resistant strains (88). Causes of relapse include inappropriate drugs, failure of patients to comply with prolonged antibiotic therapy, or localized foci of infection requiring surgical drainage. Most of these patients are cured by another course of treatment.

Chronic Brucellosis

Perhaps no aspect of the disease is more controversial and difficult to manage than chronic brucellosis. Although there is no universally accepted definition, many adopt Spink's arbitrary criteria of symptoms persisting for more than a year after the original diagnosis (89). Using this definition, Spink found that patients could be divided into three categories. The first two included patients with *relapse* and *localized infection*, in whom objective evidence of infection were present, titers of antibodies remained elevated, and on occasion, brucellae could be recovered from blood or other tissues. Patients in the third category, accounting for about 20% of cases, lacked objective signs of infection, had low or absent titers of antibodies, and remained bacteriologically sterile. Spink concluded that patients in the third category suffered from psychoneurosis. Emboden et al. studied a group of patients with laboratory-acquired brucellosis and compared those with delayed convalescence to those who recovered without sequelae (90). On the basis of psychological tests and psychiatric interviews, it was concluded that delayed convalescence was an emotional disorder related to personality traits that preceded the infection but were exacerbated by it.

The complaints voiced by patients with delayed convalescence from brucellosis resemble those of patients with chronic fatigue syndrome (CFS). In the decade following World War II, CFS then termed neuromyasthenia, was believed to be caused by brucellosis (91). It has even been suggested that chronic brucellosis can exist without specific antibodies in the serum, the diagnosis being made by a positive Coomb's test (92). Evidence against such a concept is the observation that Coomb's test reactivity persists in a high percentage of patients who have recovered from brucellosis without evidence of persistent infection or delayed convalescence (68).

The management of patients with delayed convalescence from brucellosis in the absence of objective evidence of continued infection is similar to the treatment of CFS. Despite assurances that repeated courses of antibiotics will not improve their symptoms, such patients are reluctant to abandon the notion that chronic brucellosis is the cause of their ill health. The situation is made more complex when such patients have litigation or workman's compensation claims pending. This is not to say that such patients are not ill or are malingering; rather, it is possible that brucellosis is one of many causes of the CFS and its attendant immunologic alterations.

REFERENCES

1 **Texas Department of Health**. Under-reporting of four infectious diseases by Texas hospitals. Disease Prevention News 1993;No. 7:53.

2 **Dajani YF, Masoud AA, Barakat HF.** Epidemiology and diagnosis of brucellosis in Jordan. Eastern Mediterranean Region Epidemiol Bull 1988;No. 9:13–22.

3 **Lulu AR, Araj GF, Khateeb MI, Mustafa MY, Yusuf AR, Fenech FF.** Human brucellosis in Kuwait: a prospective study of 400 cases. Q J Med 1988;66:39–54.

4 **Ismaily SIN, Harby HAM, Nicoletti P.** Prevalence of brucella antibodies in four animal species in the Sultanate of Oman. Trop Animal Health Prod 1988;20:269–271.

5 **Escalante JA, Held JR.** Brucellosis in Peru. J Am Vet Med Assoc 1969;155:2146–2152.

6 **Young EJ, Suvannoparrat U.** Brucellosis outbreak attributed to ingestion of unpasteurized goat cheese. Arch Intern Med 1975;135:240–243.

7 **Thapar MK, Young EJ.** Urban outbreak of goat cheese brucellosis. Pediatr Infect Dis 1986;5:640–643.

8 **Eckman MR.** Brucellosis linked to Mexican cheese. JAMA 1975;232:636–637.

9 **Taylor PM, Perdue JN.** The changing epidemiology of human brucellosis in Texas, 1977–1986. Am J Epidemiol 1989;130:160–165.

10 **Arnow PM, Smaron M, Ormiste V.** Brucellosis in a group of travellers to Spain. JAMA 1984;251:505–507.

11 **Buchanan TM, Hendricks SL, Patton CM, Feldman RA.** Brucellosis in the United States, 1960–1972: an abattoir-associated disease. III. Epidemiology and evidence for acquired immunity. Medicine 1974;53:427–439.

12 **Kaufmann AF, Fox MD, Boyce JM, et al.** Airborne spread of brucellosis. Ann NY Acad Sci 1980;353:105–114.

13 **Lenard D.** Perspectives on brucellosis in domestic swine. Proc Brucellosis Epidemi-ology Conference, U.S. Department of Agriculture, Memphis, TN, April 22–24, 1991.

14 **Davis DS.** Role of wildlife in transmitting brucellosis. In: Adams LG, ed. Advances in brucellosis research. College Station, TX: Texas A & M University Press, 1990:373–385.

15 **Becker HN, Belden RC, Breault T, Burridge MJ, Frankenberger WB, Nicoletti P.** Brucellosis in feral swine in Florida. J Am Vet Med Assoc 1978;173:1181–1182.

16 **Robinson JM, Harrison MW, Wood RN, Tilse MH, McKay AB, Brodribb TR.** Brucellosis: re-emergence and changing epidemiology in Queensland. Med J Aust 1993;159:153–158.

17 **Chan J, Baxter C, Wenman WM.** Brucellosis in an Inuit child, probably related to caribou meat consumption. Scand J Infect Dis 1989;21:337–338.

18 **Xin X.** Orally administrable brucellosis vaccine: *Brucella suis* strain 2 vaccine. Vaccine 1986;4:212–216.

19 **Carmichael LS.** Contagious abortion in Beagles. Hounds and Hunting 1967;64:14–18.

20 **Swenson R, Carmichael LS, Cundy KP.** Human infection with *Brucella canis*. Ann Intern Med 1972;76:435–438.

21 **Polt SS, Dismukes WE, Flint A, Schaefer J.** Human brucellosis caused by *Brucella canis*. Ann Intern Med 1982;97:717–719.

22 **Polt SS, Schaefer J.** A microagglutination test for human *Brucella canis* antibodies. Am J Clin Pathol 1982;77:740–744.

23 **Badakhsh FF, Carmichael LE, Douglass JA.** Improved rapid slide agglutination test for presumptive diagnosis of canine brucellosis. J Clin Microbiol 1982;15:286–289.

24 **Graves RR.** The story of John M. Buck's and Matilda's contribution to the cattle in-

dustry. J Am Vet Med Assoc 1943;102: 193–195.

25 **Young EJ.** Clinical manifestations of human brucellosis. In: Young EJ, Corbel MJ, eds. Brucellosis: clinical and laboratory aspects. Boca Raton, Fla: CRC Press, 1989: 114–116.

26 **Young EJ.** *Brucella* antibodies in veterinarians exposed to strain 19. In: Adams LG, ed. Advances in brucellosis research. College Station, TX: Texas A & M University Press, 1990:465.

27 **Meyer KF, Eddie B.** Laboratory infections due to brucella. J Infect Dis 1941;68:24–32.

28 **Miller CD, Songer JR, Sullivan JF.** A twenty-five year review of laboratory-acquired human infections at the National Animal Disease Center. Am Ind Hyg Assoc J 1987;48:271–275.

29 **Olle-Goig JE, Canela-Solar J.** An outbreak of *Brucella melitensis* infection by airborne transmission among laboratory workers. Am J Public Health 1987;77:335–338.

30 **Al-Aska AK, Chagla AH.** Laboratory-acquired brucellosis. J Hosp Infect 1989; 14:69–71.

31 **Kiel FW, Khan MY.** Brucellosis among hospital employees in Saudi Arabia. Infect Control Hosp Epidemiol 1993;14:268–272.

32 **Staszkiewicz J, Lewis CM, Colville J, Zervos M, Band J.** Outbreak of *Brucella melitensis* among microbiology laboratory workers in a community hospital. J Clin Microbiol 1991;29:287–290.

33 **Luzzi GA, Brindle R, Sockett PN, Solera J, Klenerman P, Warrell DA.** Brucellosis: imported and laboratory-acquired cases, and an overview of treatment trials. Trans Roy Soc Trop Med Hyg 1993;87:138–141.

34 **Porreco RP, Haverkamp AD.** Brucellosis in pregnancy. Obstet Gynecol 1974;44:597–602.

35 **Poole PM, Whitehouse DB, Gilchrist MM.** A case of abortion consequent upon infection with *Brucella abortus* biotype 2. J Clin Pathol 1972;25:882–884.

36 **Schreyer P, Caspi E, Leiba Y, Eshchar Y, Sompolinsky D.** Brucella septicemia in pregnancy. Eur J Obstet Gynecol Reprod Biol 1980;10:99–107.

37 **Spink WW.** The nature of brucellosis. Minneapolis: University of Minnesota Press, 1956.

38 **Economidou J, Kalafatas P, Vatopoulou T, Petropoulou D, Kattamis C.** Brucellosis in two thalassaemic patients infected by blood transfusions from the same donor. Acta Haematol 1976;55:244–249.

39 **Naparstek E, Block CS, Slavin S.** Transmission of brucellosis by bone marrow transplantation. Lancet 1982;1:574–575.

40 **Vandercam B, Zech F, deCooman S, Bughin C, Gigi J, Wauters G.** Isolation of *Brucella melitensis* from human sperm. Eur J Clin Microbiol Infect Dis 1990;9:303–304.

41 **Ruben B, Band JD, Wong P, Colville J.** Person-to-person transmission of *Brucella melitensis*. Lancet 1991;337:14–15.

42 **Lindberg J, Larsson P.** Transmission of *Brucella melitensis*. Lancet 1991;337:848–849.

43 **Eyre JWH.** Melitensis septicemia (Malta or Mediterranean fever). Lancet 1908;1:1747–1752.

44 **Young EJ.** Human brucellosis. Rev Infect Dis 1983;5:821–842.

45 **Mousa ARM, Muhtaseb SA, Almudallal DS, Khodeir SM, Marafie AA.** Osteoarticular complications of brucellosis: a study of 169 cases. Rev Infect Dis 1987; 9:531–543.

46 **McLean DR, Russell N, Khan MY.** Neurobrucellosis: clinical and therapeutic features. Clin Infect Dis 1992;15:582–590.

47 **Jacobs F, Abramowicz D, Vereerstraeten P, LeClerc JL, Zech F, Thys JP.** Brucella endocarditis: the role of combined medical and surgical treatment. Rev Infect Dis 1990;12:740–744.

48 **Ibrahim AIA, Awad R, Shetty SD, Saad M, Bilal NE.** Genitourinary complications of brucellosis. Br J Urol 1988;6:294–298.

49 **Lubani MM, Lulu AR, Araj GF, Khateeb MI, Qurtom MAF, Dudin KI.** Pulmonary brucellosis. Q J Med 1989;71:319–324.

50 **Al Aska AK.** Gastrointestinal manifestations of brucellosis in Saudi Arabian patients. Trop Gastroenterol 1989;10:217–219.

51 **Ariza J, Servitje O, Pallares R, et al.** Characteristic cutaneous lesions in patients with brucellosis. Arch Dermatol 1989;125:380–383.

52 **Spink WW.** Suppuration and calcification of the liver and spleen due to long standing infection with *Brucella suis*. N Engl J Med 1957;257:209–210.

53 **Martin WJ, Nichols DR, Beahrs OH.** Chronic localized brucellosis. Arch Intern Med 1961;107:143–148.

54 **Walker J, Sharma OP, Rao NA.** Brucellosis and uveitis. Am J Ophthalmol 1992;114: 374–375.

55 **Madkour MM.** Brucellosis. Boston: Butterworths, 1989.

56 **Crosby E, Llosa L, Quesada MM, Carrillo C, Gotuzzo E.** Hematologic changes in brucellosis. J Infect Dis 1984;150:419–424.

57 **Martin-Moreno S, Soto-Guzman O, Bernaldo-de-Quiros J, Reverte-Cejudo D, Bascones-Casas C.** Pancytopenia due to hemophagocytosis in patients with brucellosis: a report of four cases. J Infect Dis 1983;147:445–447.

58 **Zimmerman SJ, Gillikin S, Sofat N, Bartholomew WR, Amsterdam D.** Case report and seeded blood culture study of *Brucella* bacteremia. J Clin Microbiol 1990; 28:2139–2141.

59 **Solomon HM, Jackson D.** Rapid diagnosis of *Brucella melitensis* in blood: some operational characteristics of the BACT/ALERT. J Clin Microbiol 1992;30:222–224.

60 **Kolman S, Maayan MC, Gotesman G, Rozenszajn LA, Wolach B, Lang R.** Comparison of the Bactec and lysis concentration methods for recovery of *Brucella* species from clinical specimens. Eur J Clin Microbiol Infect Dis 1991;10:647–648.

61 **Peiris V, Fraser S, Fairhurst M, Weston D, Kaczmarski E.** Laboratory diagnosis of brucella infection: some pitfalls. Lancet 1992;1:1415–1416.

62 **Barham WB, Church P, Brown JE, Paparello S.** Misidentification of *Brucella* species with use of rapid bacterial identification systems. Clin Infect Dis 1993;17: 1068–1069.

63 **Herman L, De Ridder H.** Identification of *Brucella* spp. by using the polymerase chain reaction. Appl Environ Microbiol 1992; 58:2099–2101.

64 **Young EJ.** Serologic diagnosis of human brucellosis: analysis of 214 cases by agglutination tests and review of the literature. Rev Infect Dis 1991;13:359–372.

65 **Reddin JL, Anderson RK, Jenness R, Spink WW.** Significance of 7S and macroglobulin brucella agglutinins in human brucellosis. N Engl J Med 1965;272:1263–1267.

66 **Anderson RK, Jenness R, Brumfield HP, Gough P.** Brucella-agglutinating antibodies: relation of mercaptoethanol stability to complement fixation. Science 1964;143: 1334–1335.

67 **Klein GC, Behan KA.** Determination of brucella immunoglobulin G agglutinating antibody titer with dithiothreitol. J Clin Microbiol 1981;14:24–25.

68 **Farrell ID, Robertson L, Hinchliffe PM.** Serum antibody response in acute brucellosis. J Hyg Camb 1975;74:23–28.

69 **Pellicer T, Ariza J, Foz A, Pallares R, Gudiol F.** Specific antibodies detected during relapse of human brucellosis. J Infect Dis 1988;157:918–924.

70 **Gazapo E, Lahoz JG, Subiza JL, Baquaro M, Gil J, de la Concha EG.** Changes in IgM and IgG antibody concentrations in brucellosis over time: importance for diagnosis and follow-up. J Infect Dis 1989;159: 219–225.

71 **Ariza J, Pellicer T, Pallares R, Foz A, Gudiol F.** Specific antibody profile in human brucellosis. Clin Infect Dis 1992;14: 131–140.

72 **Buchanan TM, Faber LC.** 2-Mercaptoethanol brucella agglutination test: usefulness for predicting recovery from brucellosis. J Clin Microbiol 1980;11:691–693.

73 **Cooper CW.** Prevalence of antibody to brucella in asymptomatic well individuals in Saudi Arabia. J Trop Med Hyg 1992; 95:140–142.

74 **Smith LD, Ficht TA.** Pathogenesis of brucellosis. Crit Rev Microbiol 1990;17: 209–230.

75 **Hall WH.** Modern chemotherapy for brucellosis in humans. Rev Infect Dis 1990;12:1060–1099.

76 **Lang R, Dagan R, Potasman I, Einhorn M, Raz R.** Failure of ceftriaxone in the treatment of acute brucellosis. Clin Infect Dis 1992;14:506–509.

77 **Richardson M, Holt JN.** Synergistic action of streptomycin with other antibiotics on intracellular *Brucella abortus* in vitro. J Bacteriol 1962;84:638–646.

78 **Mortensen JE, Moore DG, Clarridge JE, Young EJ.** Antimicrobial susceptibility of clinical isolates of *Brucella*. Diagn Microbiol Infect Dis 1986;5:163–169.

79 **Rubinstein E, Lang R, Shasha B, et al.** In vitro susceptibility of *Brucella melitensis* to antibiotics. Antimicrob Agents Chemother 1991;35:1925–1927.

80 **Colmenero Castillo JD, Hernandez Marquez S, Reguera Iglesias JM, Cabrera Franquelo F, Ruis Diaz F, Alonso A.** Comparative trial of doxycycline plus streptomycin versus doxycycline plus rifampin for the therapy of human brucellosis. Chemotherapy 1989;35:146–152.

81 **Ariza J, Gudiol F, Pallares R, Rufi G, Fernandez-Viladrich P.** Comparative trial

of rifampin-doxycycline versus tetracy-cline-streptomycin in the therapy of human brucellosis. Antimicrob Agents Chemother 1985;28:548–551.

82   Cisneros JM, Viciana P, Colmenero J, Pachon J, Martinez C, Alarcon A. Multicenter prospective study of treatment of *Brucella melitensis* brucellosis with doxycycline for 6 weeks plus streptomycin for 2 weeks. Antimicrob Agents Chemother 1990;34:881–883.

83   Ariza J, Gudiol F, Pallares R, et al. Treatment of human brucellosis with doxycycline plus rifampin or doxycycline plus streptomycin. Ann Intern Med 1992;117:25–30.

84   Lubani MM, Dudin KI, Sharda DC, et al. A multicenter therapeutic study of 1100 children with brucellosis. Pediatr Infect Dis 1989;8:75–78.

85   Lang R, Rubinstein E. Quinolones for the treatment of brucellosis. J Antimicrob Chemother 1992;29:357–363.

86   Bouza E, Garcia de la Torre M, Parras F, Guerrero A, Rodriguez-Creixems M, Gobernado J. Brucellar meningitis. Rev Infect Dis 1987;9:810–822.

87   Flugelman MY, Galun E, Ben-Chetrit E, Caraco J, Rubinow A. Brucellosis in patients with heart disease: when should endocarditis be diagnosed? Cardiology 1990;77:313–317.

88   Ariza J, Bosch J, Gudiol F, Linares J, Fernandez-Viladrich P, Martin R. Relevance of in vitro antimicrobial susceptibility of *Brucella melitensis* to relapse rate in human brucellosis. Antimicrob Agents Chemother 1986;30:958–960.

89   Spink WW. What is chronic brucellosis? Ann Intern Med 1951;35:358–374.

90   Emboden JB, Canter A, Cluff LE, Trever RW. Brucellosis: III. Psychologic aspects of delayed convalescence. Arch Intern Med 1959;103:406–414.

91   Cluff LE. Medical aspects of delayed convalescence. Rev Infect Dis 1991;13(suppl 1):S138–S140.

92   Lagra F, Raptopoulou-Gigi M, Orphanou-Koumerkeridou H, Goulis G. In vitro effect of interferon alpha-2b on T lymphocyte transformation and leukocyte migration inhibition in patients with chronic brucellosis. Immunopharmacol Immunotoxicol 1989;11:223–232.

Chancroid: New Developments in an Old Disease

JEANNE M. MARRAZZO
H. HUNTER HANDSFIELD

Chancroid is one of the five classical venereal diseases, along with gonorrhea, syphilis, lymphogranuloma venereum, and granuloma inguinale. The disease was first described by Brassereau as "le chancre mou" (soft chancre) in 1852. Chancroid is caused by *Haemophilus ducreyi* and is characterized by genital ulceration and regional lymphadenopathy. Considerable variation in the proportion of genital ulcer disease attributable to *H. ducreyi* exists across geographical areas, but chancroid remains the most common cause of genital ulceration in many developing countries. In North America, the incidence of chancroid declined to very low levels after the Vietnam and Korean wars, but a remarkable resurgence of the disease occurred in the 1980s. Advances in culture methods for *H. ducreyi* in the late 1970s led to major improvements in our understanding of the pathogenesis, epidemiology, antimicrobial susceptibility, and treatment of the disease. Several recent studies have documented a close association between genital ulcer disease, especially chancroid, and transmission of the human immunodeficiency viruses (HIV).

MICROBIOLOGY

Microbiologic and Molecular Characterization

Auguste Ducrey first described the causative bacillus in chancroid ulcer exudate in 1889 (1). The organism was initially placed in the family Pasteurellaceae and the genus *Haemophilus* due to its requirement for blood-enriched culture media (2), but ribosomal RNA typing indicates a closer relationship to *Actinobacillus* than to other *Haemophilus* species (3). For the moment, however, the name *H. ducreyi* remains in general usage.

Haemophilus ducreyi is a small, gram-negative rod without an extracellular capsule. The classically described "school of fish" or "railroad track" morphol-

129

ogy describes a tendency for the organism to form long parallel strands; this pattern is observed primarily in broth culture and occasionally in clinical specimens. Biochemically, the organism is cytochrome oxidase positive and catalase negative, produces alkaline phosphatase, reduces nitrate, and requires hemin (X factor). Its lipooligosaccharide is unique (4) but shares several biologic and immunochemical features with that of *Neisseria gonorrhoeae* (5). Little is known about the chromosomal genetics of *H. ducreyi*, but its plasmid content has been studied extensively (2,6,7). Several plasmids confer and transfer antibiotic resistance, most notably to β-lactam drugs and sulfonamides.

Growth Requirements and Isolation

Media optimal for growth of *H. ducreyi* were not developed until the late 1970s, when the successful use of a modified gonococcal agar base containing bovine hemoglobin and a nutritional supplement was reported by Hammond et al. (8). In general, enriched media for isolation of *H. ducreyi* contain a source of hemin, a growth supplement such as IsoVitaleX®, and serum, most commonly fetal bovine serum. Vancomycin (3 mg/L) usually is added as a selective agent. Several successful variations using Mueller-Hinton agar, gonococcal agar base, or modified heart infusion agar as the base have been described (2). A recent report suggests that activated charcoal may be substituted for serum, resulting in substantial cost savings without a decrement in performance (9). Cultures require incubation in a high humidity environment with 5% CO_2 at 33° to 35°C; these conditions are achieved in a candle-extinction jar that contains a wet sponge. Growth is relatively slow; colonies may appear heterogeneous, but typical ones are small (1 to 2 mm at 48 to 72 hours), nonmucoid, translucent, and tan or gray-yellow, and are easily pushed intact across the agar surface (2). On horse blood agar, colonies may initially appear nonhemolytic, but weak β or α hemolysis may be seen after several days.

Studies in the 1980s demonstrated a wide range (47 to 94%) of recovery of *H. ducreyi* in culture from clinically typical chancroid ulcers or lymph node aspirates. Determining which media are most sensitive for isolation has not been straightforward because there is no "gold standard" for the presence of *H. ducreyi*. The development of more sensitive diagnostic tools, such as polymerase chain reaction (PCR), may clarify this issue in the future.

Several factors may contribute to the generally low yield of *H. ducreyi* in culture and perhaps to the range of performance among various media. *H. ducreyi* is nutritionally fastidious, and differences may exist in nutritional requirements among strains (2,10). The presence of vancomycin in selective media may inhibit isolation of some strains for which this antibiotic has relatively low minimal inhibitory concentrations (11). In addition, self-administered antibiotic use, which may be prevalent in some populations with high rates of chancroid, may interfere with isolation of the organism (12). For these reasons, recovery of *H. ducreyi* is maximized by concurrent use of more than one type of medium, such as enriched gonococcal agar base and Mueller-Hinton agar. In the hands of experienced investigators, this approach typically results in estimated sensitivities of 75 to 90% (10,13,14). Unfortunately, use of multiple media may be impractical outside research settings, and the performance of all media probably is substantially lower in clinical laboratories without extensive experience in isolating *H. ducreyi*. Transport media for *H. ducreyi* have not been perfected or comprehensively studied.

PATHOLOGY AND PATHOGENESIS

The chancroid ulcer has been described as having three distinct histologic zones (15). Necrosis predominates in the most superficial zone; erythrocytes, fibrin, and degenerating neutrophils are prominent. The middle zone consists of inflammatory tissue edema with microvascularization and endothelial cell stranding. The deepest zone is characterized by a dense infiltrate of plasma cells and lymphocytes.

Whether *H. ducreyi* exists as a nonpathogenic colonizer of the human genital tract is a matter of debate (16,17). Although insensitivity of culture may underestimate the presence of asymptomatic *H. ducreyi* carriage, most investigators agree that human infection with *H. ducreyi* usually results in overt ulceration and that most asymptomatic cases result from infection in less sensate locations, such as the cervix or the proximal vaginal mucosa.

Experimental Infection

The animal models most frequently used to assess virulence of *H. ducreyi* have been intradermal inoculation in the rabbit or mouse, but both exhibit substantial differences compared with human infection (18). A recently described primate model using genital inoculation of pigtailed macaques may more closely approximate human infection in clinical course and histopathology (19). This model offers the additional advantage of facilitating assessment and study of regional lymphadenopathy, and it may prove useful in assessing the effects of retrovirus-induced immunodeficiency. Experimental human challenge with *H. ducreyi* or with exudate from genital ulcers was used in past decades, but the results were compromised by limitations in knowledge of the microbiology and pathogenesis of the disease. Spinola et al. (20) recently described the first such studies in the modern era. This approach appears safe because systemic manifestations and serious complications are rare, and it holds great promise for future studies.

Correlates of Virulence

Virulent strains of *H. ducreyi* are generally characterized by their ability to adhere to human epithelial cells (21). The surface component mediating adherence is not known, but pili, demonstrated on some strains, may be important (22). Whether *H. ducreyi* invades epithelial cells is controversial (19,21,23). There is evidence for the importance of both lipooligosaccharide and an as yet uncharacterized cytotoxin in the cell death and tissue necrosis that lead to ulcer formation (18,23,24).

Immunologic Response

The immunologic response to infection with *H. ducreyi* is not well understood. Human infection is followed by development of antibodies to several antigenic components of the organism, including heat shock proteins, various outer membrane proteins, and lipooligosaccharide (18,25,26). In the recently described primate model, evidence of induced systemic immunity to *H. ducreyi* was seen; this response will require further characterization (19). It is unknown whether these responses confer immunity, although chancroid reinfections are known to occur in endemic areas.

EPIDEMIOLOGY

Efforts to characterize the epidemiology of chancroid have been complicated by several factors. The lack of widespread availability of suitable culture media and the technical difficulties in isolating *H. ducreyi* probably have contributed to an underestimation of the disease; only about 10% of 5409 cases reported in U.S. outbreaks from 1981 to 1990 were confirmed by culture (27). In 1990, only 16 (14%) of 115 sexually transmitted disease (STD) clinics in the United States had culture media for *H. ducreyi* available. Moreover, only nine of these clinics had the ability to perform a comprehensive diagnostic evaluation of genital ulcer disease, that is, to isolate *H. ducreyi* and herpes simplex virus (HSV) and to perform darkfield microscopy and syphilis serology (27). According to the Centers for Disease Control and Prevention (CDC), several outbreaks in the United States since the mid-1980s went unreported due to lack of culture confirmation (27).

The effect of the poor predictive performance of clinical diagnosis on incidence statistics is more difficult to estimate, resulting in either over- or underascertainment of disease. Clinicians may be less likely to presumptively diagnose chancroid if it is not known to be regionally common. On the other hand, Schmid (28) has described the equally confounding tendency of clinicians to presumptively diagnose atypical genital lesions as chancroid when culture confirmation is not available. Until 1990, no standard clinical definition for presumptive diagnosis of chancroid existed; surveillance definitions (Table 6.1) were published recently by the CDC (29). On balance, it is probable that surveillance for chancroid in the United States substantially underestimates total morbidity.

Chancroid in the United States

Prior to the 1980s, the peak recorded numbers of chancroid cases in the United States occurred in 1947, when 9515 cases were documented. Reported cases then declined until 1978, when the trend reversed, leading to a second peak in 1987, when 5035 cases were reported (Figure 6.1). From 1979 to 1987, the incidence of reported cases rose tenfold, from 0.2 to 2.1/100,000 population (28). Most reported cases in the past decade occurred in localized outbreaks. Indeed, a handful of states have consistently accounted for most of the cases reported to the CDC in the past decade. New York, California, Texas, Florida, and Georgia together accounted for 92% of all reported cases from 1981 to 1986, and in 1990 Texas and New York accounted for 68% of all cases (2,11,27).

Chancroid outbreaks in the United States and Canada have generally involved the traditional STD core populations (30) but with special foci of disease

Table 6.1. Surveillance Definitions of the Centers for Disease Control and Prevention for Chancroid

---

Definite Chancroid
Isolation or definitive identification of *Haemophilus ducreyi*

Probable Chancroid
A clinically compatible case with one or more painful genital ulcers, plus:
　No evidence of *Treponema pallidum* infection by darkfield examination of ulcer
　　exudate or by a serologic test for syphilis performed at least 7 d after onset of
　　ulcer
　and
　Clinical presentation not typical of disease caused by herpes simplex virus (HSV);
　　or negative culture for HSV

SOURCE: Centers for Disease Control and Prevention. Case definitions for public health surveillance. MMWR 1990;39(RR-13):8–9.

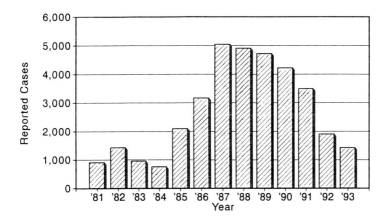

Figure 6.1. Reported cases of chancroid in the United States, 1981–1993. (Data from the Division of STD/HIV Prevention, Centers for Disease Control and Prevention. Sexually Transmitted Disease Surveillance, 1992 [for 1981–1993].

in drug users and in female sex workers and their clients. In nine discrete outbreaks in the United States summarized by Schmid et al. (28), most cases occurred in African Americans or Hispanics, and almost all affected individuals were heterosexual. In all outbreaks, cases in men greatly outnumbered those in women, with male:female ratios varying from 3:1 to 25:1; this probably is due largely to difficulties in identifying and bringing female sex workers to treatment. In eight of the nine outbreaks, sex workers played a central role in transmission. In a 1988–1991 outbreak in San Francisco, the exchange of drugs for money or sex was the major risk marker for acquisition of chancroid, and prostitution was a secondary factor (14). Substance abuse, especially of alkaloidal cocaine (crack), also was strongly associated with chancroid in the 1989–1993 outbreak in New Orleans (31).

Reported cases of chancroid began to fall after 1987, and the decline accelerated from 1990 to 1993 (see Figure 6.1), when the incidence rate was 0.5 cases/100,000 population (32). The reasons for the decline are unclear, and it remains to be seen whether this trend will be sustained.

Chancroid in Developing Countries

Numerous studies have documented the predominance of chancroid as a cause of genital ulcer disease in sub-Saharan Africa. From studies in STD clinics and general health centers in Kenya, Rwanda, Zimbabwe, South Africa, and elsewhere, estimates of the percentage of genital ulcer disease attributable to chancroid have ranged from 12 to 70% in women and from 22 to 60% in men (33–40). In general, the epidemiology of chancroid in Africa closely approximates that of most outbreaks in the United States, with a high proportion of infected men reporting intercourse with female sex workers.

The incidence of chancroid in Southeast Asia has been studied in Thailand, Malaysia, and Singapore (41). Contact with sex workers is consistently reported. In Bangkok in 1982, *H. ducreyi* was isolated from 38% of 120 genital ulcers in men who were also cultured for HSV (42). *H. ducreyi* was isolated from 9% of genital ulcers in 249 patients in Kuala Lumpur; however, only one type of culture medium was used, no pathogen was isolated in 62%, and 41% of the patients had treated themselves with antibiotics before evaluation (12).

Reliable data are even more difficult to obtain for Central Asia, South America, Central America, and the Caribbean. Using official reports from 1987 to 1991, Betts and Zacarías (43) noted an increasing trend in the number of reported cases of chancroid in the Caribbean and Latin America despite an apparent decline in gonorrhea. Chancroid is generally believed to be a common cause of genital ulceration in the Indian subcontinent. In most developing countries in all continents, the clinical appearance of lesions, the usual absence of evidence of syphilis or HSV infection, and the therapeutic response suggest that chancroid accounts for most of the culture-negative cases of genital ulcer disease. Thus, the prevalence of chancroid among STD clinic patients with genital ulcer disease may approach 90% in some developing countries.

Commercial Sex and Substance Abuse

Haemophilus ducreyi has an historical association with commercial sex work. Female sex workers may constitute a sustained source of disease for several reasons. Continuation of sex work even in the presence of painful ulcers appears to be common in some settings (44). Intravaginal ulcers may be asymptomatic and are difficult to detect, especially in settings in which vaginal speculum examinations are not the norm. Limited access to affordable health care may be an important factor that sustains chancroid in sex workers. Finally, contact tracing of sex workers may be difficult. Most of these factors are consistent in all societies and all geographical areas. However, in North America—and perhaps also in the Caribbean and Latin America—the association between prostitution and chancroid is strongly modified by addiction to drugs, especially crack cocaine. Such relationships have been documented in New York City (45) and New Orleans (31,46).

In summary, throughout the world chancroid appears to be associated more closely with prostitution and substance abuse than any other traditional STD, including syphilis and gonorrhea. We hypothesize that this occurs because asymptomatic carriage of *H. ducreyi* is uncommon, so that maintenance of chancroid in a community requires a population of infected persons who continue sexual activity in the presence of painful genital ulcers. Drug addiction and the economic imperatives of prostitution may provide the necessary incentives. By contrast, most other STDs are transmitted primarily by asymptomatic persons or those with relatively trivial symptoms.

Male Circumcision

In addition to the association of HIV transmission and acquisition with lack of circumcision in men, the presence of an intact foreskin has been epidemiologically associated with chancroid itself (17,47). In the recent San Francisco outbreak, the circumcision status of 20 men with chancroid was known; 15 (75%) were uncircumcised (14). The physiologic explanation for this association is uncertain, but it is plausible that the less-cornified epithelium of the glans and foreskin is more susceptible to invasion by *H. ducreyi* than fully cornified skin. In addition, the preputial sac may act as a reservoir that prolongs exposure of uncircumcised men to their partners' genital secretions.

Association of Chancroid with HIV Infection

Genital ulcer disease has been closely and consistently linked with HIV acquisition in both case-control and cohort studies. In a powerful landmark study, Cameron et al. (48) followed 422 HIV-seronegative men attending a Nairobi STD clinic for a mean of 14 weeks and found that initial presentation to the clinic with a genital ulcer and being uncircumcised were independent (and the strongest) predictors of HIV-1 seroconversion. The same investigators also followed 124 female sex workers for 2 years (49). Eighty-three (67%) of these women acquired HIV-1 during 2 years of prospective evaluation; both the occurrence and frequency of genital ulcer episodes during the study period both were strong and independent risk factors for seroconversion (49). In a New York City STD clinic, the risk of HIV-1 acquisition in 462 patients who presented with genital ulcer disease was 2.4 times that in those without ulceration (95% confidence interval [CI_{95}], 1.1 to 5.4); the relative risk was 3.5 (CI_{95} 1.01 to 8.98) among patients whose only other risk behavior was heterosexual activity (50).

Numerous other studies have assessed the association between genital ulcer disease and HIV acquisition and transmission. Chancroid has been more prominently implicated in HIV transmission than either genital herpes or syphilis. However, most studies, including the best-designed cohort studies, have been carried out where chancroid is the predominant cause of genital ulcer. In addition, it is likely that the population-attributable risk of genital ulcer disease varies widely between geographical areas, risk groups, and the dominant risk behaviors in the population. In the New York City study (50), a clinical diagnosis of chancroid was significantly associated with HIV seroconversion, but most cases were not confirmed by culture and no attempt was made to isolate HSV. Other STDs and genital anatomic factors that have been associated with HIV transmission or acquisition include genital herpes, syphilis, gonorrhea, chlamydial infection, and cervical ectopy (51).

The mechanisms by which ulceration or other genital inflammation might enhance transmission of HIV are unknown, but it is plausible that ulceration (whether macroscopic or microscopic) simply increases exposure to blood or other infected secretions. In addition, activated T lymphocytes and macrophages, which are present in large numbers in chancroid ulcers, might serve as a site of accelerated HIV replication and high burden titers in an HIV-infected person. Similarly, in an individual not infected with HIV, such cells in the base of an ulcer could provide susceptible viral targets. Whether alterations in local or systemic immunity in HIV-infected persons play a role in these interactions is not yet known. Bolstering the epidemiologic links between genital ulceration and HIV infection, HIV-1 has been identified by culture and DNA amplification in genital ulcers, some of which were confirmed as chancroid on culturing (44,52).

CLINICAL MANIFESTATIONS

Although the classical presentation of the chancroid ulcer is common, it is important to appreciate the wide variation in lesion presentation. Culture-proven chancroid lesions commonly are confused with those of primary syphilis, genital herpes, squamous cell carcinoma, and other conditions, and erroneous diagnosis of inguinal buboes occasionally leads to attempted herniorrhaphy. Several studies have shown the lack of specificity if clinical examination is relied on as the sole diagnostic method for genital ulceration, especially in settings where chancroid is not common.

Figures 6.2 through 6.4 illustrate typical cases of chancroid. The incubation period, best characterized in men, usually is 4 to 10 days, with a range of 2 to 35 days (2). The initial lesion, a painless papule on an erythematous base, is infrequently seen by clinicians. It rapidly evolves to a pustule, the precursor to the soft, painful ulcer. Most chancroid ulcers are 1 to 2 cm in diameter, but lesions can vary from as little as 1 to 2 mm to several centimeters in size. The margins are sharp and tend to be slightly raised and sometimes are undermined. The shape may be round, oval, or irregular. The base of the ulcer is frequently coated with an overtly purulent yellow or gray exudate. The most common sites of ulcers in men are the prepuce, coronal sulcus, and glans, and two or more ulcers are found in about two thirds of cases. Local autoinoculation to an opposing skin or mucosal surface ("kissing lesions") sometimes occurs, for example, between the glans and foreskin.

In women, ulcers occur most commonly on the labia majora and minora, the vaginal introitus, the periurethral area, and often the perianal area. Cervical and internal vaginal ulcers also are common. Ulcers in women may tend to be more numerous than in men; in 43 sex workers with chancroid in Nairobi, the mean number was 4.5, with most lesions observed on the labia and fourchette

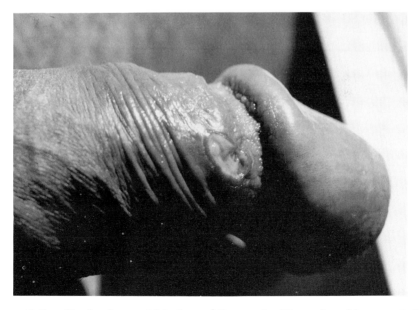

Figure 6.2. Single chancroidal ulcer of the penis. (Reproduced by permission from Handsfield HH. Color atlas and synopsis of sexually transmitted diseases. New York: McGraw-Hill, 1992.)

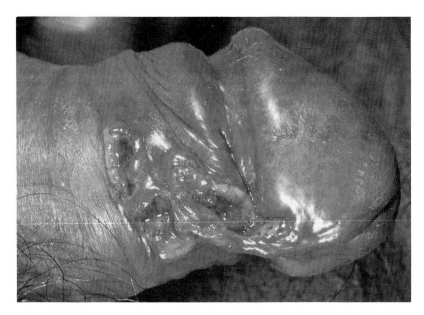

Figure 6.3. Multiple irregularly shaped penile ulcers due to chancroid in an uncircumcised man. (Reproduced by permission from Handsfield HH. Color atlas and synopsis of sexually transmitted diseases. New York: McGraw-Hill, 1992.)

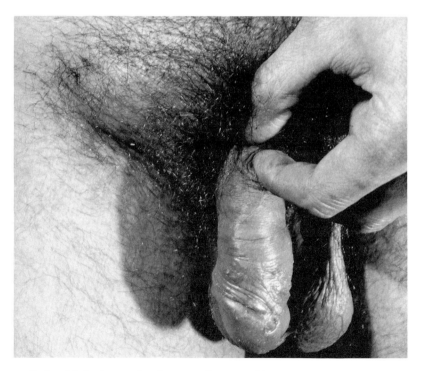

Figure 6.4. Multiple penile ulcers and inguinal bubo in a patient with chancroid. The dark spots adjacent to the bubo mark the sites of needle aspiration. (Reproduced by permission from Handsfield HH. Color atlas and synopsis of sexually transmitted diseases. New York: McGraw-Hill, 1992.)

(34). The clinical presentation in women may not be straightforward, particularly with intravaginal or cervical lesions, and presenting complaints of dyspareunia, dysuria, and hematochezia have been noted (53). No adverse effects of chancroid on the course of pregnancy or the health of the fetus have been reported.

Inguinal lymphadenitis occurs in about half the men with chancroid, often with central necrosis and liquefaction (bubo) (see Figure 6.4). Buboes have been reported somewhat less commonly in women, perhaps because lymphatic drainage from the posterior wall of the vagina is to the sacral lymph nodes. However, inguinal buboes were present in 35% of the women studied by Plummer et al. (34). Clinically apparent lymphadenitis typically appears one to two weeks after the primary lesion and has an acute, painful onset; it is unilateral in about two thirds of cases and bilateral in the remainder. The bubo may be confused with an incarcerated inguinal hernia. Buboes untreated for one to two weeks may spontaneously rupture, especially if their size exceeds 5 cm. Although overt pus is present, it does not frequently yield *H. ducreyi* on culture. The bubo often follows a course independent of the ulcer, occasionally developing or worsening as the ulcer responds to antibiotic treatment; such an occurrence does not necessarily denote treatment failure. Systemic manifestations such as fever or malaise are almost always absent, even in cases characterized by aggressive ulceration and bilateral buboes, and disseminated infection with *H. ducreyi* occurs rarely, if ever.

Urethritis is an uncommon manifestation of *H. ducreyi* infection in men. In a prospective review of 456 men with culture-documented chancroid ulcers, symptomatic urethritis was diagnosed in 16 (3.5%); in 7 of these (1.9% of the total), *H. ducreyi* was isolated from urethral culture (54). *N. gonorrhoeae* also was isolated in two of the men with urethritis. Among 57 men without urethritis who were evaluated for asymptomatic urethral carriage, none had a positive urethral culture for *H. ducreyi*. The same investigators also isolated *H. ducreyi* from the urethra of one man among 106 who had urethritis without genital ulceration (54). These findings suggest that *H. ducreyi* can colonize the urethra but it is an uncommon cause of symptomatic urethritis.

The natural history of chancroid in HIV-infected individuals may differ from that in the immunocompetent host. Atypical presentations have been reported, including multiple genital or extragenital ulcerations, systemic symptoms, and perhaps delayed healing (55,56). However, the individual ulcers seem not to differ in appearance compared with those in HIV-negative persons (55). All of these observations are anecdotal, however, and require confirmation in controlled studies. It is possible that HIV infection also increases susceptibility to *H. ducreyi*. Cameron et al. (57) reported that although condom use helped prevent acquisition of genital ulcer disease in female sex workers in Nairobi, HIV-seropositive women acquired genital ulcers at a substantially higher rate than HIV-seronegative women, negating the protective effect of condoms.

DIAGNOSIS

Diagnostic techniques for chancroid are rapidly evolving. New developments, most notably DNA amplification using PCR or perhaps the ligase chain reaction, may lead to more accurate assessment of genital ulcer disease and more precise contributions to the study of the epidemiology and natural history of chancroid.

Clinical Recognition and Differential Diagnosis

Throughout the world, great regional and local variations exist in the diseases responsible for genital ulceration. Unfortunately, although several studies (cited above) have systematically assessed the differential diagnosis of genital ulcer disease in developing countries, often using sophisticated diagnostic tests, no similar studies in industrialized countries have been published in the past two decades. Table 6.2 summarizes the approximate proportions of the main diagnoses in sexually active young adults presenting to STD clinics with discrete genital ulcers (without systemic dermatoses) in industrialized and developing countries, based on published studies, anecdotal reports, and the authors' experience (58).

In evaluating a sexually active person with genital ulceration, clinicians should consider the local prevalence and incidence of the major causes, as well as the patient's sexual and social history, including illicit drug use by the patient and his or her partner(s), prostitution, sexual exposure to sex workers, and travel, in addition to the clinical history and physical examination findings. As summarized in Table 6.3, a clinical diagnosis of genital herpes, without a requirement for laboratory confirmation, may be warranted in some highly typical cases, for example, in the presence of classical vesiculopustular lesions or clusters of tender, superficial ulcers. Virtually all other patients

Table 6.2. Etiology of Genital Ulcer Disease*

Diagnosis	North America	Tropical Developing Countries
Genital herpes	60–70%	0–10%
Syphilis	10–20%	10–20%
Chancroid	0–10%	50–60%
Other/unknown	10–20%	20–30%

* For young patients (15–40 years old) at risk for sexually transmitted disease who present with discrete cutaneous or mucosal genital ulcers that are not part of a generalized dermatosis. Based on published and unpublished studies, anecdotal reports, and the authors' clinical experience.
SOURCE: Adapted from Handsfield HH. The clinical approach to genital ulcer disease. STD-2000 1994;1:3–11.

Table 6.3. Laboratory Diagnosis of Genital Ulcer Disease*

Clinically Typical Genital Herpes Lesions
Optional: Culture or other sensitive and specific assay (e.g., direct fluorescent antibody test) of lesion for herpes simplex virus (HSV)
Screening tests for other common STDs, including serologic tests for syphilis and HIV infection and tests for *Neisseria gonorrhoeae* and *Chlamydia trachomatis*
Other Cases
Culture or other test of lesion for HSV
Darkfield microscopy or direct fluorescent antibody test for *Treponema pallidum*
Syphilis serology
Culture for *H. ducreyi*, if available and indicated by case history, local epidemiology, or clinical appearance
Selected Cases†
Repeat syphilis serology and other tests, as indicated
Routine bacterial culture for pyogenic infection
Type-specific HSV antibody test, if available
Biopsy

* Authors' recommendations, adapted from Handsfield HH. The clinical approach to genital ulcer disease. STD-2000 1994;1:3–11.
† For example, when the diagnosis remains obscure following the preceding evaluation.

should have specific diagnostic tests to assess genital herpes and syphilis, including a culture of the lesion for HSV, darkfield microscopy, and syphilis serology.

Chancroid should be considered in all patients with clinically typical lesions or fluctuant inguinal lymphadenopathy, especially if chancroid is known to be locally prevalent or if the patient has recently been sexually active in a city or country where the disease is common. Unfortunately, the clinical diagnosis of chancroid is not reliable, especially in settings where the disease is uncommon (59–61). In Malaysia, where chancroid accounted for 9% of genital ulcer disease cases in men, the accuracy of a clinical diagnosis of chancroid was 47% (12). By contrast, in a South Africa study in which the culture-documented prevalence of chancroid among 210 cases of genital ulcer disease was 70%, a clinical diagnosis of chancroid had a positive predictive value of 97% (35). Ten patients with clinical diagnoses of syphilis actually had culture-positive chancroid, leading to a negative predictive value of only 55%; however, the overall accuracy of the clinical diagnosis for chancroid was 80% (35). These results are in accord with our clinical experience: chancroid is rare in our clinic, and most patients with clinically typical chancroid in fact have genital herpes (Figure 6.5). Primary syphilis also can mimic chancroid (Figure 6.6).

Accordingly, isolation of *H. ducreyi* should be attempted, especially in settings where chancroid is an uncommon cause of genital ulcer disease. Unfortunately, media for *H. ducreyi* may not be readily available or experience with culture may be limited. In such settings, the CDC's standard clinical definition

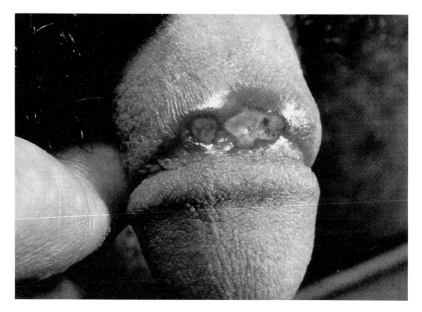

Figure 6.5. Penile ulcers due to genital herpes, mimicking chancroid; herpes simplex virus was isolated and culture for *H. ducreyi* was negative. (Reproduced by permission from Handsfield HH. Color atlas and synopsis of sexually transmitted diseases. New York: McGraw-Hill, 1992.)

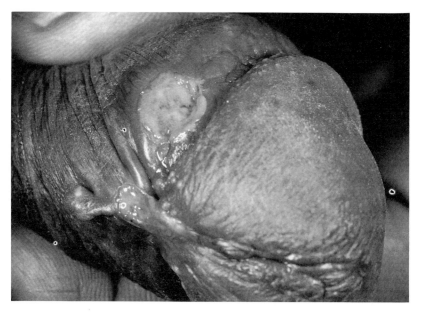

Figure 6.6. Primary syphilis with two nonindurated penile ulcers with purulent bases, mimicking chancroid. Darkfield examination was positive for *Treponema pallidum* and a culture for *H. ducreyi* was negative. (Reproduced by permission from Handsfield HH. Color atlas and synopsis of sexually transmitted diseases. New York: McGraw-Hill, 1992.)

for a "probable" case of chancroid (see Table 6.1) should be used, along with knowledge of the local epidemiology of genital ulcer disease. Certain features of an ulcer, in combination, may more specifically suggest chancroid, including undermined borders, tenderness, and a purulent base (see Figures 6.2–6.4). Herpetic ulcers tend to be more shallow than those due to chancroid, usually have clean bases, and often are multiple; additional lesions more typical of herpes (e.g., vesicles or pustules) may also be present. Syphilitic chancres usually are indurated and minimally tender, but exceptions are common (see Figure 6.6), and the base of the lesion may be either clean or purulent.

The nature of inguinal lymphadenopathy, if present, also is helpful. Syphilitic nodes typically are firm, only mildly tender, and usually occur bilaterally. Herpetic lymphadenopathy usually is bilateral and more tender than that of syphilis, but the nodes are not fluctuant. Among these diseases, only chancroidal lymphadenopathy becomes fluctuant or is accompanied by overlying cutaneous erythema. Fluctuant lymphadenopathy without genital ulceration should alert the clinician to the possibility of lymphogranuloma venereum, which usually presents without overt genital ulceration.

Laboratory Diagnosis

Gram-Stained Smear   Stained smears have been used with variable success to identify *H. ducreyi* morphotypes (i.e., small, pleomorphic, gram-negative rods, sometimes with the classical "school of fish" appearance) to diagnose chancroid. The sensitivity of gram-stained smears of exudate from the base of the ulcer in the diagnosis of culture-proven chancroid has been reported to range from 10% to over 90% in several small studies; most authorities believe the sensitivity to be 50% or less (2,62). Specificity also is a problem, and most experts agree that Gram stain has limited utility in either diagnosing or excluding chancroid (2,62). Some authorities believe smears of lymph node aspirates to be somewhat more reliable, especially if typical organisms are seen and no other bacteria are found. However, the sensitivity clearly is low and specificity has not been assessed.

Culture   The difficulties presented by relative insensitivity of the available media for isolation of *H. ducreyi*, their expense and general unavailability, and the poor performance of culture outside highly experienced laboratories have been addressed above. Nevertheless, culture diagnosis should be attempted if available. Specimens from genital ulcers should be obtained from the base after any overlying exudate has been removed and directly inoculated onto growth medium. Although most cultures will be positive in 48 hours, the plates should be held for 5 days to optimize recovery of *H. ducreyi*. Because vancomycin-sensitive strains have in fact been responsible for chancroid outbreaks (11), repeated culture-negative results in a suspicious clinical setting should prompt the use of vancomycin-free medium.

Antigenic and Genetic Diagnosis Nonculture tests to detect *H. ducreyi* antigens or genetic material appear promising for clinical application but are not yet commercially available. A direct fluorescence antibody test has been investigated (63) but has not yet been refined for routine clinical use. DNA probes appear to be quite sensitive, detecting *H. ducreyi* in concentrations of 10^3 to 10^4 organisms/mL, with specificity that approaches 100% (64,65). PCR appears to offer an especially promising alternative for more sensitive diagnosis of chancroid, with performance characteristics that may exceed those of culture (66).

Serology Serologic testing for antibody to *H. ducreyi* has been useful for epidemiologic studies (2,62,67), but the inability to distinguish acute from past exposure precludes routine clinical application of the currently available tests.

TREATMENT

The management of chancroid has been complicated in the past decade by two major developments: the emergence of antimicrobial resistance in *H. ducreyi* and the effect of HIV on the therapeutic response. These developments have narrowed the spectrum of effective drugs and prolonged the duration of therapy necessary for cure in many settings.

Assessing treatment efficacy is not always straightforward. Until recent years, many studies did not account for coinfection with HIV. In addition, variable definitions of clinical response to treatment have been used, a particular problem in assessment of culture-negative cases (which often outnumber those with microbiologic documentation). In addition, treatment efficacy may be affected by the site and size of the lesion and the presence of lymphadenopathy (68), characteristics that often were not described in published studies. Recommendations to include these parameters and other suggestions for the design of future therapeutic studies have been published (69).

Antimicrobial Susceptibility

Substantial geographical variation exists in the antimicrobial susceptibility of *H. ducreyi*. In the past two decades, resistance to ampicillin and amoxicillin has become highly prevalent in most of the world, mediated by the same plasmid-borne TEM-1 gene that is the most common determinant of β-lactamase production in *N. gonorrhoeae* (2,62,70). Resistance to combinations of β-lactam drugs with β-lactamase inhibitors also may be increasing; for example, 32% of strains from a recent outbreak in San Francisco were resistant to amoxicillin/clavulanate (71,72). The same is true for trimethoprim with sulfonamide, especially in the United States and Southeast Asia, although this combination remains active against most strains in a few geographical areas. Resistance to erythromycin, a drug with long-standing reliability in the treatment of chancroid, has been documented in Southeast Asia, but it remains generally effective (70,71). Ceftriaxone is highly active in all parts of the globe, although clinical failures (apparently unrelated to antimicrobial susceptibility) may be increasing in parts of Africa (55). Resistance to the fluoroquinolones has been documented in Southeast Asia but not elsewhere (70). The tetracyclines and aminoglycosides were useful in past years, but their use is now precluded by widespread resistance.

Antimicrobial Treatment

A substantial number of clinical studies of various antibiotics against chancroid have been reported in recent years. Comprehensive reviews are available (70,73).

β-Lactam Antibiotics   Ceftriaxone in a single dose of 250 mg intramuscularly has proven to be highly effective in the treatment of chancroid (70,73,74). However, despite continued in vitro sensitivity to ceftriaxone, increased clinical failures recently were reported in Nairobi (55). Some features of this study raise concerns about its generalization, and similar results have not been reported by other investigators; more studies are needed. Cefotaxime also has been effective (70), but no other third-generation cephalosporins have been systematically evaluated in clinical studies. Amoxicillin 500 mg combined with clavulanic acid 125 mg, given orally three times daily for 7 days, has been reported to be effective (70,75), but no new studies have been reported in the past several years.

Macrolides and Azalides   Erythromycin, in a dose of 500 mg orally four times daily for 7 days, has been widely recommended for two decades and remains reliable therapy for chancroid in most of the world (70,73). Erythromycin-resistant strains were reported in Singapore and Malaysia over a decade ago (76), but this appears to be the exception and both in vitro resistance and clinical failures remain rare in most settings. Efforts to shorten the course of erythromycin therapy have proven frustrating; Ballard et al. reported success with a 5-day course (68), but most authorities continue to recommend 7 days of therapy.

Azithromycin is a new azalide antibiotic (chemically related to the macrolides, with a similar mechanism of action) with a long serum half-life (68 hours) and excellent tissue penetration, and is active against *H. ducreyi* in vitro (71,72). In New Orleans, a single oral dose of 1.0 g gave a 100% cure rate in 71 patients with culture-proven chancroid (77). In Nairobi, the same regimen cured 73 (89%) of 82 patients, including 78% of those with HIV-infection and 93% of patients without HIV (78). The advantages of single-dose oral therapy have led to the recommendation of azithromycin as one of the drugs of choice for chancroid, despite the modest numbers of cases treated to date, the high cost of the drug, and occasional gastrointestinal intolerance.

Fluoroquinolones   The fluoroquinolones have shown great promise in the treatment of chancroid (70,73). Ciprofloxacin has been most extensively studied, with reported cure rates of 95 to 100% for 3-day courses, usually in a dose of 500 mg orally three times daily (70,79). Single-dose regimens of ciprofloxacin, ofloxacin, or other fluoroquinolones have resulted in somewhat reduced cure rates, typically around 90% (70,80). Other fluoroquinolones that have been investigated in clinical studies include fleroxacin, enoxacin, and rosaxacin (70,73); all were effective, but these drugs have no particular advantages and none is available in the United States. Resistance of *H. ducreyi* to ciprofloxacin has been documented in Thailand (71); in view of the ability of some gram-negative pathogens to rapidly develop high-level resistance to the quinolones and the widespread use of these drugs for a variety of indications, close monitoring of susceptibility is indicated.

Other Drugs   Although the combination of trimethoprim with sulfamethoxazole or other sulfonamides was once highly effective in both single- and multiple-dose regimens and was recommended by the CDC for treatment of chancroid, widespread resistance now precludes this option in the United States (70–72). Spectinomycin is notable for its single-dose efficacy in an intramuscular dose of 2.0 g, and it has been reported to be more effective in the treatment of buboes than other antimicrobials (70,81). However, treatment failures have been reported and resistance appears to be increasing (70,71). Rifampin is active against *H. ducreyi* and is effective alone or in combination with trimethoprim (17,70), but concerns about induction of resistance, as well as potential effects of widespread use on the drug's activity against *Mycobacterium tuberculosis*, have precluded widespread usage.

Response to Treatment

The clinical response usually is prompt in immunocompetent patients. Relief of pain usually occurs within 48 hours; reepithelialization is complete within 7 days in 50% of patients and within 14 days in 80% (62,69). Failure of reepithelialization, persistent purulence, or continued pain after 7 days or continued isolation of *H. ducreyi* any time after therapy denotes treatment failure, and an alternative regimen should be instituted (69,82). Relapse occurs in about 3% of patients, usually at the site of the initial lesion.

The response to antimicrobial treatment appears to be impaired in HIV-infected persons, especially after single-dose or 3-day regimens using drugs with relatively brief serum half-lives. Schulte and Schmid (70) summarized six published and unpublished studies that assessed the relationship between HIV infection and the results of single-dose or 3-day treatment with ceftriaxone, trimethoprim/sulfamethoxazole, or fluoroquinolones. For all regimens combined, cure was documented in 96 (55%) of 173 HIV-infected patients, compared with 519 (81%) of 643 HIV-negative patients ($P < .0001$) (70). More recently, the Nairobi investigators reported that erythromycin (2.0 g daily for 7 days) or single-dose azithromycin (1.0 g) cured 30 (79%) of 38 HIV-infected chancroid patients compared with 84 (94%) of 89 HIV-seronegative patients ($P = .02$); the results were similar for both azithromycin and erythromycin (78). Thus, it is clear that single-dose or three-day therapy with short-acting antibiotics is associated with substantially reduced cure rates in the presence of HIV infection, and it seems likely that the response is impaired to a lesser degree following 7 days of erythromycin or single-dose azithromycin.

Recommendations for Antimicrobial Treatment

The 1993 CDC recommendations for the treatment of chancroid (83) are summarized in Table 6.4. According to these guidelines, close follow-up is indicated for HIV-infected patients, especially after single-dose therapy with ceftriaxone or, because experience is limited, single-dose azithromycin. Many experts prefer the 7-day course of erythromycin in HIV-infected patients. Alternatively, a longer course of ciprofloxacin or another fluoroquinolone may be effective, but regimens longer than 3 days in duration have not been systematically evaluated.

Other Management Considerations

Traditionally, it has been recommended that fluctuant lymph nodes be aspirated to prevent inguinal ulcer formation and spontaneous rupture. It has been said that closed-needle aspiration is superior to incision and drainage, which

Table 6.4. Recommendations of the Centers for Disease Control and Prevention for Treatment of Chancroid

---

Recommended Regimens
   Azithromycin 1.0 g orally (single dose)
   or
   Ceftriaxone 250 mg IM (single dose)
   or
   Erythromycin 500 mg orally q.i.d. for 7 d
Alternative Regimens
   Amoxicillin/clavulanate (Augmentin®) 500/125 mg orally t.i.d. for 7 d
   or
   Ciprofloxacin 500 mg orally b.i.d. for 3 d

SOURCE: Dangor Y, Ballard RC, Miller SD, Koornhof HJ. Treatment of chancroid. Antimicrob Agents Chemother 1990;34:1308–1311.

were believed to increase the risk of superinfection and chronic sinus formation. On the other hand, needle aspiration often must be repeated, and incision
and drainage probably are safe when used in conjunction with currently recommended antibiotics. Buboes under 5 cm in diameter may resolve without drainage and are less likely to suppurate spontaneously (8).

The need for careful follow-up cannot be overemphasized. Patients should be
reevaluated three to seven days after initiation of therapy. Failure to improve
on the initial antibiotic regimen by 7 days warrants an alternative medication
because a resistant strain of *H. ducreyi* may be responsible. Other explanations
for failure to improve include misdiagnosis, poor bioavailability of medication,
and concomitant HIV infection.

Patient education and counseling about the nature of STD, HIV infection and
risks, and protective methods should be strongly emphasized at the initial
encounter and at follow-up. After counseling, HIV and syphilis serologies
should be performed at the initial visit and three months later. Contact tracing,
discussed below, is a crucial tool in containing outbreaks. Some authorities
recommend repeating the syphilis serology at follow-up (73).

PREVENTION AND CONTROL

Prevention of chancroid has assumed a new urgency because of epidemiologic
synergy between HIV infection and other STDs, especially genital ulcer disease
and chancroid, as described by Wasserheit (51). Targeted intervention programs aimed at the sexual contacts of cases of chancroid appear to have been
successful in containing local outbreaks in North America, although the actual
contribution of such case-finding efforts has been difficult to quantitate. Efficacy of identifying and treating sex workers implicated as infection sources was
reported in conjunction with two outbreaks in Winnipeg, Canada (53) and in an
outbreak in Pennsylvania in 1985–1986 (28). The relatively short incubation
period of *H. ducreyi* suggests that sexual contacts within the preceding 10 days
should be intensively sought.

Although the efficacy of barrier methods in preventing chancroid has not
been formally studied, there is little doubt that substantial protection results
from their use. From the perspective of prevention at the individual level, use
of barrier methods, particularly condoms, should be strongly urged. Although
the efficacy of the female condom in preventing acquisition of chancroid has
not been studied, it offers an alternative method of self-protection for women.

The clinician who encounters a suspected case of chancroid can contribute to
disease control by attempting to confirm the diagnosis, using a CDC-recom-
mended treatment regimen, arranging follow-up, urging condom use, screening for other STDs, urging the patient to refer his or her sexual partner(s) for
diagnosis and treatment, and immediately telephoning a report to the local
health department (which in most communities will assume responsibility for
partner notification).

FUTURE DIRECTIONS

Substantial advances have been made in the understanding of *H. ducreyi* and chancroid in the past decade, but much remains unknown. Pathogenesis in humans needs to be further defined. Characterization of the inflammatory process at the level of the ulcer and studies to understand local and systemic immunity will be important, including both humoral and cellular elements of the immune response. Such studies will be especially vital in defining interactions between chancroid and HIV infection; new animal models may prove useful in this arena. There is an urgent public health need to understand the epidemiology shared by *H. ducreyi* and HIV and to interrupt the potential synergy for transmission of the latter in the setting of genital ulcer disease; improved diagnosis, perhaps based on DNA amplification technologies, will be central to this effort. The clinical course of chancroid and the response to treatment in persons infected with HIV need to be better defined. Efforts to halt the spread of chancroid in difficult-to-reach populations is a high priority. With the continuing evolution of antimicrobial resistance, research in mechanisms of resistance and drug development will remain important, as will careful surveillance for the detection of resistant strains.

ACKNOWLEDGMENTS

The authors gratefully acknowledge the assistance of Dr. Patricia Totten in the preparation of this chapter.

REFERENCES

1 **Ducrey A.** Experimentelle Untersuchungen über den Ansteckungsstoff des weichen Schankers und über die Bubonen. Monatsh Prakt Dermatol 1889;9:387–405.

2 **Morse SA.** Chancroid and *Haemophilus ducreyi*. Clin Microbiol Rev 1989;2:137–157.

3 **Dewhirst FE, Paster BJ, Olsen I, Fraser GJ.** Phylogeny of 5 representative strains of species in the family Pasteurellaceae as determined by comparison of 16S rRNA sequences. J Bacteriol 1992;174:2002–2013.

4 **Melaugh W, Phillips NJ, Campagnari AA, et al.** Partial characterization of the major lipooligosaccharide from a strain of *Haemophilus ducreyi*, the causative agent of chancroid, a genital ulcer disease. J Biol Chem 1992;267:1343–1349.

5 **Campagnari AA, Spinola SM, Lesse AJ, et al.** LOS epitopes shared among gram-negative non-enteric mucosal pathogens. Microb Pathog 1990;8:353–362.

6 **McNicol PJ, Ronald AR.** The plasmids of *Haemophilus ducreyi*. J Antimicrob Chemother 1984;14:561–573.

7 **Handsfield HH, Totten PA, Fennel CL, et al.** Molecular epidemiology of *Haemophilus ducreyi* infections. Ann Intern Med 1981; 95:315–318.

8 **Hammond GW, Lian CJ, Wilt JC, Ronald AR.** Comparison of specimen collection and laboratory techniques for isolation of *Haemophilus ducreyi*. J Clin Microbiol 1978; 7:39–43.

9 **Lockett AE, Dance DA, Mabey DCW, Drasar BS.** Serum-free media for isolation of *Haemophilus ducreyi*. Lancet 1991;338:326.

10 **Nsanze H, Plummer FA, Maggwa AB, et al.** Comparison of media for primary isolation of *Haemophilus ducreyi*. Sex Transm Dis 1984;11:6–9.

11 **Jones C, Rosen T, Clarridge J, Collins S.** Chancroid: results from an outbreak in

Houston, Texas. South Med J 1990;83: 1384–1389.

12 **Zainah S, Cheong YM, Sinniah M, et al.** A microbiological study of genital ulcers in Kuala Lumpur. Med J Malaysia 1991;46: 274–282.

13 **Macdonald KC, Cameron DW, D'Costa LJ, et al.** Evaluation of fleroxacin (RO23-6240) as single dose therapy of culture-proven chancroid in Nairobi, Kenya. Antimicrob Agents Chemother 1989;33: 612–614.

14 **Flood JM, Sarafian SK, Bolan GA, et al.** Multistrain outbreak of chancroid in San Francisco, 1989–1991. J Infect Dis 1993;167: 1106–1111.

15 **Freinkel AL.** Histological aspects of sexually transmitted genital lesions. Histopathology 1987;11:819–831.

16 **McEntegart MG, Hafiz S, Kinghorn GR.** *Haemophilus ducreyi* infections: time for reappraisal. J Hyg (London) 1982;89:467–478.

17 **Plummer FA, Nsanze H, D'Costa LJ, et al.** Short-course and single-dose antimicrobial therapy for chancroid in Kenya: studies with rifampin alone and in combination with trimethoprim. Rev Infect Dis 1983; 5(suppl):565–572.

18 **Lagergård T.** The role of *Haemophilus ducreyi* bacteria, cytotoxin, endotoxin and antibodies in animal models for study of chancroid. Microb Pathog 1992;13:203–217.

19 **Totten PA, Morton WR, Knitter GH, et al.** A primate model for chancroid. J Infect Dis 1994;169:1284–1290.

20 **Spinola S, Wild L, Apicella M, Campagnari A.** Experimental human challenge with *Haemophilus ducreyi*. Sex Transm Dis 1994;21(suppl):S112–S113. Abstract.

21 **Alfa MJ, Degagne P, Hollyer T.** *Haemophilus ducreyi* adheres to but does not invade cultured human foreskin cells. Infect Immun 1993;61:1735–1742.

22 **Castellazzo A, Shero M, Apicella MA, Spinola SM.** Expression of pili by *Haemophilus ducreyi*. J Infect Dis 1992;165 (suppl 1):S198–S199.

23 **Lammel CJ, Dekker NP, Palefsky J, Brooks GF.** In vitro model of *Haemophilus ducreyi* adherence to and entry into eukaryotic cells of genital origin. J Infect Dis 1993; 167:642–650.

24 **Purvén M, Lagergård T.** *Haemophilus ducreyi*, a cytotoxin-producing bacterium. Infect Immun 1992;60:1156–1162.

25 **Brown TJ, Ison CA.** Non-radioactive ribotyping of *Haemophilus ducreyi* using a digoxigenin labeled cDNA probe. Epidemiol Infect 1993;110:289–295.

26 **Roggen E, De Breucker S, Van Dyck E, Piot P.** Antigenic diversity in *Haemophilus ducreyi* as shown by Western blot (immunoblot) analysis. Infect Immun 1992; 60:590–595.

27 Centers for Disease Control and Prevention. Chancroid in the United States, 1981–1990: evidence for underreporting of cases. MMWR 1992;41(SS-3):57–61.

28 **Schmid GP.** Chancroid in the United States: reestablishment of an old disease. JAMA 1987;258:3265–3268.

29 **Centers for Disease Control and Prevention.** Case definitions for public health surveillance. MMWR 1990;39(RR-13):8–9.

30 **Yorke JA, Hethcote HW.** Dynamics and control of the transmission of gonorrhea. Sex Transm Dis 1978;5:51–58.

31 **Martin DH.** Recent changes in the epidemiology of genital ulcer disease in the United States: the crack cocaine connection. Sex Transm Dis 1994;21(suppl):S76–S80.

32 **Division of STD/HIV Prevention.** Sexually transmitted disease surveillance, 1993. U.S. Department of Health and Human Services, Public Health Service. Atlanta: Centers for Disease Control and Prevention, October 1994.

33 **Nsanze H, Fast MV, D'Costa LJ, et al.** Genital ulcers in Kenya: clinical and laboratory study. Br J Vener Dis 1981;57:378–381.

34 **Plummer FA, D'Costa LJ, Nsanze H, et al.** Clinical and microbiological studies of genital ulcers in Kenyan women. Sex Transm Dis 1985;12:193–197.

35 **Dangor Y, Ballard RC, da L'Exposto F, et al.** Accuracy of clinical diagnosis of genital ulcer disease. Sex Transm Dis 1990;17:184–189.

36 **Bogaerts J, Ricart CA, Van Dyck E, et al.** The etiology of genital ulceration in Rwanda. Sex Transm Dis 1989;16:123–126.

37 **O'Farrell N, Hoosen AA, Coetzee KD, van den Ende J.** Genital ulcer disease in men in Durban, South Africa. Genitourin Med 1991;67:327–330.

38 **O'Farrell N, Hoosen AA, Coetzee KD, van den Ende J.** Genital ulcer disease in women in Durban, South Africa. Genitourin Med 1991;67:322–326.

39 **Kreiss JK, Koech D, Plummer FA, et al.** AIDS virus infection in Nairobi prostitutes: spread of the epidemic to East Africa. N Engl J Med 1986;314:414–418.

40 **LeBacq F, Mason PR, Gwanzura L, et al.** HIV and other sexually transmitted diseases at a rural hospital in Zimbabwe. Genitourin Med 1993;69:352–356.

41 **Tan T, Rajan VS, Koe SL, et al.** Chancroid: a study of 500 cases. Asian J Infect Dis 1977;1:27–28.

42 **Taylor DN, Duangmani C, Suvongse C, et al.** The role of *Haemophilus ducreyi* in penile ulcers in Bangkok, Thailand. Sex Transm Dis 1984;11:148–151.

43 **Betts C, Zacarías F.** Regional Assessment of STD trends in Latin America and the Caribbean. Sex Transm Dis 1994;21(suppl): S108. Abstract.

44 **Kreiss JK, Coombs R, Plummer F, et al.** Isolation of human immunodeficiency virus from genital ulcers in Nairobi prostitutes. J Infect Dis 1989;160:380–384.

45 **Chirgwin K, DeHovitz JA, Dillon S, McCormack WM.** HIV infection, genital ulcer disease, and crack cocaine use among patients attending a clinic for sexually transmitted diseases. Am J Public Health 1991;82:1576–1579.

46 **DiCarlo RP, Martin DH.** Risk factors for genital ulcer disease (abstract 497). Program and Abstracts, 33rd Interscience Conference on Antimicrobial Agents and Chemotherapy. Washington, DC: American Society for Microbiology, 1993:210.

47 **Hammond GW, Slutchuk M, Scatliff J, et al.** Epidemiologic, clinical, laboratory, and therapeutic features of an urban outbreak of chancroid in North America. Rev Infect Dis 1980;2:867–879.

48 **Cameron DW, Simonsen JN, D'Costa LJ, et al.** Female to male transmission of human immunodeficiency virus type 1: risk factors for seroconversion in men. Lancet 1989;2:403–407.

49 **Plummer FA, Simonsen JN, Cameron DW, et al.** Co-factors in male to female transmission of HIV. J Infect Dis 1991; 163:233–239.

50 **Telzak EE, Chiasson MA, Bevier PJ, et al.** HIV-1 seroconversion in patients with and without genital ulcer disease: a prospective study. Ann Intern Med 1993;119:1181–1186.

51 **Wasserheit JN.** Epidemiological synergy: interrelationships between human immunodeficiency virus and other sexually transmitted diseases. Sex Transm Dis 1992; 19:61–77.

52 **Plummer FA, Wainberg MA, Plourde P, et al.** Detection of HIV-1 in genital ulcer exudate of HIV-1 infected men by culture and gene amplification. J Infect Dis 1990;161: 810–811. Letter.

53 **Jessamine PG, Ronald AR.** Chancroid and the role of genital ulcer disease in the spread of human retroviruses. Med Clin North Am 1990;74:1417–1431.

54 **Kunimoto DY, Plummer FA, Namaara W, et al.** Urethral infections with *Haemophilus ducreyi* in men. Sex Transm Dis 1988;15:37–39.

55 **Tyndall M, Malisa M, Plummer FA, et al.** Ceftriaxone no longer predictably cures chancroid in Kenya. J Infect Dis 1993;167: 469–471.

56 **Quale J.** Atypical presentation of chancroid in a patient infected with HIV. Am J Med 1990;88(5N):43N–44N.

57 **Cameron DW, Ngugi EN, Ronald AR, et al.** Condom use prevents genital ulcer disease and therapy reduces HIV-1 infection in women working as prostitutes in Nairobi, Kenya. Sex Transm Dis 1991;18: 188–191.

58 **Handsfield HH.** The clinical approach to genital ulcer disease. STD-2000 1994;1:3–11.

59 **Chapel TA, Brown WJ, Jeffries C, Stewart JA.** How reliable is the morphologic diagnosis of penile ulcerations? Sex Transm Dis 1977;4:150–152.

60 **Fast MV, D'Costa LJ, Nsanze H, et al.** The clinical diagnosis of genital ulcer disease in men in the tropics. Sex Transm Dis 1984; 11:72–76.

61 **Sturm AW, Stolting GJ, Cormane RH, Zanen HC.** Clinical and microbiological evaluation of 46 episodes of genital ulceration. Genitourin Med 1987;63:98–101.

62 **Ronald AR, Albritton W.** Chancroid and *Haemophilus ducreyi*. In: Holmes KK, et al., eds. Sexually transmitted diseases, 2nd ed. New York: McGraw-Hill, 1990:263–271.

63 **Karim QN, Finn GY, Easmon CS, et al.** Rapid detection of *Haemophilus ducreyi* in clinical and experimental infections using monoclonal antibody: a preliminary evaluation. Genitourin Med 1989;65:361–365.

64 **Parsons LM, Shayegani M, Waring AL, et al.** DNA probes for the identification of *Haemophilus ducreyi*. J Clin Microbiol 1989; 27:1441–1445.

65 **Rossau R, Duhamel M, Jannes G, et al.** The development of specific rRNA-derived oligonucleotide probes for *Haemophilus ducreyi*, the causative agent of chancroid. J Gen Microbiol 1991;137:277–285.

66 Chui L, Albritton W, Paster B, et al. Development of the polymerase chain reaction for diagnosis of chancroid. J Clin Microbiol 1993;31:659–664.

67 Pepin J, Quigley M, Todd J, et al. Association between HIV-2 infection and genital ulcer diseases among male sexually transmitted disease patients in The Gambia. AIDS 1992;6:489–493.

68 Ballard RC, Duncan MO, Fehler HG, et al. Treating chancroid: summary of studies in southern Africa. Genitourin Med 1989;65: 54–57.

69 Ronald AR, Corey L, McCutchan JA, Handsfield HH. Evaluation of new antiinfective drugs for the treatment of chancroid. Clin Infect Dis 1992;15(suppl 1): S108–S114.

70 Schulte JM, Schmid GP. Treatment of chancroid, 1993. Clin Infect Dis, in press.

71 Knapp JS, Back AF, Babst AF, et al. In vitro susceptibilities of isolates of Haemophilus ducreyi from Thailand and the United States to currently recommended and newer agents for treatment of chancroid. Antimicrob Agents Chemother 1993;37:1552–1555.

72 Aldridge KE, Cammarata C, Martin DH. Comparison of the in vitro activities of various parenteral and oral antimicrobial agents against endemic Haemophilus ducreyi. Antimicrob Agents Chemother 1993;37:1986–1988.

73 Schmid GP. Treatment of chancroid, 1989. Rev Infect Dis 1990;12(suppl 6):S580–S589.

74 Bowmer MI, Nsanze H, D'Costa LJ, et al. Single-dose ceftriaxone for chancroid. Antimicrob Agents Chemother 1987;31:67–69.

75 Ndinya-Achola JO, Nsanze H, Karasira P, et al. Three day oral course of augmentin to treat chancroid. Genitourin Med 1986;62: 202–204.

76 Sanson-Le Pors MJ, Casin I, Ortenberg M, et al. In vitro susceptibility of 30 strains of Haemophilus ducreyi to several antibiotics including six cephalosporins. J Antimicrob Chemother 1983;11:271–280.

77 Martin DH, Sargent S, Wendel GD, et al. Azithromycin versus ceftriaxone for the treatment of chancroid (abstract 931). Program and Abstracts, 32nd Interscience Conference on Antimicrobial Agents and Chemotherapy. Washington, DC: American Society for Microbiology, 1992:265.

78 Tyndall MW, Agoki E, Plummer FA, et al. Single dose azithromycin for the treatment of chancroid: a randomized comparision with erythromycin. Sex Transm Dis 1994; 21:231–234.

79 Naamara W, Plummer FA, Greenblatt RM, et al. Treatment of chancroid with ciprofloxacin: a prospective, randomized clinical trial. Am J Med 1987;82(suppl 4A): 317–320.

80 Ballard RC, Radebe F, Mampuru M, et al. A comparison of ofloxacin and ciprofloxacin in the treatment of chancroid. Sex Transm Dis 1994;21(suppl):S135. Abstract.

81 Ballard RC, da L'Exposto F, Dangor Y, et al. A comparative study of spectinomycin and erythromycin in the treatment of chancroid. J Antimicrob Chemother 1990; 26:429–434.

82 Dangor Y, Ballard RC, Miller SD, Koornhof HJ. Treatment of chancroid. Antimicrob Agents Chemother 1990;34: 1308–1311.

83 Centers for Disease Control and Prevention. 1993 sexually transmitted diseases treatment guidelines. MMWR 1993;42(RR-14):20–22.

Cholangitis: Pathogenesis, Diagnosis, and Treatment

LAWRENCE H. HANAU
NEAL H. STEIGBIGEL

Cholangitis comprises several different disease entities (1), including acute cholangitis, recurrent cholangitis, sclerosing cholangitis related to acquired immunodeficiency syndrome (AIDS), and primary or idiopathic sclerosing cholangitis (2). This review concentrates on acute cholangitis.

Acute cholangitis is caused by infection in an obstructed biliary system, especially at the level of the common bile duct (3–20), and is caused most commonly by stones. It may also be due to benign strictures, resulting from prior surgery or endoscopy; other bile duct abnormalities, such as cysts, diverticula, choledochocoeles; congenital abnormalities; parasites (ascaris, clonorchis, echinococcus); pancreatitis; neoplasm of the pancreas or bile ducts; sclerosing cholangitis; or from a blockage in a previously placed drainage tube (3–15,17–26). The obstruction may be complete or partial and because the infected material lacks an adequate route of drainage, intraductal pressure increases and may lead to bacteremia sometimes accompanied by septic shock and death (3–20).

PATHOGENESIS

The steps required for cholangitis to occur are 1) infection of the bile, also known as bactibilia (27–30); 2) partial or complete obstruction of the common bile duct (3–20), with increased intraluminal pressures (31–34); 3) multiplication of the organisms within the duct (35), which often results in seeding of the bloodstream (36,37).

Bile is normally sterile (38–43). However, the presence of biliary pathology, for example, stones or benign strictures, is associated with bile duct infection (28,38–48) in about 50 to 75% and 80 to 100% of cases, respectively (38). Although partial obstruction due to neoplasm also often results in biliary tract infection (29), complete obstruction due to malignancy only rarely leads to

153

bactibilia (28,46). How bacteria reach the biliary tract is not known, but several routes have been proposed: via the portal venous system (27); via secretion from the liver (27,28), perhaps seeded by portal blood (27); via the lymphatics (45); ascension from the duodenum (29,35); or from an infected gallbladder (28).

Evidence for a portal source derives from animal studies. Dineen showed that the biliary tract of guinea pigs, whose common bile duct had been ligated, could be infected when bacteria were inoculated into systemic veins or via the portal vein (27). However, lymphatic flow was away from the biliary tree, and infection could not be established via the duodenal lymphatics (27). Similarly, Sung et al. showed that biliary infection could be introduced in cats with chronic bile duct obstruction when organisms were introduced into the portal system (30). Although the portal system of some animals may often harbor bacteria, it is unclear if that is the case in human beings (49). In one study of patients undergoing abdominal surgery for conditions in which infection was felt to play no role, no significant isolate was found in the portal blood in 101 samples; three isolates were considered contaminants (49).

Nevertheless, if portal blood were the source of infection, incomplete clearance by the reticuloendothelial system would be responsible for allowing organisms to enter the biliary tree (27,28). Studies on hepatic uptake of labeled microaggregated human albumin did show abnormal reticuloendothelial clearance in patients with obstructive jaundice (50). Similarly, rats with experimentally induced biliary obstruction have impaired hepatic clearance of bacteria (51). However, if hepatic secretion were a common mechanism of biliary infection, patients with totally obstructed bile ducts as in pancreatic carcinoma would be expected to have a high rate of bactibilia rather than the low rate encountered.

Another proposed route of infection is ascent from the duodenum (29,35). This mechanism is consistent with the low rate of biliary infection found in patients with complete biliary obstruction. Both partial biliary obstruction and reduction in biliary motility probably lead to stasis and decreased bacterial clearance from the biliary tree. In addition, patients with bactibilia are usually older, and host immune defenses and clearance decrease with age (29). Lygidakis demonstrated that patients with choledochoduodenostomies who had positive bile cultures had delayed emptying of the biliary tree as shown by stasis of contrast; those with negative bile cultures had normal emptying times (35). Engstrom et al. showed that cultures of bile obtained at surgery correlated with duodenal aspirates in cases where intestinal levels of enterobacteriaceae and enterococci were above 10^3/mL (47).

Objections to the proposed mechanism of ascending infection include the rarity of bactibilia in those with total obstruction, because, it has been argued (28), that partial obstruction must have been present before the blockage became complete, giving organisms ample time to colonize the biliary tree. In addition, the duodenum or jejunum are inconsistently colonized with coliforms (52,53), organisms frequently involved in cholangitis. Significant growth of bacteria from the jejunum is unusual (53), and the organisms isolated are often mouth flora (52,53). However, changes with age, such as hypo-chlorhydria, or disease could change the bacteriology of the duodenum and jejunum (15,29).

Once the bile is colonized by bacteria, biliary stasis favors multiplication (32,33), and increased biliary pressure often allows organisms to enter the bloodstream. Patients with high biliary pressures measured during surgery have higher rates of bacteremia, morbidity, and mortality than those in whom ductal pressures are less elevated (33). Moreover, although biliary pressures are higher in those with choledocholithiasis than in controls, patients with cholangitis have significantly higher pressures than either group (34).

Studies in experimental animals show that infection in the presence of complete biliary obstruction is more likely to cause hepatic damage (31). In addition, studies in dogs have shown that endotoxin injected into an intrahepatic bile duct is much more likely to reach the systemic circulation when intrabiliary pressure is higher (15). High biliary pressure also enables bacteria to enter both the lymphatics and the bloodstream of experimental animals (32). In one study, bacteria were found in the lymphatics at a lower pressure than that which enabled them to reach the systemic circulation (32). Others have found that bacteria were present in the venous system before they reached the thoracic duct (37). Raper et al. (36), working with rats, suggested that bacteria may reach the bloodstream from the biliary tract by penetrating into or between hepatocytes. They showed that in the presence of complete obstruction of the common bile duct, there was bile duct proliferation, distortion of tight junctions between hepatocytes, and blunting of the microvillus border of the hepatocytes (36). When bacteria were injected into the obstructed biliary system, they were found between hepatocytes as well as in vacuoles within hepatocytes (36). Thus, the increased pressure found in biliary obstruction may lead to hepatocellular changes that could allow colonizing organisms to reach the bloodstream.

CLINICAL MANIFESTATIONS

The great preponderance of cholecystitis in women compared to men is not found with cholangitis. In various reports, men make up between 25 and 100% of those with cholangitis (3–10,12–15,17–19). Most studies show median ages of patients to be 50 to 60 years. Many patients have had previous episodes of cholangitis or other biliary diseases (3–15,17–19,21–23,33,34).

Acute cholangitis has a broad spectrum of clinical manifestations (3,8). Traditionally the syndrome had been divided into two groups (3,8): those with acute cholangitis who manifested Charcot's triad (54) of fever and chills, right upper quadrant abdominal pain, and jaundice, and those with acute obstructive suppurative cholangitis, whose biliary tree contained pus under pressure, and who also exhibited altered mental status and were in shock. The combination of Charcot's triad with shock and altered mental status constitutes Reynolds' pentad (18). These divisions are arbitrary, however, and cases occur in which pus is present in the biliary tree without shock, and in which shock has occurred in the absence of purulence (3).

Charcot's triad is present in 50 to 100% of cases of cholangitis (3–8,11,13,19, 20,55). Fever is the most common sign, found in over 90% of patients (3,4,7– 9,11–13,17,18,33,34,55), and jaundice has generally been detected in more than 60% (3–5,7,9,12–14,17,19,33,34,55). Abdominal pain is also noted by more than 70% of patients (3,5,7,12–14,19,33,34) but is not always localized to the right upper quadrant (3,4,13). Abdominal tenderness is found in more than 59% of those studied (3–5,13), but peritoneal signs are less frequent (14 to 45%) (3,5,8,13,17,19), except in one report (13). In reports including all forms of cholangitis, altered mental status and hypotension are exhibited by 10 to 20% and up to 30% of patients, respectively (3–5,8,33,34,55), whereas Reynolds' pentad is rare (less than 14%) (3,6,8,55).

Among common laboratory findings is an elevated leukocyte count (3,5,7,8,10,11,13,14), although some may only have a "left shift" (3). Liver function tests are consistent with a cholestatic pattern; expected values in cholestasis are summarized in Table 7.1 (56). In cholangitis, hyperbilirubinemia is found in 88 to 100% of patients (4–7,10,11,13–15,55); alkaline phosphatase is increased in more than 78% of patients (5,7,9,13,55); and transaminases are usually only mildly elevated (3–5,55), although there are rare reports of values greater than 1000 very early in cholangitis due to a sudden increase in intraductal pressure (57). Amylase is usually within normal limits (3,5,13,14), and measurements of the prothrombin time have been provided infrequently (3,9). In our experience, the rise in bilirubin or alkaline phosphatase sometimes lags behind the symptoms of cholangitis by one to 2 days.

Plain film radiography plays a limited role in the diagnosis of cholangitis. In one study, x-rays of the abdomen were abnormal in only 15% of patients (5). As expected, since few calculi are radiopaque, only 2 of 52 patients had calculi visualized; one had air in the biliary tree (5).

Cholescintigraphy (with a ^{99m}Tc-labeled imino diacetic acid derivative) can be used to demonstrate the presence or absence of obstruction but is less useful in determining its cause (58). It is also useful in distinguishing cholangitis from cholecystitis (59) and is more sensitive than ultrasound in detecting obstruction

Table 7.1.   Liver Function Tests in Cholestatic Disease

Test	Result
Bilirubin	6–20 mg/dL (102–340 µmol/L)
Alkaline phosphatase	2–5 times normal
Transaminases (units/mL)	< 200*

*Rarely patients may have markedly elevated transaminases (57).
SOURCE: Modified from Lamont JT. Cholestasis: medical or surgical? Hosp Pract 1985; 82A–82EE.

within the first day after it has occurred but before biliary dilatation is detectible (60).

Ultrasound has become increasingly useful in the management of cholangitis and obstructive jaundice. The value of sonography in detecting biliary duct dilatation has been known for some time (61–63). It was initially noted to be less useful in determining the etiology of obstructive jaundice (63–70), with differing conclusions regarding its ability to determine the level of obstruction (63,67,70). With improvement in imaging modalities, recent reports have indicated increased sensitivity and specificity in elucidating both the site and cause of obstruction (71–74), although not with the degree of accuracy found with invasive cholangiography (73,74). Ultrasound may be particularly useful in diagnosing cholangitis resulting from the rupture of an echinococcal cyst (21–23). Recently, it has been proposed that the presence of a hypoechoic stripe in the common bile duct may be indicative of cholangitis (75).

Computerized tomography (CT) offers an additional level of sensitivity beyond ultrasound in determining the etiology and level of obstruction (69,70); a recent study has also demonstrated its usefulness in cholangitis (76). Most studies suggest that it be reserved for those in whom ultrasound has been nonrevealing (70,77), although not all would agree (78).

Finally, percutaneous and endoscopic cholangiography have leading roles in the evaluation of obstructive jaundice (77). These procedures can elucidate the site and cause of the obstruction, delineate the anatomy of the biliary tree, detect those cases where obstruction is present without dilatation, and drain the obstructed system (77). In patients with or without cholangitis, these procedures may lead to bacteremia (59,79–81).

When a patient presents with signs and symptoms of cholangitis, a reasonable interpretation of the above information suggests that the initial radiologic evaluation include a plain film of the abdomen and an abdominal ultrasound study. If the ultrasound examination shows dilated ducts but does not indicate the cause or site of the obstruction, an abdominal CT study may be useful. Cholescintigraphy should be reserved for patients who are suspected of having cholangitis but do not have dilated ducts on ultrasound or CT, or in whom both cholangitis and cholecystitis are being considered as alternative diagnoses. Endoscopic cholangiography should generally be performed before surgery but often may obviate surgery when calculi can be removed endoscopically.

MICROBIOLOGY

The microbiology of the biliary tract of patients both with (3–9,13–15,17,82–88) and without cholangitis (35,38,41,42,45,46,82,89–99) has been elucidated (Table 7.2). Bile cultures are positive in 80 to 100% of patients with cholangitis and infections are polymicrobial in 30 to 83% of the episodes (3,6,7,9,13,17,83–88). Anaerobes have been isolated from the bile infrequently in most studies; however, more recent investigations of patients with biliary diseases not limited to cholangitis have detected anaerobes in up to 40% of patients (42,94) but only rarely as the sole isolate (43,94). *Bacteroides* species are the most common anaerobic isolate, followed by *Clostridium* species (42,92,94). Improvements in transportation and anaerobic culturing techniques are probably responsible for the increased rate of detection of these organisms in recent years (92,93). Consistent with this hypothesis is the fact that clostridial species, which are more tolerant of oxygen than other anaerobes, were the most frequent anaerobic isolates in the past (92,93).

Candida are rarely isolated. Morris et al. (96) reviewed data on 31 patients with biliary candidiasis, most of whom did not have the syndrome of acute cholangitis. They found that these patients had similar predisposing risk factors for candidal infection as did those with candidemia. Patients had syndromes including uncomplicated or gangrenous cholecystitis, common or hepatic duct obstruction, cholangitis, or intra-abdominal abscesses. When the candida were limited to the gallbladder or biliary tract, patients recovered from the acute episode after surgical treatment or drainage, but without antifungal therapy and remained free of candidal infection during the follow-up period. If there was candidemia or any extrabiliary focus, antifungal therapy was indicated.

Bacteremia is documented in 21 to 71% of patients with cholangitis (3–9,17,83,84–88). The organisms isolated reflect a similar distribution to that of biliary cultures (see Table 7.2). Blood isolates and bile isolates are identical in 33 to 84% of episodes of cholangitis. Bacteremia due to anaerobes is uncommon (94). Of 60 patients in one study who had anaerobes isolated as part of their biliary flora, only 3 had anaerobic bacteremia; a fourth was bacteremic with *Bacteroides fragilis* even though no anaerobes were found in the biliary cultures (94).

DIFFERENTIAL DIAGNOSIS

The differential diagnosis of cholangitis has been well summarized by Nahrwold (59). The entity most difficult to distinguish from cholangitis is acute cholecystitis. Both conditions can present with right upper quadrant pain, fever, and jaundice, along with an increased leukocyte count. However, the abdominal pain is frequently more severe in cholecystitis and is much less likely to be absent; peritoneal signs are also more likely to be associated with cholecystitis. Transaminases and alkaline phosphatase are generally normal or slightly elevated in uncomplicated cholecystitis (100). They are more likely to be elevated in the presence of choledocholithiasis or cholangitis (3–5,55,100). Dumont (101) found that bilirubin levels in patients with cholecystitis and a normal common bile duct were between 1.4 and 4.1 mg/dL; in the presence of choledocholithiasis, they ranged from 1.9 to 11.3 mg/dL. The mechanism for hyperbilirubinemia in cholecystitis unaccompanied by common duct stones or cholangitis is unknown. Hypotheses include compression of the common bile duct by the inflamed gallbladder, intrahepatic cholestasis, or increased

Table 7.2. Microbiology of Bile and Blood in Patients with Cholangitis

Organism	Percent of Isolates*	
	Bile[†]	Blood[‡]
Escherichia coli	38.5	51.5
Klebsiella species[§]	16.5	16.0
Enterococci	8.0	5.0
Pseudomonas species	5.0	6.0
Enterobacter and *Aerobacter* species[§]	5.0	4.0
Proteus species	4.5	3.0
Citrobacter, Serratia, and *Morganella* species	3.0	0.5
Staphylococci	0.5	3.5[ǁ]
Viridans streptococci	0.5	2.0
Unspecified streptococci	2.0	0.0
Bacteroides species[¶]	1.5	0.5
Clostridium species[¶]	2.5	1.5
Candida species	0.5	0.5
Other organisms	9.0[#]	5.5**

* Rounded to the nearest 0.5%.
[†] 578 total isolates; see references 3, 5, 7, 13, 17, 55, 82–84, 87.
[‡] 145 total isolates; see references 3, 7, 17, 85–87, 111.
[§] An additional 3.5% of the isolates were a combined group of *Klebsiella* and *Enterobacter/Aerobacter* species.
[ǁ] 1.5% *Staphylococcus aureus* and 2.0% coagulase-negative staphylococci.
[¶] See text for additional information on more recent studies of anaerobes in biliary tract disease, not limited to cholangitis.
[#] Includes one "beta streptococcus," one *Hafnia*, 3 paracolon bacilli, 7 unspecified gram-positive organisms, and 39 unidentified organisms.
** One paracolon bacillus and 7 unidentified organisms.

permeability of the gallbladder epithelium, allowing the bilirubin in bile to enter the bloodstream (101,102). Cholescintigraphy and ultrasound studies often help to differentiate acute cholecystitis from choledocholithiasis or cholangitis (59).

Hepatic abscesses, which may be a complication of cholangitis, are distinguishable by ultrasound, CT, or sometimes by cholescintigraphy (59). Both viral and drug-induced hepatitis usually produce higher aminotransferase levels than cholangitis (59). In addition, in hepatitis the entire liver is often tender, which can be recognized on palpation of the lateral aspect of the intercostal spaces or by soliciting punch tenderness in the same area (103). Pancreatitis is accompanied by a higher amylase and more "striking pain" (59) than is cholangitis. Other diagnoses such as perforated duodenal ulcer, right-sided pyelonephritis, acute appendicitis, right lower lobe pneumonia, and pulmonary infarcts, should be identified based on history, serial physical examinations, and laboratory investigations (59).

An important entity in the differential diagnosis of cholangitis is the abnormal liver function encountered in some cases of localized gram-negative infection, as well as in bacteremias due to both gram-positive as well as gram-negative organisms (the "hepatopathy of sepsis") (104–107). The abnormal liver function is primarily due to a defect in the excretion of conjugated bilirubin (104) by the hepatocyte into the bile canaliculi, a step mediated by the membrane Na^+-K^+ ATPase (108). Generally, there is a significantly elevated conjugated bilirubin level, which may precede recognition of the bacteremia, and the patient may be jaundiced (105,106,109). Unlike cholangitis, alkaline phosphatase and aminotransferases are usually only minimally elevated (104–106,109), although significant elevations may occur (105). Rarely, patients may have an elevated alkaline phosphatase, with normal bilirubin levels (110). Histologically, cholestasis may be seen along with Kupffer cell hyperplasia, but hepatocyte necrosis is absent. Bacterial products probably play a role in causing these changes (105,106). Often, cholangitis will be distinguishable from the hepatopathy associated with infection by the presence in the latter of an obvious focus of serious infection outside of the hepatobiliary system and the absence of pain. An imaging modality may help in the differentiation (59).

TREATMENT

Most patients with cholangitis can be managed medically during the acute episode, with a definitive invasive procedure performed later if necessary (3–5,7,111). In addition, acute episodes of cholangitis may resolve spontaneously (3,5,12). Medical management includes the use of intravenous fluids and antibiotics, careful monitoring, correction of any coagulopathy, and possible nasogastric tube suction (3–5,7,111). Blood cultures should be obtained prior to beginning antimicrobial therapy, and the antibiotic chosen should be active against the expected organisms. Although some antibiotics achieve higher levels in the bile than others (112–114), it is unclear if biliary excretion of an antimicrobial agent is important. Keighly et al. found that the postoperative infection rate in patients undergoing biliary surgery was lower in those who received gentamicin, a drug that achieves poor biliary levels, than in those who received rifamide, which is mainly excreted in bile. They concluded that serum levels were more important than biliary levels (115). Moreover, secretion of antibiotics into the biliary tree is markedly diminished when intrabiliary pressure is increased (112,114,116,117), with the concentrations often being below effective levels (114,116). Thus, successful treatment with an antimicrobial sometimes may have to do more with the reduction of systemic infection than with sterilization of the bile. However, although the requirements for high biliary levels are uncertain, it seems reasonable to favor agents that may achieve good levels in bile.

In the recent past, cholangitis was frequently treated with a combination of a penicillin—usually ampicillin—and an aminoglycoside (114,118), to achieve activity against facultative gram-negative bacilli and enterococci. This combination now has the disadvantage of limited anaerobic coverage, frequent resistance of gram-negative bacilli to ampicillin, and the risk of nephrotoxicity of the aminoglycoside. Recently, the ureidopenicillins, piperacillin (118,119) and mezlocillin (120), which have a spectrum of activity that includes many anaerobes, were compared to ampicillin and gentamicin or tobramycin. In one study mezlocillin was superior in effecting a cure (120); in two other studies, piperacillin was not (118,119). It would seem unlikely that the difference in the results could be attributed to a difference in spectrum or potency of the two similar ureidopenicillins; the differences in outcome were more likely due to other factors, attributable to different patient populations and times and places of treatment. Whether an increased response to the ureidopenicillins could be achieved by adding an aminoglycoside or an agent more active against anaerobes (e.g., metronidazole) has not been evaluated, although some recommend those regimens (116). It is likely that other agents with similar or broader coverage would also be efficacious (116), and choice of therapy should consider local antibiotic sensitivity patterns (121). The recent recognition of an increasing number of isolates of enterococci that are multiply resistant to antibiotics (122) suggests that the use of cephalosporins be decreased because they may select out enterococci from the patient's endogenous flora (123,124).

For initial use in a patient with acute cholangitis, we favor the use of a ureidopenicillin plus an aminoglycoside and metronidazole. The use of the aminoglycoside with the penicillin may be synergistic in some patients with severe gram-negative sepsis and would be useful as well when a sensitive enterococcal species is involved. The ureidopenicillins also achieve good levels in bile (125). Ampicillin/sulbactam, ticarcillin/clavulanic acid or piperacillin/tazobactam, each used together with an aminoglycoside, are reliable alternative regimens.

Invasive Therapy

The need for relief of obstruction of the biliary tree in cholangitis has been appreciated since the early years of this century (126). If the obstruction remains, even if there is initial clinical improvement, cholangitis is likely to recur at increasing frequency (3), and the continued obstruction may lead to multiple hepatic abscess formation or, much later, to secondary biliary cirrhosis with its associated complications (3,12,127). Those who respond to medical therapy may be treated electively to relieve the obstruction. Emergent invasive therapy is reserved for the 15% who fail to show a clinical response to medical treatment within 12 to 24 hours (5,11), or those who deteriorate after an initial clinical improvement (11). In the past, intervention to relieve the obstruction was surgical. At present, endoscopic and percutaneous techniques are also available, and these may be definitive or temporizing. The procedure used will depend on availability and on whether it is emergent or elective.

Surgery Surgery has been used to treat cholangitis since Rogers tried to decompress an obstructed biliary system by inserting a glass tube into an obstructed hepatic duct (126). The goals of surgery remain similar today, specifically, "to remove or bypass the obstruction, and establish free drainage between the duct and the gut" (3). In emergencies, all that may be possible is decompression with insertion of a T tube into the common bile duct, the definitive procedure being deferred until the patient is more stable (3,4,10,59,111). The type of procedure chosen depends on the cause of the obstruction (4,7,14), and the timing of surgery depends on the initial response to antibiotics (3,5). Complications (4,7,8,14) may not only be due to the presence of infection in the biliary tree, but also may result from the presence of obstructive jaundice (111,128–134). Morbidity includes but is not limited to recurrent cholangitis (3,4,8,9) and other infectious sequelae, for example, abscesses, wound infections, and systemic bacteremias (3,4,8,9,14,19). Occasionally recurrent cholangitis occurs even though the biliary system appears patent and free draining. These cases are felt to be due to bactibilia accompanying intrahepatic bile stasis due to a damaged duct (135). Surgical mortality varies widely among reports and depends on the underlying disease, the urgency and timeliness of the procedure, the clinical status of the patient, the effectiveness of the decompression, and whether infection has spread into the liver (3–5,7–14,17–19).

Percutaneous Drainage Transhepatic percutaneous biliary drainage has been used to decompress the biliary systems of patients with obstructive jaundice (133,136–145). Decompression usually leads to a reduction in serum bilirubin levels and other elevated liver function tests (133,136–144). Some reports noted improvement in morbidity and mortality of subsequent surgical procedures (136,138), but others did not (141,142). The procedure has significant complication rates, including cholangitis (137–144,146,147), and patients who had long-term drainage had an infection rate of approximately 40% regardless of whether the drainage was internal or external (147). Nevertheless, percutaneous drainage has been used in cholangitis both with and without subsequent definitive procedures (15,55,84,144,148–150). Patients not only had improvements in laboratory parameters, but most also had clinical improvement as well (55,84,144,148,150). The overall morbidity and mortality of percutaneous drainage in patients with cholangitis is similar to that in patients with biliary pathology, but without infection, although the incidence of postprocedure bacteremia was higher in those with cholangitis (149). Percutaneous drainage often makes it possible for the patient to be more stable clinically when definitive surgery is performed and also may allow enough time to elapse so that inflammation is reduced in and around the bile ducts (55). In addition, percutaneous drainage may provide access for nonsurgical procedures such as stone retrieval (146) and dissolution (151–153).

Endoscopic Procedures Endoscopy offers the opportunity to do either a definitive or a temporizing procedure to relieve biliary obstruction. Patients with choledocholithiasis may be treated with endoscopic sphincterotomy followed by stone extraction (154,155). Occasionally, the increased size of the orifice allows the stones to pass into the duodenum (156–159). Although sphincterotomy has complications, including infection (154,155,160–163), it has had great success in treating cholangitis (86,155,157–159,162,164–169). Comparing the morbidity and mortality rates of endoscopic stone extraction to surgery has been difficult because patient demographics and data collected were not always comparable (170,171). Despite these limitations, sphincterotomy has been found in retrospective reviews to have fewer complications in patients with (86,168) and without (160) cholangitis. However, one group found greater complications than with surgery, but their success rate of sphincterotomy was below that of other investigators (169). Nevertheless, surgery may be required in some patients in whom endoscopic decompression has either been unsuccessful (172), or whose anatomy limits its efficacy (170). Endoscopy generally compares favorably to a percutaneous approach (158) because it offers an opportunity to do a definitive procedure with less trauma (74).

An alternative to sphincterotomy is endoscopic placement of an indwelling prosthesis (157,173), for example, stents (145,154–156,171,174) or nasobiliary drains (86,145,154–156,165,166,172,174–176). Stents may be placed as temporary or long-term therapy (145,157) and have been used to treat various biliary pathologies: malignancy (74,145,174,177,178); obstruction due chronic pancreatitis (145,163); benign strictures (179–182); fistulas (181,182); and choledocholithiasis (157,174,183,184), where the stent functions not as a drain but by keeping calculi from occluding the ampulla of Vater (157). Stents have also been placed for treatment of cholangitis (145,158,163). Complications include obstruction (145,163,178,181), migration of the stent (163,181), and recurrent cholangitis (145,157,178,183–185). Endoscopic placement of stents is considered superior to percutaneous methods (145) because it has fewer complications (174,186) and provides continual access to the prosthesis (174).

Endoscopically placed nasobiliary drains have been used after sphincterotomy in patients who have retained stones (145,157,173,183), and occasionally for stenosis or obstruction (174). It not only relieves obstruction, but also provides access to the biliary tree for obtaining cultures (145) and therapeutic dissolution procedures (86,145,174). In addition, nasobiliary drainage has been useful in the therapy of cholangitis (86–88,145,156,165–167,183,186–189) particularly in patients with choledocholithiasis who do not respond to antibiotic therapy (86–88,156,165–167,187–189). In a prospective study, it had a mortality rate that was significantly lower than emergency surgery and also had less morbidity (88). The authors recommended that nasobiliary drainage be used in patients who need relief of obstruction emergently. In addition, it has recently been shown that endoscopic placement of nasobiliary drains may be performed under ultrasound guidance, enabling them to be placed at the bedside of patients who require intensive care monitoring (189). A limitation of nasobiliary catheters is that they serve only as a temporary measure (145,157); they are uncomfortable and can be accidentally displaced (183).

Choice of Procedure

In patients who present with cholangitis, initial management should be noninvasive. Good cooperation among the primary physician, surgeon, gastro-enterologist, infectious diseases consultant, and radiologist will optimize the ensuing management. Both the gastroenterologist and the surgeon should advise as to the best approach to rectify the underlying biliary pathology. Both should also be readily available should the patient be among the approximately 15% who do not show substantial clinical improvement on antibiotic therapy within 12 to 24 hours, or among those who deteriorate after an initial clinical improvement. In emergent situations, an endoscopic approach should be used if possible, and the procedure limited to only that necessary to relieve obstruction. Often this will simply be the placement of a nasobiliary drain or a stent. Occasionally, the biliary pathology of those patients whose obstruction is due to calculi will be such that sphincterotomy and stone extraction may be performed rapidly. Surgery or percutaneous drainage should be reserved for patients in whom an endoscopic method is not efficacious.

Once the acute episode has resolved, the underlying abnormality can be corrected. The procedure chosen will be determined by the underlying pathology, but it should be the least invasive possible. An endoscopic procedure frequently may be all that is needed, but surgery will still be required in some patients.

PROGNOSIS

The prognosis of patients with cholangitis depends on several factors. Clinical presentation and response to initial antibiotic therapy are significant prognostic indicators. Those who present with Reynolds' pentad have a higher mortality rate (3,5,6,8), and mortality approaches 100% in patients who fail to respond to initial conservative measures if intervention is not performed in a timely fashion (9,12,14,17). Increased mortality is also associated with the presence of pus in the common bile duct (8,15), first attacks (3), and the presence of associated conditions, such as hepatic abscess (5,12,17) or biliary cirrhosis (3). The etiology of the obstruction also is significant. Malignant obstruction is associated with a worse prognosis than other etiologies (3,4,8). Death not only results from biliary or abdominal sepsis, but also from the malignancy itself (8). Similarly, the presence of underlying medical conditions also portends a worse prognosis (88,111,128). Several workers have tried to identify clinical or laboratory traits that are predictive of a poor outcome (6,86,88,111,128,190). Although no group had identical findings, several factors were common to all studies: renal insufficiency (6,86,88,128,190), concomitant medical problems (88,111,128), abnormal platelet counts (88,111), hypoalbuminemia (86,88,111), and older age (6,128). The mode of drainage may also affect mortality (88). Morbidity also depends on many of the same factors and is affected by the interventional procedure chosen (88).

RECURRENT PYOGENIC OR ORIENTAL CHOLANGITIS

Also known as oriental infestational cholangitis (191) or intrahepatic pigmented stone disease (192), the disease, as the name implies, is common in eastern Asia, although with increased immigration it is becoming more common in western nations (192,193).

Patients have recurrent episodes of fever and chills, abdominal pain, and jaundice. Pathologic studies (191,192,194–197) may reveal both stricture and dilatation of the intrahepatic bile ducts. Extrahepatic ducts may be dilated, but they rarely contain strictures. The common bile duct is often thickened with external fibrosis and may also be dilated. The papilla of Vater may be hypertrophied, fibrosed, and rigid but is usually patent. The gallbladder may be involved as well, and its mucosa may be flattened or the epithelial layer denuded. The liver may be enlarged, scarred, with nonvascular adhesions between the surface and the diaphragm, but after multiple attacks the liver may be shrunken, particularly the lateral segment of the left lobe. The stones, which are of differing consistencies, are found in approximately 75 to 80% of patients and are mainly composed of bile pigment and calcium.

Two theories have been offered to explain the pathogenesis of recurrent pyogenic cholangitis (RPC). The first (191–193,195) invokes a pivotal role for parasitic infection due to clonorchis, ascaris, or perhaps fasciola. Because opisthorchus causes disease in a similar manner to clonorchus, it can be assumed that it also could cause RPC (193). These parasites induce ductal injury and strictures, which lead to stone formation and then obstruction. Infection then develops in the obstructed system; the bacteria may be brought into the biliary system by the worm itself (191). In favor of this hypothesis (192,193), many of these patients are infected with clonorchis and ascaris and microscopic sections of stones reveal the presence of eggs or fragments of those worms. However, the incidence of clonorchis infection in patients with RPC is not significantly different from that in the indigenous population as a whole (192–195), and the disease occurs in localities where clonorchis is not found (195). It should be noted that cholangitis kills the intraductal parasites (192).

A second theory (192–195) emphasizes poor nutrition and portal bacteremia as playing a pivotal role in pathogenesis. It is proposed that bacteria reach the biliary tree via the portal circulation. When biliary obstruction occurs, either due to stones, tumor, or parasites, bacterial multiplication may occur. These bacteria induce stone formation by deconjugating bilirubin, which may occur because glucaric acid, a β-glucuronidase inhibitor, is absent from the diet.

The incidence of RPC in men and women is nearly equal (191, 192,194,196,198). Patients are generally of a low socioeconomic status (192) and are usually also younger than those in the West who have cholangitis (191,192,198). There are recurrent attacks and remissions of fever, abdominal pain with nausea and vomiting, and jaundice (192). Physical examination often reveals epigastric tenderness and rigidity (192) and the liver, gallbladder, or spleen may be palpable (194). Occasionally the patient is in shock and exhibits mental confusion (192). Other entities that need to be distinguished from RPC include acute cholangitis, clonorchiasis, tumor, sclerosing cholangitis, and cystic diseases of the biliary system (192,196).

Laboratory values are similar to those in western cholangitis (192,194,196), as is the microbiology of the biliary system (150,191,192,194,198,199). Clonorchis eggs have also been found in the bile (199). Blood cultures are positive in 15 to 47% of patients (194,198).

Ultrasonography (192,196) is useful in demonstrating biliary dilatation, whether it is extrahepatic or intrahepatic, and will usually detect calculi as well (196). CT (192,200,201) will also demonstrate ductal dilatation but is less efficacious than ultrasound for stones, particularly scans done with intravenous contrast. It may be useful in planning hepatic resection or complex drainage procedures (200,201). Cholangiography has the potential to reveal ductal changes, stones, and abscesses or fistulas (192,202). A limitation of cholangiography is that when a stone completely obstructs the bile duct it may be missed (192,202).

Like western cholangitis, RPC may resolve spontaneously, respond to antibiotic therapy, or require a procedure to decompress the biliary system (192,195). Even with successful decompression the disease may still recur (194). Occasionally a hepatic lobectomy will be required in patients who have hemobilia or strictures and retained stones with marked destruction of the hepatic parenchyma (191,195,197,203).

The mortality rate of RPC is usually low for an individual episode and has been reported to be between 8 and 11% (191,194). Patients who require emergent surgery or who present in shock have higher mortality rates—12% (198) and 18% (191), respectively. Overall the prognosis depends on the stage of the disease (191).

CHOLANGIOPATHY OR SCLEROSING CHOLANGITIS IN AIDS PATIENTS

The presence of biliary tract disease in patients with human immunodeficiency virus (HIV) infection has been reported since the early years of the epidemic (204–207) and has been the subject of a recent review (208) as well as several case reports (204–207,209–230). Biliary disease usually occurs after the patient has had an AIDS-defining illness (231–234). Occasionally biliary manifestations are found in patients who have otherwise been asymptomatic (222,234) and may even occur shortly after seroconversion (223). There is also a recent report of cholangiopathy associated with HIV-2 (235).

The terms AIDS sclerosing cholangitis is based on findings seen on cholangiography that are similar to primary sclerosing cholangitis (231, see also 2), but gallbladder involvement also occurs and may be the major site of disease (204,205,209–213,226,227,229).

Cello has identified four morphologic forms of AIDS cholangiopathy (208,233): papillary stenosis; sclerosing cholangitis; both papillary stenosis and sclerosing cholangitis; and long, extrahepatic bile duct strictures. The pathogenesis of these changes is not known (208). Cryptosporidium (204–207,210, 212,220,221,224–227,229–233,236–239), cytomegalovirus (CMV) (205,209,210, 219,222,224,227,229,231,234,236,238–243) and more recently microsporidia (215–217,232) have been associated with these lesions and are the pathogens most often isolated. There are occasional reports of cholangiopathy associated with *Campylobacter fetus* (211), candida (225,244), lymphoma (213), and Kaposi's sarcoma (207), and in some cases no organisms are detected (224,231,233). However, it is not known whether CMV, cryptosporidia, or microsporidia induce these changes or are simply colonizing a damaged biliary tree induced by HIV or a process related to HIV infection (212,220,233). Nonetheless, it has been shown that CMV viremia may induce a cholestatic pattern of liver function tests (245), and recently, there has been a report of squamous metaplasia of bile duct mucosa in association with cryptosporidial infection (221).

Patients usually have fever (221,233,236) and right upper quadrant (231–233,236,242,246,247) or epigastric pain (231,232,236,246). They may also note diarrhea (231,232,242); nausea, with or without vomiting (215,217,220,221,246); and weight loss (231,232). Physical examination may reveal hepatic (217) or abdominal (210,219,220,233) tenderness, guarding (209), and should the gallbladder be involved, a positive Murphy's sign may be present (209).

Liver function abnormalities are most notable for an elevated alkaline phosphatase (231–233,242,246,247), which is frequently at least two times normal (231). Transaminases are usually less elevated (208,232,233), and may be within the normal range (216,217,219). Serum bilirubin is elevated in only a minority of patients (231–233,236,247). Some patients will present with entirely normal liver function tests (231,242).

Ultrasonography, CT, cholescintigraphy, and cholangiography may all be useful in the evaluation of a patient with AIDS cholangiopathy. On ultrasound (231,233,234,236,237,242,246–252), the common bile duct or the intrahepatic ducts may be dilated, with or without thickening of the walls, and ductal strictures may also be seen. Edema of the ampulla may be visualized as a hypoechoic nodule. The gallbladder walls may be thickened, and sludge may be visualized in the lumen. Occasional findings include an enlarged liver (230) and a distended gallbladder (211), and in some cases the sonogram may be normal (220,233,246).

Findings on CT (228,233,248,251,252) generally parallel those seen on ultrasonography; however, CT is more useful in demonstrating thickening of the wall of the common bile duct and the dilatation and irregular arborization of the intrahepatic ducts.

Three patterns have been noted on cholescintigraphy (253): focal duct dilatation with focal or diffuse parenchymal retention, diffuse dilatation of the biliary tree with diffuse parenchymal retention, and parenchymal retention without ductal abnormality.

Endoscopic cholangiography may be useful in diagnosing AIDS cholangiopathy (208,222,228,231–236,246,248,251–253) and may reveal abnormalities even when ultrasonography and CT are unremarkable. Findings include common bile duct dilatation, with or without papillary stenosis; delayed drainage of contrast; stones or strictures in the distal common bile duct; "pruning" and focal dilatation of the intrahepatic ducts; intrahepatic strictures; extrahepatic duct dilatation with mural abnormalities; extrahepatic strictures; and pancreatic duct dilatation. The cholangiogram may also be normal, even in the presence of an abnormal ultrasound or CT (233).

Treatment of AIDS cholangiopathy is directed at relieving pain (231,233) and if possible relieving biliary obstruction. There has been little success in treating the organisms that may be involved. Use of anti-CMV drugs results in limited improvement (208,231), and there is only one report of a successful outcome with anticryptosporidial therapy (230). Some patients may improve spontaneously (231); others may achieve relief with analgesics (231,233). In patients with gallbladder involvement cholecystectomy may be indicated (232,234,238,243,244). Endoscopic sphincterotomy has been used in patients with papillary stenosis (206,208,231,233,236,248). Pain may decrease, but there is little decrease in the alkaline phosphatase (208,233,236,248), and pain may recur (233). The procedure may be complicated by acute cholangitis (248). Surgery may be performed for patients who have papillary stenosis and who are not suitable candidates for endoscopy (252).

The prognosis of patients with AIDS who have cholangiopathy is poor (231). Patients usually die from causes unrelated to biliary disease (231,233,234,237,248). It would seem that the goal of therapy should be to obtain symptomatic relief.

ACKNOWLEDGMENT

We thank Leslie H. Bernstein, M.D., Head of the Division of Gastroenterology at Montefiore Medical Center and the Albert Einstein College of Medicine for reviewing the manuscript and for his helpful suggestions.

REFERENCES

1 **Sinanan MN.** Acute cholangitis. Infect Dis Clin North Am 1992;6:571–599.

2 **Martin M.** Primary sclerosing cholangitis.

Annu Rev Med 1993;44:221–227.

3 **Boey JH, Way LW.** Acute cholangitis. Ann Surg 1980;191:264–270.

4 Thompson JE Jr, Tompkins RK, Longmire WP Jr. Factors in management of acute cholangitis. Ann Surg 1982;195: 137–145.

5 Saharia PC, Cameron JL. Clinical management of acute cholangitis. Surg Gynecol Obstet 1976;142:369–372.

6 Gigot JF, Leese T, Dereme T, Coutinho J, Castaing D, Bismuth H. Acute cholangitis: multivariate analysis of risk factors. Ann Surg 1989;209:435–438.

7 Saik RP, Greenburg AG, Farris JM, Peskin GW. Spectrum of cholangitis. Am J Surg 1975;130:143–150.

8 O'Connor MJ, Schwartz ML, McQuarrie DG, Sumner HW. Acute bacterial cholangitis: an analysis of clinical manifestations. Arch Surg 1982;117:437–441.

9 Hinchey EJ, Couper CE. Acute obstructive suppurative cholangitis. Am J Surg 1969;117:62–68.

10 Glenn F, Moody FG. Acute obstructive suppurative cholangitis. Surg Gynecol Obstet 1961;113:265–273.

11 Ostermiller W, Thompson RJ, Carter R, Hinshaw DB. Acute obstructive cholangitis. Arch Surg 1965;90:392–395.

12 Dow RW, Lindenauer SM. Acute obstructive suppurative cholangitis. Ann Surg 1969;169:272–276.

13 Haupert AP, Carey LC, Evans WE, Ellison EH. Acute suppurative cholangitis: experience with 15 consecutive cases. Arch Surg 1967;94:460–468.

14 Welch JP, Donaldson GA. The urgency of diagnosis and surgical treatment of acute suppurative cholangitis. Am J Surg 1976; 131:527–532.

15 Kinoshita H, Hirohashi K, Igawa S, Nagata E, Sakai K. Cholangitis. World J Surg 1984;8:963–969.

16 Nahrwold DL. Acute cholangitis. Surgery 1992;112:487–488.

17 Andrew DJ, Johnson SE. Acute suppurative cholangitis, a medical and surgical emergency: a review of ten years experience emphasizing early recognition. Am J Gastroenterol 1970;54:141–154.

18 Reynolds BM, Dargan EL. Acute obstructive cholangitis: a distinct clinical syndrome. Ann Surg 1959;150:299–303.

19 O'Connor MJ, Schwartz ML, McQuarrie DG, Sumner HW. Cholangitis due to malignant obstruction of biliary outflow. Ann Surg 1981;193:341–345.

20 Scully RE, Mark EJ, McNeely WF, McNeely BU. Case records of the Massachusetts General Hospital. N Engl J Med 1990;323:467–475.

21 Uflacker R, Wholey MH, Amaral NM, Lima S. Parasitic and mycotic causes of biliary obstruction. Gastrointest Radiol 1982;7:173–179.

22 Ovnat A, Peiser J, Avinoah E, Barki Y, Charuzi I. Acute cholangitis caused by ruptured hydatid cyst. Surgery 1984;95: 497–500.

23 Lygidakis NJ. Septic cholangitis as a complication of intrabiliary rupture of hydatid cysts of the liver. Br J Clin Pract 1984;38: 57–61.

24 Robert J-Y, Bretagne J-F, Raoul J-L, Siproudhis L, Heresbach D, Gosselin M. Recurrent cholangitis caused by the migration of pancreatic calculi associated with pancreas divisum. Gastrointest Endosc 1993;39:452–454.

25 Harris AI, Korsten MA. Acute suppurative cholangitis secondary to calcific pancreatitis. Gastroenterology 1976;71: 847–850.

26 Irani M, Truong LD. Candidiasis of the extrahepatic biliary tract. Arch Pathol Lab Med 1986;110:1087–1090.

27 Dineen P. The importance of the route of infection in experimental biliary tract obstruction. Surg Gynecol Obstet 1964;119: 1001–1008.

28 Scott AJ, Khan GA. Origin of bacteria in bileduct bile. Lancet 1967;2:790–792.

29 Cetta F. The route of infection in patients with bactibilia. World J Surg 1983;7:562. (Editorial).

30 Sung JY, Shaffer EA, Olson ME, Leung JWC, Lam K, Costerton JW. Bacterial invasion of the biliary system by way of the portal-venous system. Hepatology 1991; 14:313–317.

31 Williams RD, Fish JC, Williams DD. The significance of biliary pressure. Arch Surg 1967;95:374–379.

32 Huang T, Bass JA, Williams RD. The significance of biliary pressure in cholangitis. Arch Surg 1969;98:629–632.

33 Lygidakis NJ, Brummelkamp WH. The significance of intrabiliary pressure in acute cholangitis. Surg Gynecol Obstet 1985;161:465–469.

34 Csendes A, Sepulveda A, Burdiles P, et al. Common bile duct pressure in patients with common bile duct stones with or without acute suppurative

cholangitis. Arch Surg 1988;123:697–699.

35 Lygidakis NJ. Incidence of bile infection in patients with choledocholithiasis. Am J Gastroenterol 1982;77:12–17.

36 Raper SE, Barker ME, Jones AL, Way LW. Anatomic correlates of bacterial cholangiovenous reflux. Surgery 1989; 105:352–359.

37 Mackie R, Sievert C, Thorson B, Gerding D, Vennes JA. Quantitation of bacteremia secondary to retrograde biliary flow. Gastrointest Endosc 1982;28:138. (Abstract).

38 Jackaman FR, Hilson GRF, Marlow LS. Bile bacteria in patients with benign bile duct stricture. Br J Surg 1980;67:329–332.

39 Scott AJ. Bacteria and disease of the biliary tract. Gut 1971;12:487–492.

40 Edlund YA, Mollstedt BO, Ouchterlony O. Bacteriological investigation of the biliary system and liver in biliary tract disease correlated to clinical data and microstructure of the gallbladder and liver. Acta Chir Scand 1958/1959;116:461–476.

41 Dye M, MacDonald A, Smith G. The bacterial flora of the biliary tract and liver in man. Br J Surg 1978;65:285–287.

42 Nielsen ML, Justesen T. Anaerobic and aerobic bacteriological studies in biliary tract disease. Scand J Gastroenterol 1976; 11:437–446.

43 Shimada K, Urayama K, Noro T, Inamatsu T. Biliary tract infection with anaerobes and the presence of free bile acids in bile. Rev Infect Dis 1984;6:S147–S151.

44 Fukunaga FH. Gallbladder bacteriology, histology, and gallstones: study of unselected cholecystectomy specimens in Honolulu. Arch Surg 1973;106:169–171.

45 Anderson RE, Priestley JT. Observations of the bacteriology of choledochal bile. Ann Surg 1951;133:486–489.

46 Flemma RJ, Flint LM, Osterhout S, Shingleton WW. Bacteriologic studies of biliary tract infection. Ann Surg 1967; 166:563–572.

47 Engstrom J, Hellstrom K, Hogman L, Lonnqvist B. Microorganisms of the liver, biliary tract and duodenal aspirates in biliary diseases. Scand J Gastroenterol 1971; 6:177–182.

48 Elkeles G, Mirizzi PL. A study of the bacteriology of the common bile duct in comparison with the other extrahepatic segments of the biliary tract. Ann Surg 1942;116:360–366.

49 Orloff MJ, Peskin GW, Ellis HL. A bacteriologic study of human portal blood: implications regarding hepatic ischemia in man. Ann Surg 1958;148:738–746.

50 Drivas G, James O, Wardle N. Study of reticuloendothelial phagocytic capacity in patients with cholestasis. Br Med J 1976; 1:1568–1569.

51 Katz S, Grosfeld JL, Gross K, et al. Impaired bacterial clearance and trapping in obstructive jaundice. Ann Surg 1984;199: 14–20.

52 Plaut AG, Gorbach SL, Nahas L, Weinstein L, Spanknebel G, Levitan R. Studies of intestinal microflora. III. The microbial flora of human small intestinal mucosa and fluids. Gastroenterology 1967;53:868–873.

53 Kalser MH, Cohen R, Arteaga I, et al. Normal viral and bacterial flora of the human small and large intestine. N Engl J Med 1966;274:500–505;558–563.

54 Charcot JM. Lecons sur les maladies du foie des voices bilars et des reins. Faculte de Medicine de Paris. Recueillies et publiees par Bournville et Sevestre, 1877.

55 Pessa ME, Hawkins IF, Vogel SB. The treatment of acute cholangitis: percutaneous transhepatic biliary drainage before definitive therapy. Ann Surg 1987;205: 389–392.

56 Lamont JT. Cholestasis: medical or surgical? Hosp Pract 1985;82A–82EE.

57 Kalser MH. Cholangitis: clinical aspects and medical management. In: Berl JE, ed. Bockus, Gastroenterology, 4th ed. Philadelphia: WB Saunders, 1985:3717–3724.

58 Taylor TV, Sumerling MD, Carter DC, McLoughlin GP, Miller AM. An evaluation of ^{99}Tc^m-labelled HIDA in hepatobiliary scanning. Br J Surg 1980;67:325–328.

59 Nahrwold DL. Cholangitis. In: Sabiston DC Jr. Textbook of Surgery—the Biological Basis of Modern Surgical Practice, 14th ed. Philadelphia: WB Saunders, 1991: 1064–1069.

60 Kaplun L, Weissmann HS, Rosenblatt RR, Freeman LM. The early diagnosis of common bile duct obstruction using cholescintigraphy. JAMA 1985;254:2431–2434.

61 Taylor KW, Rosenfield AT. Grey-scale ultrasonography in the differential diag-

nosis of jaundice. Arch Surg 1977;112: 820–825.

62 Taylor KJW, Rosenfield AT, Spiro HM. Diagnostic accuracy of gray scale ultrasonography for the jaundiced patient: a report of 275 cases. Arch Intern Med 1979;139:60–63.

63 Berk RN, Cooperberg PL, Gold RP, Rohrmann CA, Ferrucci JT Jr. Radiography of the bile ducts: a symposium on the use of new modalities for diagnosis and treatment. Radiology 1982;145:1–9.

64 Cronan JJ, Mueller PR, Simeone JF, et al. Prospective diagnosis of choledocholithiasis. Radiology 1983;146:467–469.

65 Gross BH, Harter LP, Gore RM, et al. Ultrasonic evaluation of common bile duct stones: prospective comparison with endoscopic retrograde cholangiopancreatography. Radiology 1983;146:471–474.

66 Laing FC, Jeffrey RB Jr. Choledocholithiasis and cystic duct obstruction: difficult ultrasonographic diagnosis. Radiology 1983;146:475–479.

67 Honickman SP, Mueller PR, Wittenberg J, et al. Ultrasound in obstructive jaundice: prospective evaluation of site and cause. Radiology 1983;147:511–515.

68 Einstein DM, Lapin SA, Ralls PW, Halls JM. The insensitivity of sonography in the detection of choledocholithiasis. Am J Roentgenol 1984;142:725–728.

69 Mitchell SE, Clark RA. A comparison of computed tomography and sonography in choledocholithiasis. Am J Roentgenol 1984;142:729–733.

70 Baron RL, Stanley RJ, Lee JKT, et al. A prospective comparison of the evaluation of biliary obstruction using computed tomography and ultrasonography. Radiology 1982;145:91–98.

71 Tobin MV, Mendelson RM, Lamb GH, Gilmore IT. Ultrasound diagnosis of bile duct calculi. Br Med J 1986;293:16–17.

72 Gibson RN, Yeung E, Thompson JN, et al. Bile duct obstruction: radiologic evaluation of level, cause, and tumor resectability. Radiology 1986;160:43–47.

73 Laing FC, Jeffrey RB, Wing VW. Improved visualization of choledocholithiasis by sonography. Am J Roentgenol 1984;143:949–952.

74 Cronan JJ. US diagnosis of choledocholithiasis: a reappraisal. Radiology 1986;161:133–134.

75 Gaines P, Markham N, Leung J, Metreweli C. The thick common bile duct in pyogenic cholangitis. Clin Radiol 1991; 44:175–177.

76 Balthazar EJ, Birnbaum BA, Naidich M. Acute cholangitis: CT evaluation. J Comput Assist Tomogr 1993;17:283–289.

77 Mueller PR. Imaging in obstructive jaundice. In: Taveras JM, Ferrucci JT, eds. Radiology, Diagnosis-Imaging-Intervention, vol. 4. Philadelphia: JB Lippincott, 1991;69:1–13.

78 Summerfield JA. Biliary obstruction is best managed by endoscopists. Gut 1988; 29:741–745.

79 Lai ECS, Lo C-M, Choi T-K, Cheng W-K, Fan S-T, Wong J. Urgent biliary decompression after endoscopic retrograde cholangiopancreatography. Am J Surg 1989;157:121–125.

80 Deviere J, Motte S, Dumonceau JM, Serruys E, Thys JP, Cremer M. Septicemia after endoscopic retrograde cholangiopancreatography. Endoscopy 1990;22: 72–75.

81 Harbin WP, Mueller PR, Ferrucci JT Jr. Transhepatic cholangiography: complications and use patterns of the fine-needle technique. Radiology 1980;135:15–22.

82 Lewis RT, Goodall RG, Marien B, Park M, Lloyd-Smith W, Wiegand FM. Biliary bacteria, antibiotic use, and wound infection in surgery of the gallbladder and common bile duct. Arch Surg 1987;122: 44–47.

83 Lau WY, Chu KW, Yuen WK, Poon GP, Hwang JST, Li AKC. Operative choledochoscopy in patients with acute cholangitis: a prospective, randomized study. Br J Surg 1991;78:1226–1229.

84 Gould RJ, Vogelzang RL, Neiman HL, Pearl GJ, Poticha SM. Percutaneous biliary drainage as an initial therapy in sepsis of the biliary tract. Surg Gynecol Obstet 1985;160:523–527.

85 Pitt HA, Postier RG, Cameron JL. Consequences of preoperative cholangitis and its treatment on the outcome of operation for choledocholithiasis. Surgery 1983;94: 447–452.

86 Leese T, Neoptolemos JP, Baker AR, Carr-Locke DL. Management of acute cholangitis and the impact of endoscopic sphincterotomy. Br J Surg 1986;73:988–992.

87 Lai ECS, Paterson IA, Tam PC, Choi TK, Fan ST, Wong J. Severe acute cholangitis:

the role of emergency nasobiliary drainage. Surgery 1990;107:268–272.

88   Lai ECS, Mok FPT, Tan ESY, et al. Endoscopic biliary drainage for severe acute cholangitis. N Engl J Med 1992; 326:1582–1586.

89   Maddocks AC, Hilson GRF, Taylor R. The bacteriology of the obstructed biliary tree. Ann Roy Coll Surg Engl 1973;52:316–319.

90   Pitt HA, Postier RG, Cameron JL. Biliary bacteria: significance and alterations after antibiotic therapy. Arch Surg 1982;117:445–449.

91   Siegman-Igra Y, Schwartz D, Konforti N, Perluk C, Rozin RR. Septicemia from biliary tract infection. Arch Surg 1988;123:366–368.

92   Shimada K, Inamatsu T, Yamashiro M. Anaerobic bacteria in biliary disease in elderly patients. J Infect Dis 1977;135:850–854.

93   England DM, Rosenblatt JE. Anaerobes in human biliary tracts. J Clin Microbiol 1977;6:494–498.

94   Bourgault A-M, England DM, Rosenblatt JE, Forgacs P, Bieger RC. Clinical characteristics of anaerobic bactibilia. Arch Intern Med 1979;139:1346–1349.

95   Brook I, Altman RP. The significance of anaerobic bacteria in biliary tract infection after hepatic portoenterostomy for biliary atresia. Surgery 1984;95:281–283.

96   Morris AB, Sands ML, Shiraki M, Brown RB, Ryczak M. Gallbladder and biliary tract candidiasis: nine cases and review. Rev Infect Dis 1990;12:483–489.

97   Mason GR. Bacteriology and antibiotic selection in biliary tract surgery. Arch Surg 1968;97:533–537.

98   Armstrong CP, Dixon JM, Duffy SW, Elton RA, Taylor TV, Davies GC. Choledochotomy and sepsis in benign biliary disease. J Royal Coll Surg Edinb 1985;30:343–347.

99   Engstrom J, Groth C-G, Lundh G, Lonnqvist B. Infectious complications after surgery for biliary calculus: the significance of bacteria in the biliary tract. Acta Chir Scand 1972;138:357–361.

100   Jarvinen H. Abnormal liver function tests in acute cholangitis; the predicting of common duct stones. Ann Clin Res 1978; 10:323–327.

101   Dumont AE. Significance of hyperbilirubinemia in acute cholecystitis. Surg Gynecol Obstet 1976;142:855–857.

102   Nolan DJ, Espiner HJ. Compression of the common bile duct in acute cholecystitis. Br J Radiol 1972;45:821–824.

103   Silen W. Cope's Early Diagnosis of the Acute Abdomen, 16th ed. New York: Oxford University Press, 1983:132.

104   Miller DJ, Keeton GR, Webber BL, Saunders SJ. Jaundice in severe bacterial infection. Gastroenterology 1976;71:94–97.

105   Zimmerman HJ, Fang M, Utili R, Seeff LB, Hoofnagle J. Jaundice due to bacterial infection. Gastroenterology 1979;77:362–374.

106   Franson TR, Hierholzer WJ Jr, LaBrecque DR. Frequency and characteristics of hyperbilirubinemia associated with bacteremia. Rev Infect Dis 1985;7:1–9.

107   Sikuler E, Guetta V, Keynan A, Neumann L, Schlaeffer F. Abnormalities in bilirubin and liver enzyme levels in adult patients with bacteremia: a prospective study. Arch Intern Med 1989;149:2246–2248.

108   Utili R, Abernathy CO, Zimmerman HJ. Inhibition of Na^+, K^+-adenosine-triphosphatase by endotoxin: a possible mechanism for endotoxin-induced cholestasis. J Infect Dis 1977;136:583–587.

109   Franson TR, LaBrecque DR, Buggy BP, Harris GJ, Hoffmann RG. Serial bilirubin determinations as a prognostic marker in clinical infections. Am J Med Sci 1989; 297:149–152.

110   Fang MH, Ginsberg AL, Dobbins WO III. Marked elevation in serum alkaline phosphatase activity as a manifestation of systemic infection. Gastroenterology 1980;78:592–597.

111   Lai ECS, Tam P-C, Paterson IA, et al. Emergency surgery for severe acute cholangitis; the high-risk patients. Ann Surg 1990;211:55–59.

112   Schoenfield LJ. Biliary excretion of antibiotics. N Engl J Med 1971;284:1213–1214. (Editorial).

113   Nagar H, Berger SA. The excretion of antibiotics by the biliary tract. Surg Gynecol Obstet 1984;158:601–607.

114   Keighley MRB, Drysdale RB, Quoraishi AH, Burdon DW, Alexander-Williams J. Antibiotic treatment of biliary sepsis. Surg Clin North Am 1975;55:1379–1390.

115   Keighley MRB, Drysdale RB, Quoraishi AH, Burdon DW, Alexander-Williams J. Antibiotics in biliary disease: the relative importance of antibiotic concentra-

tions in the bile and serum. Gut 1976; 17:495–500.

116   Dooley JS, Hamilton-Miller JMT, Brumfitt W, Sherlock S. Antibiotics in the treatment of biliary infection. Gut 1984; 25:988–998.

117   Leung JWC, Chan RCY, Ling TKW, Chung SCS, French GL. The role of antibiotic prophylaxis in biliary obstruction. Gastrointest Endosc 1987;33:155. (Abstract).

118   Muller EL, Pitt HA, Thompson JE, Doty JE, Mann LL, Manchester B. Antibiotics in infections of the biliary tract. Surg Gynecol Obstet 1987;165:285–292.

119   Thompson JE Jr, Pitt HA, Doty JE, Coleman J, Irving C. Broad spectrum penicillin as an adequate therapy for acute cholangitis. Surg Gynecol Obstet 1990; 171:275–282.

120   Gerecht WB, Henry NK, Hoffman WW, et al. Arch Intern Med 1989;149:1279–1284.

121   French GL, Chan RCY, Chung SCS, Leung JWC. Antibiotics for cholangitis. Lancet 1989;2:1271–1272. (Letter).

122   Handwerger S, Raucher B, Altarac D, et al. Nosocomial outbreak due to *Enterococcus faecium* highly resistant to vancomycin, penicillin, and gentamicin. Clin Infect Dis 1993;16:750–755.

123   Moellering RC Jr. Emergence of *Enterococcus* as a significant pathogen. Clin Infect Dis 1992;14:1173–1176.

124   Graninger W, Ragette R. Nosocomial bacteremia due to *Enterococcus faecalis* without endocarditis. Clin Infect Dis 1992; 15:49–57.

125   Norris S, Nightingale CH, Mandell GL. Tables of antimicrobial agent pharmacology. In: Mandell GL, Douglas RG Jr, Bennett JE, eds. Principles and Practice of Infectious Diseases, 3rd ed. New York: Churchill Livingstone, 1990:434–460.

126   Rogers L. Biliary abscesses of the liver: with operation. Br Med J 1903;2:706–707.

127   Scobie BA, Summerskill WHJ. Hepatic cirrhosis secondary to obstruction of the biliary system. Am J Digest Dis 1965;10: 135–146.

128   Csendes A, Diaz JC, Burdiles P, Maluenda F, Morales E. Risk factors and classification of acute suppurative cholangitis. Br J Surg 1992;79:655–658.

129   Thompson JN, Edwards WH, Winearls CG, Blenkharn JI, Benjamin IS, Blumgart LH. Renal impairment following biliary tract surgery. Br J Surg 1987; 74:843–847.

130   Pitt HA, Cameron JL, Postier RG, Gadacz TR. Factors affecting mortality in biliary tract surgery. Am J Surg 1981;141:66–72.

131   Blamey SL, Fearon KCH, Gilmour WH, Osborne DH, Carter DC. Prediction of risk in biliary surgery. Br J Surg 1983;70: 535–538.

132   Dixon JM, Armstrong CP, Duffy SW, Davies GC. Factors affecting morbidity and mortality after surgery for obstructive jaundice: a review of 373 patients. Gut 1983;24:845–852.

133   Armstrong CP, Dixon JM, Taylor TV, Davies GC. Surgical experience of deeply jaundiced patients with bile duct obstruction. Br J Surg 1984;71:234–238.

134   Greig JD, Krukowski ZH, Matheson NA. Surgical morbidity and mortality in one hundred and twenty-nine patients with obstructive jaundice. Br J Surg 1988;75: 216–219.

135   Goldman LD, Steer ML, Silen W. Recurrent cholangitis after biliary surgery. Am J Surg 1983;145:450–454.

136   Nakayama T, Ikeda A, Okuda K. Percutaneous transhepatic drainage of the biliary tract. Technique and results in 104 cases. Gastroenterology 1978;74:554–559.

137   Pollock TW, Ring ER, Oleaga JA, Freiman DB, Mullen JL, Rosato EF. Percutaneous decompression of benign and malignant biliary obstruction. Arch Surg 1979;114:148–151.

138   Denning DA, Ellison EC, Carey LC. Preoperative percutaneous transhepatic biliary decompression lowers morbidity in patients with obstructive jaundice. Am J Surg 1981;141:61–65.

139   Berquist TH, May GR, Johnson CM, Adson MA, Thistle JL. Percutaneous biliary decompression: internal and external drainage in 50 patients. Am J Roentgenol 1981;136:901–906.

140   Joseph PK, Bizer LS, Sprayregen SS, Gliedman ML. Percutaneous transhepatic biliary drainage: results and complications in 81 patients. JAMA 1986; 255:2763–2766.

141   Hatfield ARW, Terblanche J, Fataar S, et al. Preoperative external biliary drainage in obstructive jaundice. A prospective controlled clinical trial. Lancet 1982;2: 896–899.

142   McPherson GAD, Benjamin IS, Hodgson HJF, Bowley NB, Allison DJ, Blumgart LH. Preoperative percutaneous

biliary drainage: the results of a controlled trial. Br J Surg 1984;71:371–375.

143 **Audisio RA, Bozzetti F, Severini A, et al.** The occurrence of cholangitis after percutaneous biliary drainage: evaluation of some risk factors. Surgery 1988;103:507–512.

144 **Ferrucci JT Jr, Mueller PR, Harbin WP.** Percutaneous transhepatic biliary drainage: technique, results, and applications. Radiology 1980;135:1–13.

145 **Classen M, Hagenmuller F.** Biliary drainage. Endoscopy 1983;15:221–229.

146 **Mueller PR, vanSonnenberg E, Ferrucci JT Jr.** Percutaneous biliary drainage: technical and catheter-related problems in 200 procedures. Am J Roentgenol 1982;138:17–23.

147 **Szabo S, Mendelson MH, Mitty HA, Bruckner HW, Hirschman SZ.** Infections associated with transhepatic biliary drainage devices. Am J Med 1987;82:921–926.

148 **Kadir S, Baassiri A, Barth KH, Kaufman SL, Cameron JL, White RI Jr.** Percutaneous biliary drainage in the management of biliary sepsis. Am J Roentgenol 1982;138:25–29.

149 **Lois JF, Gomes AS, Grace PA, Deutsch L-S, Pitt HA.** Risks of percutaneous transhepatic drainage in patients with cholangitis. Am J Roentgenol 1987;148:367–371.

150 **Huang M-H, Ker C-G.** Ultrasonic guided percutaneous transhepatic bile drainage for cholangitis due to intrahepatic stones. Arch Surg 1988;123:106–109.

151 **Palmer KR, Hofmann AF.** Intraductal mono-octanoin for the direct dissolution of bile duct stones: experience in 343 patients. Gut 1986;27:196–202.

152 **Hellstern A, Rubesam D, Leuschner M, Wendt T, Fuchs H, Leuschner U.** Percutaneous transhepatic gallstone dissolution with methyl tert-butyl ether in complicated stone diagnosis and gallbladder anomalies. Endoscopy 1990;22:254–258.

153 **Janssen D, Bommarito A, Lathrop J.** A new technique for the rapid dissolution of retained ductal gallstones with monoctanoin in T-tube patients. Am Surg 1992;58:141–145.

154 **Vaira D, Ainley C, Williams S, et al.** Endoscopic sphincterotomy in 1000 consecutive patients. Lancet 1989;2:431–433.

155 **Sivak MV.** Endoscopic management of bile duct stones. Am J Surg 1989;158:228–240.

156 **Gogel HK, Runyon BA, Volpicelli NA, Palmer RC.** Acute suppurative obstructive cholangitis due to stones: treatment by urgent endoscopic sphinterotomy. Gastrointest Endosc 1987;33:210–213.

157 **Cairns SR, Dias L, Cotton PB, Salmon PR, Russell RCG.** Additional endoscopic procedures instead of urgent surgery for retained common bile duct stones. Gut 1989;30:535–540.

158 **Worthley CS, Toouli J.** Endoscopic decompression for acute cholangitis due to stones. Aust N Z J Surg 1990;60:355–359.

159 **Siegel JH.** Endoscopic papillotomy: a definitive treatment for cholangitis. Gastroenterology 1978;78:1259. (Abstract).

160 **Cotton PB, Lehman G, Vennes J, et al.** Endoscopic sphincterotomy complications and their management: an attempt at consensus. Gastrointest Endosc 1991;37:383–393.

161 **Kracht M, Thompson JN, Bernhoft RA, Tsang V, Gibson RN, Blumgart LH.** Cholangitis after endoscopic sphincterotomy in patients with stricture of the biliary duct. Surg Gynecol Obstet 1986;163:324–326.

162 **Davidson BR, Neoptolemos JP, Carr-Locke DL.** Endoscopic sphincterotomy for common bile duct calculi in patients with gall bladder in situ considered unfit for surgery. Gut 1988;29:114–120.

163 **Deviere J, Devaere S, Baize M, Cremer M.** Endoscopic biliary drainage in chronic pancreatitis. Gastrointest Endosc 1990;36:96–100.

164 **Ditzel H, Schaffalitsky de Muckadell OB.** Endoscopic sphincterotomy in acute cholangitis due to choledocholithiasis. Hepatogastroenterology 1990;37:204–207.

165 **Vallon AG, Shorvon PJ, Cotton PB.** Duodenoscopic treatment of acute cholangitis. Gut 1982;23:A915. (Abstract).

166 **Leung JWC, Chung SCS, Sung JY, Li MKW, Li AKC.** Mortality is reduced by early endoscopic drainage in patients with acute calculous cholangitis with shock. Gastrointest Endosc 1988;34:190. (Abstract).

167 **Leung JWC, Chung SCS, Li AKC.** Urgent endoscopic drainage in acute suppurative cholangitis. Gut 28:A1384. (Abstract).

168 **Siegel JH, Ramsey WH, Pullano W.** Endoscopic management of 947 patients with cholangitis—proven safety and efficacy. Gastrointest Endosc 1986;32:154. (Abstract).

169 **Himal HS, Lindsay T.** Ascending cholangitis: surgery versus endoscopic or percutaneous drainage. Surgery 1990; 108:629–634.

170 **Cotton PB.** Endoscopic management of bile duct stones; (apples and oranges). Gut 1984;25:587–597.

171 **Martin DF, McGregor JC, Lambert ME, Tweedle DEF.** Stone extraction after endoscopic sphincterotomy—an active policy is best. Gut 1990;28:A1360–1361. (Abstract).

172 **Himal HS.** The role of endoscopic papillotomy in ascending cholangitis. Am Surg 1991;57:241–244.

173 **Cotton PB, Burney PGJ, Mason RR.** Transnasal bile duct catheterization after endoscopic sphincterotomy: method for biliary drainage, perfusion, and sequential cholangiography. Gut 1979;20:285–287.

174 **Siegel JH, Harding GT, Chateau F.** Endoscopic decompression and drainage of benign and malignant biliary obstruction. Gastrointest Endosc 1982;28: 79–82.

175 **Soehendra N, Reynders-Frederix V.** Palliative bile duct drainage—a new endoscopic method of introducing a transpapillary drain. Endoscopy 1980;12: 8–11.

176 **Wurbs D, Phillip J, Classen M.** Experiences with the long standing nasobiliary tube in biliary diseases. Endoscopy 1980;12:219–223.

177 **Cotton PB.** Endoscopic methods for relief of malignant obstructive jaundice. World J Surg 1984;8:854–861.

178 **Huibregtse K, Katon RM, Coene PP, Tytgat GNJ.** Endoscopic palliative treatment in pancreatic cancer. Gastrointest Endosc 1986;32:334–338.

179 **Johnson GK, Geenen JE, Venu RP, Hogan WJ.** Endoscopic treatment of biliary duct strictures in sclerosing cholangitis; follow-up assessment of a new therapeutic approach. Gastrointest Endosc 1987;33:9–12.

180 **Geenen DJ, Geenen JE, Hogan WJ, et al.** Endoscopic therapy for benign bile duct strictures. Gastrointest Endosc 1989;35: 367–371.

181 **Berkelhammer C, Kortan P, Haber GB.** Endoscopic biliary prostheses as treatment for benign postoperative bile duct strictures. Gastrointest Endosc 1989;35: 95–101.

182 **Ponchon T, Gallez J-F, Valette P-J, Chavaillon A, Bory R.** Endoscopic treatment of biliary tract fistulas. Gastrointest Endosc 1989;35:490–498.

183 **Kiil J, Kruse A, Rokkjaer M.** Large bile duct stones treated by endoscopic biliary drainage. Surgery 1989;105:51–56.

184 **Foutch PG, Harlan J, Sanowski RA.** Endoscopic placement of biliary stents for treatment of high risk geriatric patients with common duct stones. Am J Gastroenterol 1989;84:527–529.

185 **Cotton PB, Forbes A, Leung JWC, Dineen L.** Endoscopic stenting for long-term treatment of large bile duct stones: 2- to 5-year follow-up. Gastrointest Endosc 1987;33:411–412.

186 **Speer AG, Cotton PB, Russell RCG, et al.** Randomized trial of endoscopic versus percutaneous stent insertion in malignant obstructive jaundice. Lancet 1987;2:57–62.

187 **Leung JWC, Chung SCS, Sung JJY, Banez VP, Li AKC.** Urgent endoscopic drainage for acute suppurative cholangitis. Lancet 1989;1:1307–1309.

188 **Ikeda S, Tanaka M, Itoh H, Kishikawa H, Nakayama F.** Emergency decompression of bile duct in acute obstructive suppurative cholangitis by duodenoscopic cannulation: a lifesaving procedure. World J Surg 1981;5:587–593.

189 **Lin X-Z, Chang K-K, Shin J-S, Chang T-T, Lin C-Y.** Endoscopic nasobiliary drainage for acute suppurative cholangitis: a sonographically guided method. Gastrointest Endosc 1993;39:174–176.

190 **Tai DI, Shen FH, Liaw YF.** Abnormal predrainage serum creatinine as a prognostic indicator in acute cholangitis. Hepatogastroenterology 1992;39:47–50.

191 **Seel DJ, Park YK.** Oriental infestational cholangitis. Am J Surg 1983;146:366–370.

192 **Lim JH.** Oriental cholangiohepatitis: pathologic, clinical, and radiologic features. Am J Roentgenol 1991;157:1–8.

193 **Yellin AE, Donovan AJ.** Biliary lithiasis and helminthiasis. Am J Surg 1981;142: 128–136.

194 **Ong GB.** A study of recurrent pyogenic cholangitis. Arch Surg 1962;84:63–89.

195 **Turner WW Jr, Cramer CR.** Recurrent oriental cholangiohepatitis. Surgery 1983;93: 397–401.

196 **Lim JH, Ko YT, Lee DH, Hong KS.** Oriental cholangiohepatitis: sonographic findings in 48 cases. Am J Roentgenol 1990; 155:511–514.

197 **Chen H-H, Zhang W-H, Wang S-S, Caruana JA.** Twenty-two year experience with the diagnosis and treatment of intrahepatic calculi. Surg Gynecol Obstet 1984;159:519–524.

198 **Fan ST, Lai ECS, Mok FPT, Choi TK, Wong J.** Acute cholangitis secondary to hepatolithiasis. Arch Surg 1991;126:1027–1031.

199 **Wong WT, Teoh-Chan CH, Huang CT, Cheng FCY, Ong GB.** The bacteriology of recurrent pyogenic cholangitis and associated diseases. J Hyg Camb 1981;87:407–412.

200 **Fan ST, Choi TK, Chan FL, Lai ECS, Wong J.** Role of computed tomography in the management of recurrent pyogenic cholangitis. Aust N Z J Surg 1990;60:599–605.

201 **Chan F-L, Man S-W, Leong LLY, Fan S-T.** Evaluation of recurrent pyogenic cholangitis with CT: analysis of 50 patients. Radiology 1989;170:165–169.

202 **Choi TK, Wong J.** Endoscopic retrograde cholangiopancreatography and endoscopic papillotomy in recurrent pyogenic cholangitis. Clin Gastroenterol 1986;15:393–415.

203 **Fan ST, Choi TK, Wong J.** Recurrent pyogenic cholangitis: current management. World J Surg 1991;15:248–253.

204 **Pitlik SD, Fainstein V, Rios A, Guarda L, Mansell PWA, Hersh EM.** Cryptosporidial cholecystitis. N Engl J Med 1983;308:967. (Letter).

205 **Blumberg RS, Kelsey P, Perrone T, Dickersin R, Laquaglia M, Ferruci J.** Cytomegalovirus- and cryptosporidium-associated acalculous gangrenous cholecystitis. Am J Med 1984;76:1118–1123.

206 **Pitlik SD, Fainstein V, Garza D, et al.** Human cryptosporidiosis: spectrum of disease. Arch Intern Med 1983;143:2269–2275.

207 **Guarda LA, Stein SA, Cleary KA, Ordonez NG.** Human cryptosporidiosis in the acquired immune deficiency syndrome. Arch Pathol Lab Med 1983;107:562–566.

208 **Cello JP.** Human immunodeficiency virus-associated biliary tract disease. Semin Liver Dis 1992;12:213–218.

209 **Kavin H, Jonas RB, Chowdhury L, Kabins S.** Acalculous cholecystitis and cytomegalovirus infection in the acquired immunodeficiency syndrome. Ann Intern Med 1986;104:53–54.

210 **Margulis SJ, Honig CL, Soave R, Govoni AF, Mouradian JA, Jacobson IM.** Biliary tract obstruction in the acquired immunodeficiency syndrome. Ann Intern Med 1986;105:207–210.

211 **Wheeler AP, Gregg CR.** Campylobacter bacteremia, cholecystitis, and the acquired immunodeficiency syndrome. Ann Intern Med 1986;105:804. (Letter).

212 **Agha FP, Nostrant TT, Abrams GD, Mazanec M, Van Moll L, Gumucio JJ.** Cytomegalovirus cholangitis in a homosexual man with acquired immune deficiency syndrome. Am J Gastroenterol 1986;81:1068–1072.

213 **Kaplan LD, Kahn J, Jacobson M, Bottles K, Cello J.** Primary bile duct lymphoma in the acquired immunodeficiency syndrome (AIDS). Ann Intern Med 1989;110:161–162.

214 **Stillman AE, Schmid R, Howe JB.** Acquired immunodeficiency syndrome and biliary tract disease. Ann Intern Med 1987;106:634. (Letter).

215 **McWhinney PHM, Nathwani D, Green ST, Boyd JF, Forrest JAH.** Microsporidiosis detected in association with AIDS-related sclerosing cholangitis. AIDS 1991;5:1394–1395.

216 **Beaugerie L, Teilhac M-F, Deluol A-M, et al.** Cholangiopathy associated with *Microsporidia* infection of the common bile duct mucosa in a patient with HIV infection. Ann Intern Med 1992;117:401–402.

217. **Pol S, Romana C, Richard S, et al.** *Enterocytozoon bieneusi* infection in acquired immunodeficiency syndrome-related sclerosing cholangitis. Gastroenterology 1992;102:1778–1781.

218 **McWhinney PHM, Green ST, Kennedy D, Love WC.** Decline in immunoglobulins associated with AIDS-related biliary disease. AIDS 1991;6:520–522.

219 **Viteri AL, Greene JF Jr.** Bile duct abnormalities in the acquired immune deficiency syndrome. Gastroenterology 1987;92:2014–2018.

220 **Dowsett JF, Miller R, Davidson R, et al.** Sclerosing cholangitis in acquired immunodeficiency syndrome: case reports and review of the literature. Scand J Gastroenterol 1988;23:1267–1274.

221 **Kline TJ, De Las Morenas T, O'Brien M, Smith BF, Afdhal NH.** Squamous metaplasia of extrahepatic biliary system in an

AIDS patient with cryptosporidia and cholangitis. Digest Dis Sci 1993;38:960–962.

222 Keshavjee SH, Magee LA, Mullen BJ, Baron DL, Brunton JL, Gallinger S. Acalculous cholecystitis associated with cytomegalovirus and sclerosing cholangitis in a patient with acquired immunodeficiency syndrome. Can J Surg 1993;36:321–325.

223 Mercey D, Loveday C, Miller RF. Sclerosing cholangitis rapidly following anti-HIV-1 seroconversion. Genitourin Med 1991;67:239–243.

224 Iannuzzi C, Belghiti J, Erlinger S, Menu Y, Fekete F. Cholangitis associated with cholecystitis in patients with acquired immunodeficiency syndrome. Arch Surg 1990;125:1211–1213.

225 Cockerill FR III, Hurley DV, Malagelada J-R, et al. Polymicrobial cholangitis and Kaposi's sarcoma in blood product transfusion-related acquired immune deficiency syndrome. Am J Med 1986;80:1237–1241.

226 Gross TL, Wheat J, Bartlett M, O'Connor KW. AIDS and multiple system involvement with cryptosporidium. Am J Gastroenterol 1986;81:456–458.

227 Aaron JS, Wynter CD, Kirton OC, Simko V. Cytomegalovirus associated with acalculous cholecystitis in a patient with acquired immune deficiency syndrome. Am J Gastroenterol 1988;83:879–881.

228 Radin DR, Cohen H, Halls JM. Acalculous inflammatory disease of the biliary tree in acquired immunodeficiency syndrome: CT demonstration. J Comput Assist Tomogr 1987;11:775–778.

229 Hinnant K, Schwartz A, Rotterdam H, Rudski C. Cytomegaloviral and cryptosporidial cholecystitis in two patients with AIDS. Am J Surg Pathol 1989;13:57–60.

230 Hamour AA, Bonnington A, Hawthorne B, Wilkins GL. Successful treatment of AIDS-related cryptosporidial sclerosing cholangitis. AIDS 1993;7:1449–1451.

231 Forbes A, Blanchard C, Gazzard B. Natural history of AIDS related sclerosing cholangitis: a study of 20 cases. Gut 1993;34:116–121.

232 Pol S, Romana CA, Richard S, et al. Microsporidia infection in patients with the human immunodeficiency virus and unexplained cholangitis. N Engl J Med 1993;328:95–99.

233 Cello JP. Acquired immunodeficiency syndrome cholangiopathy: spectrum of disease. Am J Med 1989;86:539–546.

234 Defalque D, Menu Y, Girard P-M, Coulaud J-P. Sonographic diagnosis of cholangitis in AIDS patients. Gastrointest Radiol 1989;14:143–147.

235 Roulot D, Valla D, Brun-Vezinet F, et al. Cholangitis in the acquired immunodeficiency syndrome: report of two cases and review of the literature. Gut 1987;28:1653–1660.

236 Schneiderman DJ, Cello JP, Laing FC. Papillary stenosis and sclerosing cholangitis in the acquired immunodeficiency syndrome. Ann Intern Med 1987;106:546–549.

237 McCarty M, Choudhri AH, Helbert M, Crofton ME. Radiological features of AIDS related cholangitis. Clin Radiol 1989;40:582–585.

238 Kahn DG, Garfinkle JM, Klonoff DC, Pembrook LJ, Morrow DJ. Cryptosporidial and cytomegaloviral hepatitis and cholecystitis. Arch Pathol Lab Med 1987;111:879–881.

239 Hasan FA, Jeffers LJ, Dickinson G, et al. Hepatobiliary cryptosporidiosis and cytomegalovirus infection mimicking metastatic cancer to the liver. Gastroenterology 1991;100:1743–1748.

240 Hinnant KL, Rotterdam HZ, Bell ET, Tapper ML. Cytomegalovirus infection of the alimentary tract: a clinicopathological correlation. Am J Gastroenterol 1986;81:944–950.

241 Teixidor HS, Honig CL, Norsoph E, Albert S, Mouradian JA, Whalen JP. Cytomegalovirus infection of the alimentary canal: radiologic findings with pathologic correlation. Radiology 1987;163:317–323.

242 Thuluvath PJ, Connolly GM, Forbes A, Gazzard BG. Abdominal pain in HIV infection. Q J Med 1991;78:275–285.

243 Saraux J-L, Lenoble L, Toublanc M, Smiejan J-M, Dombret M-C. Acalculous cholecystitis and cytomegalovirus infection in a patient with AIDS. J Infect Dis 1987;155:829. (Letter).

244 Robinson G, Wilson SE, Williams RA. Surgery in patients with acquired immunodeficiency syndrome. Arch Surg 1987;122:170–175.

245 Jacobson MA, Cello JP, Sande MA. Cholestasis and disseminated cytomegalovirus disease in patients with the acquired immunodeficiency syndrome. Am J Med 1988;84:218–224.

246 **Teixidor HS, Godwin TA, Ramirez EA.** Cryptosporidiosis of the biliary tract in AIDS. Radiology 1991;180:51–56.

247 **Lebovics E, Dworkin BM, Heier SK, Rosenthal WS.** The hepatobiliary manifestations of human immunodeficiency virus infection. Am J Gastroenterol 1988; 83:1–5.

248 **Dolmatch BL, Laing FC, Federle MP, Jeffrey RB, Cello J.** AIDS-related cholangitis: radiographic findings in nine patients. Radiology 1987;163:313–316.

249 **DaSilva F, Boudghene F, Lecomte I, Delage Y, Grange J-D, Bigot J-M.** Sonography in AIDS-related cholangitis: prevalence and cause of an echogenic nodule in the distal end of the common bile duct. Am J Roentgenol 1993;160:1205–1207.

250 **Romano AJ, vanSonnenberg E, Casola G, et al.** Gallbladder and bile duct abnormalities in AIDS: sonographic findings in eight patients. AJR Am J Roentgenol 1988; 150:123–127.

251 **Wall SD.** Gastrointestinal imaging in AIDS—luminal gastrointestinal tract. Gastroenterol Clin North Am 1988;17: 523–533.

252 **Schneiderman DJ.** Hepatobiliary abnormalities of AIDS. Gastroenterol Clin North Am 1988;17:615–630.

253 **Quinn D, Pocock N, Freund J, Kelleher A, Penny R, Brew B.** Radionuclide hepatobiliary scanning in patients with AIDS-related sclerosing cholangitis. Clin Nucl Med 1993;18:417–422.

Septic Thrombophlebitis of Major Dural Venous Sinuses

FREDERICK S. SOUTHWICK

Septic thrombosis of the dural venous sinuses is rare. Several hundred cases have been reported in the English medical literature during the antibiotic era (1948 to the present). Because each clinician is likely to encounter only one case during his or her career, the possibility of this diagnosis is generally not initially considered, and the neurologic consequences of septic thrombosis of the major veins in the cerebral cortex is often misinterpreted. As a result, diagnosis is often delayed. The hallmark of septic dural sinus thrombosis is headache. This symptom combined with evidence of infection in a primary site (face, air sinuses, and middle ear) known to predispose to dural sinus thrombosis should alert the physician to this often devastating complication. Severe neurologic complications and death are too often the consequences of delayed diagnosis. With the advent of the computerized tomography (CT) scan and magnetic resonance imaging (MRI), appropriate methods are now available to rapidly and accurately diagnose dural sinus thrombosis. The major purpose of this review is to familiarize the clinician with the neuroanatomy, pathogenesis, clinical manifestations, diagnostic approach, and treatment of this rare but challenging group of diseases.

ANATOMIC CONSIDERATIONS

Understanding the anatomy of the dural sinuses and their intimate relationship to the many vital cranial nerves, as well as the importance of the superior sagittal and lateral sinuses to cerebrospinal fluid (CSF) flow, allows the physician to better appreciate the myriad of sometimes confusing manifestations associated with septic dural sinus thrombosis.

The cavernous sinuses are the most centrally located of the dural sinuses (Figures 8.1 and 8.2). These irregularly shaped sinuses contain multiple trabeculae that act as sieves trapping any particulate matter from the blood. The two

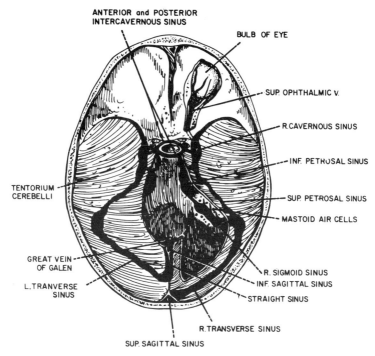

ANTERIOR and POSTERIOR
INTERCAVERNOUS SINUS

BULB OF EYE

SUP. OPHTHALMIC V.

R.CAVERNOUS SINUS

INF. PETROSAL SINUS

SUP. PETROSAL SINUS

MASTOID AIR CELLS

TENTORIUM
CEREBELLI

GREAT VEIN
OF GALEN

L.TRANVERSE
SINUS

R. SIGMOID SINUS
INF. SAGITTAL SINUS
STRAIGHT SINUS

R.TRANSVERSE SINUS

SUP. SAGITTAL SINUS

Figure 8.1.   Horizontal cross section of the skull demonstrates the locations of the major dural sinuses. The superior opthalmic vein can be seen draining into the right cavernous sinus. Also note the close proximity of mastoid air cells to the sigmoid sinus (right side).

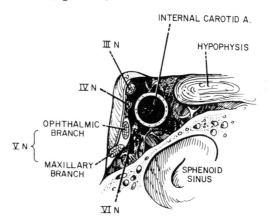

INTERNAL CAROTID A.

III N

HYPOPHYSIS

IV N

OPHTHALMIC
BRANCH

V N

MAXILLARY
BRANCH

SPHENOID
SINUS

VI N

Figure 8.2.   Anteroposterior vertical cross section through the right cavernous sinus. Multiple cranial nerves as well as the internal carotid artery pass within the sinus. Note the more medial location of the sixth nerve as compared to the other cranial nerves. Also note the proximity of the sphenoid air sinus and pituitary gland (hypophysis) to cavernous sinus.

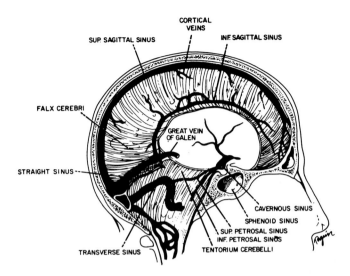

Figure 8.3. Lateral cross section of the skull demonstrates the major dural venous sinuses. Note that anterior segment of the superior sagittal sinus is near the frontal air sinus.

cavernous sinuses lie inferior to the superior sagittal sinus, positioned just lateral to the base of the sella turcica. They also lie just lateral and superior to the sphenoid air sinuses. The two cavernous sinuses are connected by intercavernous sinuses that pass anteriorly and posteriorly to the sella turcica and pituitary gland. A number of cranial nerves are attached by fibrous sheaths along the lateral wall of each cavernous sinus. The oculomotor nerve (III) is most superior followed by the trochear nerve (IV) and the opthalmic (V_1) and maxillary branches (V_2) of the trigeminal nerve. The abducens nerve (VI) is found in a more medial position near the internal carotid artery. The cavernous sinuses receive blood from the facial veins via the inferior and superior oph-thalmic veins. Blood from the cavernous sinuses normally drains into the superior and inferior petrosal sinuses, which connect to the sigmoid sinus and jugular vein, respectively (1–3).

The superior sagittal sinus is the largest venous sinus draining the brain. This sinus begins in the frontal region near the frontal air sinus, where it receives blood from the nasal septum via ethmoid veins. It also receives blood from the frontal, parietal, and occipital superior cortical veins as well as the diploic veins, which communicate with the meningeal veins (Figures 8.1 and 8.3). This sinus also plays an important role in draining the CSF. The arachnoid villi, which are responsible for CSF resorption, empty here. The superior sagittal sinus is triangular on cross section and progressively increases in diameter anastomosing with the one or both lateral (transverse) sinuses in the occipital region (1).

The lateral dural sinuses begin in the occipital protuberance and are arranged in several different configurations (see Figures 8.1 and 8.3). In 50% of people the right lateral sinus receives all the blood draining from the superior sagittal sinus. In this circumstance the left lateral sinus is smaller and receives blood from the straight sinus. This has been termed a right dominant circulation. The opposite configuration, called left dominant, is less common; a third configuration, a confluens in which all four vessels interconnect, is even rarer. Occasionally, only one lateral sinus is present and is responsible for draining both the superior sagittal and straight sinuses. Later in its course each lateral sinus passes near the middle ear and mastoid air cells where it receives blood from emissary veins draining from these sites. On leaving the tentorium, the lateral sinus becomes the sigmoid sinus, which curves inferiorly and medially draining into the jugular vein (1,4,5).

Two other important anatomic considerations must be kept in mind when trying to understand septic dural sinus thrombosis. First, the cerebral veins and venous sinuses contain no valves. Therefore, blood and infection can spread in either direction depending on pressure gradients. Secondly, in addition to the larger vessels described above there are many smaller venous channels. With time these veins may enlarge to form collateral channels that in some instances can relieve the obstructive symptoms and signs associated with acute dural sinus thrombosis (1).

SEPTIC CAVERNOUS SINUS THROMBOSIS

Septic dural sinus thrombosis occurs most frequently in the cavernous sinuses. These trabeculated venous channels can readily trap bacteria and thrombus (2,6–81).

Primary Sites of Infection

Infections of the medial third of the face including the nose, orbits, tonsils, and soft palate can spread to the cavernous sinuses via the facial veins or pterygoid plexus, which drain into the superior or inferior ophthalmic veins. Nasal furuncles caused by *Staphylococcus aureus* are among the most common infections associated with this complication, particularly if the furuncle is squeezed or drained in the absence of antibiotic coverage. Approximately 50% of cases of septic cavernous sinus thrombosis are preceded by facial infection. The second most common primary infection associated with this complication is sphenoid sinusitis (approximately 30% of cases). Infection at this site can spread via emissary veins or spread directly by breaking through the lateral air sinus wall, which lies next to the cavernous sinus (see Figure 8.2). Sphenoid sinusitis is frequently misdiagnosed and therefore treatment often delayed. The primary symptom, severe retroorbital or hemicranial headache, is frequently mistaken for a migraine headache. In addition, because this sinus lies deep below the sella turcica, routine sinus films may fail to adequately visualize the sphenoid sinus. When sphenoid sinusitis is being considered, an overpenetrated lateral sinus film should be ordered (82). Early recognition and treatment of sphenoid sinusitis is critical for preventing the high morbidity and mortality associated with cavernous sinus thrombosis (82). Dental infection is the third most common primary infection that can lead to cavernous sinus disease (approximately 10% of cases). Infection spreads to the cavernous sinus via the pterygoid venous plexus. Septic cavernous sinus thrombosis is the most common fatal infectious complication associated with dental infection (83). Although common in the preantibiotic era, otitis media now rarely results in cavernous sinus disease. In this earlier era, infection could spread unchecked from the lateral and sigmoid sinuses to the cavernous sinus via the inferior petrosal sinus.

Symptoms and History of Underlying Disease

Headache is the most common early symptom. The pain is usually described as sharp and steadily increasing in severity. The headache often interferes with sleep and is not relieved by conventional pain medication, forcing the patient to seek medical attention. The pain is generally restricted to the areas innervated by the ophthalmic and maxillary branches of the fifth nerve. The headache, therefore, is usually unilateral and involves the frontal or retroorbital regions, occasionally radiating to the occipital region. Retro-orbital pain can be associated with tearing of the eye and lead the physician incorrectly to suspect ocular migraine (81). In many instances, particularly early in the presentation, this symptom may primarily reflect sphenoid sinus infection (82).

Headache generally precedes fever and periorbital edema by several days. In rare cases of subacute cavernous sinus thrombosis, headache may persist for up to 6 months before eye signs develop (81). Initially, periorbital edema is almost always unilateral. However in acute septic cavernous sinus thrombosis, within 24 hours infection spreads via the intercavernous sinuses to the other eye, resulting in bilateral eye symptoms. In addition to periorbital edema, patients may complain of diplopia. Other less common complaints include photophobia, eye tearing, and ptosis. Change in mental status such as drowsiness, confusion and inappropriate behavior may rapidly follow eye complaints, particularly in fatal cases.

A history of predisposing illness is noted in approximately 25% of cases, diabetes mellitus and chronic sinusitis being most common.

Physical Findings

At the time of presentation nearly all patients are febrile, suggesting an infectious process. Abnormalities are generally found on examination of the face, nose, and throat. A facial cellulitis often associated with nasal furuncles is frequently noted when facial infection leads to cavernous sinus disease. Purulent exudate draining from the nose or into the posterior pharynx are commonly seen in cases caused by bacterial sinusitis. Tenderness of the frontal or maxillary sinus may also be found because sphenoid sinusitis is commonly associated with pansinusitis. Nuchal rigidity has been noted in over one third of patients, indicating inflammation of the meninges. Depression of mental status also occurs in over 50% of patients. Initial lethargy often progresses to coma during the course of treatment. Hemiparesis and seizures are less commonly observed, generally resulting from ischemic cerebral infarcts due to partial or complete occlusion of the intracavernous segment of the carotid artery.

Eye Findings   The classic constellation of ptosis, proptosis, chemosis, and ocular-muscle paralysis is also present in the majority of cases. Exophthalmos and chemosis, manifestations of periorbital edema, in all likelihood result from occlusion of the opthalmic veins (Figure 8.4). Chemosis can be marked and in one case was mistakenly diagnosed as allergic blepharitis (81).

Signs of periorbital edema are usually rapidly followed by impairment in eye movements. Generally all ocular muscles become paralyzed. Cranial nerves III, IV, and VI all pass through the cavernous sinus and suffer damage from the inflammatory exudate caused by the infection. Cranial nerve III, also called the oculomotor nerve, innervates the medial, superior, and inferior recti as well as the inferior oblique eye muscles. These muscles are critical for both vertical and horizontal gaze. In addition, cranial nerve III innervates the levator palpebrae superioris muscle, which raises the eyelid. Finally this nerve carries the para-

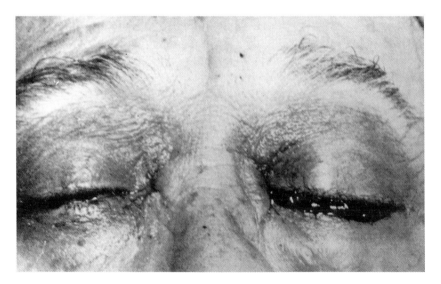

Figure 8.4.   Face of a patient with septic cavernous sinus thrombosis. Note the bilateral periorbital edema as well as chemosis and proptosis of the left eye.

sympathetic fibers to the ciliary ganglion whose postganglionic fibers innervate the sphincter muscle of the iris. Cranial nerve IV, the trochlear nerve, innervates the superior oblique muscle important for outward and downward gaze; and cranial nerve VI, the abducens nerve, innervates the lateral rectus muscle, important for lateral gaze. Dysfunction of all these nerves, therefore, results in complete ophthalmoplegia, dilatation of the pupil (mydriasis), and drooping of the eyelid (ptosis). Although ophthalmoplegia and ptosis are described in nearly all cases, dilated or sluggishly reactive pupils have been reported in only one third of patients.

In rare cases of chronic septic cavernous sinus thrombosis isolated sixth nerve dysfunction has been reported (76,81), in one case associated with Horner's syndrome (76). In some instances lateral gaze palsy may precede complete ophthalmoplegia. This increased susceptibility to damage by infection is likely to be explained by the location of the abducens nerve in the cavernous sinus. Unlike the third and fourth cranial nerves, which track along the lateral aspect of the cavernous sinus and are protected by a thick fibrous sheath, the sixth nerve is usually situated medially near the carotid artery and is surrounded on all sides by blood.

Funduscopic examination is abnormal in approximately two thirds of patients, papilledema or dilated, tortuous retinal veins being most commonly seen. Deficits in visual acuity may be present (approximately 20% of all cases) and, when present, frequently progress to blindness (approximately 15% of all cases). Causes of blindness include corneal ulceration secondary to defective lid closure (23) and occlusion of the central retinal artery due to increased pressure at the orbital apex (49,80), emboli (39), or intracavernous internal carotid arteritis (37). In addition, high intraocular pressure may compromise the blood flow to the optic nerve and lead to ischemic optic neuropathy (23).

Fifth Nerve Dysfunction   The ophthalmic (V_1) and maxillary (V_2) branches of the fifth cranial nerve, the trigeminal nerve, also pass along the lateral aspect of the cavernous sinus. It is likely that dysfunction of these nerves is common. When specifically sought, hypoesthesia or hyperesthesia of the dermatomes served by these two branches is frequently noted (81). A careful sensory examination should be performed, focusing on the forehead and dorsum of the nose (V_1) as well as regions of the upper lip, lateral nose, and upper cheek (V_2). In addition, corneal sensation (V_1) should be tested. Dysfunction of these nerves, in the appropriate setting, is strongly suggestive of inflammation in the region of the cavernous sinus.

Differential Diagnosis

Orbital cellulitis, a far more common infection, can be difficult to differentiate from cavernous sinus thrombosis. A number of clinical findings make the diagnosis of cavernous sinus thrombosis more probable: pupillary abnormalities, visual loss, papilledema, fifth cranial nerve deficits, bilateral ocular involvement and inflammatory cells in the CSF (49,81). High-resolution CT scan or MRI can most readily differentiate the two diseases. As part of the differential diagnosis other causes of periorbital edema need to be considered: intraorbital abscess (49), allergic blepharitis (81), intracavernous carotid artery aneurysm or arteriovenous fistula (84), idiopathic granulomatous inflammation of the superior orbital and cavernous sinus (Tolosa-Hunt syndrome) (85–87), polyarteritis nodosa associated with cerebral venous sinus thrombosis (Cogan syndrome) (88), nasopharyngeal tumor, meningioma, and trauma.

Laboratory Findings

The peripheral white blood cell count is elevated in over 90% of cases of septic cavernous sinus thrombosis, suggesting active bacterial infection.

Bacteriology Bacteriology is available in approximately half of cases. *Staphylococcal aureus* has been determined to be the etiologic agent in nearly 70%. Other less frequently cultured organisms include streptococcal species (including *Streptococcus pneumoniae*), gram-negative bacilli, and anaerobes (*Bacteroides* species, *Fusobacterium* species).

Lumbar Puncture Inflammatory cells are found in the CSF in approximately 75% of patients examined. Findings consistent with a parameningeal infection (moderate numbers of white blood cells, polymorphonuclear leukocytes [PMN] mixed with mononuclear cells, a normal CSF glucose, a slightly elevated or normal CSF protein, CSF culture negative) are observed in half the cases, whereas one third have findings consistent with active bacterial meningitis (increased PMN, low CSF glucose, high CSF protein, CSF culture often positive).

Radiology Use of CT and MRI can readily prove the diagnosis. Presently there has been more experience with high-resolution orbital CT scan (68,70,72,89). Early venous phase, contrast-enhanced CT scan is generally diagnostic, demonstrating regions of decreased or irregular enhancement in the cavernous sinuses as well as increased enhancement and thickening of the lateral walls of the sinuses (Figure 8.5). MRI with gadolinium enhancement has proved even more sensitive and can demonstrate similar findings (68,90). Actual blood flow within the sinus may also be assessed. In acute thrombosis, T2-weighted images demonstrate hypointense regions due to deoxyhemoglobin in entrapped red blood cells. Within 2 to 3 days thrombi become hyperintense on both T1- and T2-weighted images secondary to conversion of deoxyhemoglobin to methemoglobin, a paramagnetic substance. MRI and CT scan also allow excellent visualization of the sphenoid air sinus as

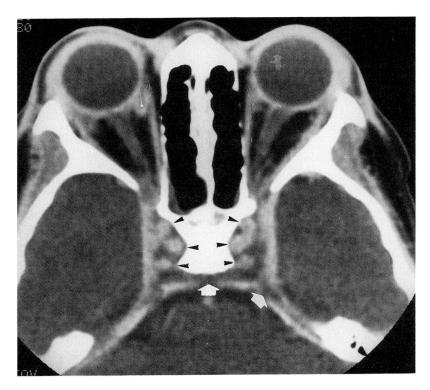

Figure 8.5. Contrast-enhanced orbital high-resolution CT scan. Coronal section shows enhancement of the intracavernous carotid artery (*black arrowheads*) and enhancement of the lateral walls of the cavernous sinus. Note the multiple black filling defects throughout both cavernous sinuses indicative of thrombus. Note also the lack of enhancement of the posterior intercavernous sinus as well as the right superior petrosal sinus indicating thrombus in these areas (*thick white arrows*).

will sinus tomograms (Figure 8.6). MRI and CT scan are also useful for demonstrating cortical regions with venous infarcts.

Other Studies Carotid angiography, when performed, demonstrates narrowing or complete obstruction of the intracavernous segment, probably secondary to spasm and thrombosis (13,15,23,24,37,54,81). Mycotic aneurysms in this region are less commonly found (70,73). With the advent of MRI and CT scans, conventional angiography as well as orbital venography are no longer necessary. On rare occasions the chest x-ray may prove abnormal, demonstrating findings consistent with pulmonary infarcts secondary to migration of thrombus from the cavernous sinus to the lung via the inferior petrosal sinus and internal jugular vein.

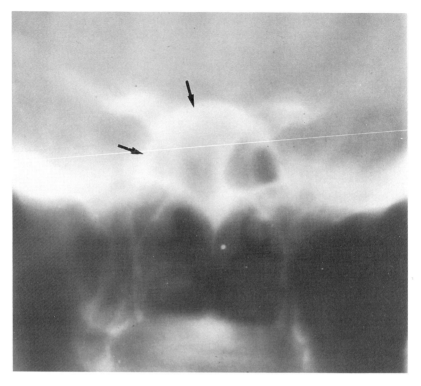

Figure 8.6.   Anteroposterior tomogram shows severe sphenoid sinusitis. Note the marked opacification of the right side of the sinus (*black arrows*).

Treatment

High-dose intravenous antibiotics should be instituted at the time of presentation. Empiric therapy should include a penicillinase-resistant penicillin such as intravenous nafcillin or oxacillin at maximal doses (3 g q6h) and a third-generation cephalosporin such as ceftriaxone (1 g q12h) or cefotaxime (2 g q4–6h). Anaerobic coverage should be considered in patients in whom the primary focus is likely to be a dental or air sinus infection. Intravenous metronidazole is the agent of choice (15 mg/kg loading dose followed by 7.5 mg/kg q6h).

In early unilateral cavernous sinus thrombosis, heparin anticoagulation should also be considered. Anticoagulation should prevent thrombus extension to the other cavernous sinus and allow recanalization to occur. In one retrospective study anticoagulation was associated with decreased mortality (81) and in a second retrospective review with decreased morbidity (74). The latter study noted a statistically significant reduction in morbidity only in those cases in which heparin was begun early in the course of the illness. Constant infusion intravenous heparin should be instituted to maintain a partial thromboplastin time of 1.5 to 2 times normal. Complications from heparin therapy of cavernous sinus thrombosis have been rare and have included gastrointestinal bleeding (67), hematuria (6), and subarachnoid hemorrhage (47). Evidence for cerebral infarction or intracerebral hemorrhage should be excluded by MRI or CT scan prior to beginning anticoagulation. Use of oral anticoagulants should be avoided because rigorous control of the degree of anticoagulation is difficult. One case of fatal intracerebral hemorrhage has been reported in association with dicumarol therapy for septic cavernous sinus thrombosis (81). In this case the prothrombin time was allowed to increase to nearly three times normal just before the onset of intracerebral hemorrhage.

Corticosteroids in some instances may prove helpful, provided the patient is being treated with appropriate antibiotics. Steroids may reverse or prevent inflammatory damage of the cranial nerves and reduce cranial nerve dysfunction (53). These agents may also be helpful in reducing persistent orbital congestion (23). Finally, in cases where infection has spread to the pituitary gland, their use in replacement doses may prevent addisonian crisis (32).

If sphenoid sinus involvement has been documented, surgical drainage should be performed emergently. Debridement of the infected sphenoid sinuses may be followed by rapid improvement. Ideally, sphenoid sinusitis should be recognized and aggressively treated medically and surgically prior to lateral spread to the cavernous sinus (82).

Mycotic aneurysms of the intracavernous region of the internal carotid are rare. In most instances conservative management is recommended, consisting of sequential MRI or conventional angiography and close clinical follow-up. Surgical repair should be considered only if ophthalmoplegia worsens and sequential MRIs or conventional angiography demonstrate progressive enlargement of the aneurysm (73).

Outcome

Even in the antibiotic era the mortality associated with septic cavernous sinus thrombosis remains high, approximately 30%. Once infection has fully developed in the cavernous sinus, injury to the intracavernous cranial nerves as well as the internal carotid artery and spread to meninges and even to the pituitary gland can occur despite appropriate antimicrobial therapy. Approximately 40% of patients fully recover, whereas the remaining 30% suffer serious sequelae including oculomotor weakness, blindness, hemiparesis, and pituitary insufficiency (30,61,78,79). Particularly high mortality (50%) and morbidity (50%) have been reported in cases of septic cavernous sinus thrombosis associated with sphenoid sinus infection (75,81). Therapy is more commonly delayed in these cases and associated with extensive involvement of the cavernous sinus at the time of presentation.

The continued poor outcome in patients with this disease emphasizes the importance of earlier recognition and treatment of primary infections associated with potential spread to the cavernous sinus. Aggressive treatment of facial infections and avoidance of manipulation of facial furuncles in the absence of appropriate antibiotic coverage need to be reemphasized. Early recognition of sphenoid sinus infection is also critical for preventing this often devastating disease.

SEPTIC LATERAL SINUS THROMBOSIS

Primary Site of Infection

In nearly all instances this disease results from spread of infection from the mastoid air cells via emissary veins or by direct spread to the lateral and sigmoid sinuses. Septic lateral sinus thrombosis is exclusively a complication of either acute or chronic otitis media (81,91–139).

Symptoms and History of Underlying Disease

As compared to septic cavernous sinus thrombosis, which is an acute disease, septic lateral sinus thrombosis has a subacute onset, symptoms generally being present for several weeks before hospitalization. Headache and earache are the most common symptoms. Ear pain generally precedes headache by several weeks. If the patient fails to seek medical attention and is not appropriately treated with systemic antibiotics, a headache may ensue. The head pain associated with lateral sinus thrombosis is generally severe and persistent. Pain is usually frontotemporooccipital in location and confined to the side of ear infection. This pain is probably a manifestation of a developing epidural abscess, irritation of the fifth cranial nerve, or septic thrombosis of the lateral sinus. Other prominent complaints may include nausea and vomiting (present in nearly half of cases), mimicking a severe gastroenteritis. This manifestation may reflect irritation of the brain stem or elevated CSF pressure. Vertigo may also develop, possibly as a result of extension of infection to the inner ear. Less common complaints may include diplopia, photophobia, neck stiffness, and cough associated with bloody sputum.

Septic lateral sinus thrombosis is generally a disease of young otherwise healthy individuals. Other than chronic otitis media, a history of a chronic predisposing illness is uncommon in this disorder.

Physical Findings

Fever is present in the majority of cases (80%); however, absence of fever does not exclude the possibility of this diagnosis. Patients often appear toxic. Evidence of ear infection and persistent fever despite the administration of antibiotics should always raise the possibility of lateral sinus thrombosis.

Otologic Examination   Examination of the ears is almost always abnormal. Purulent drainage from a ruptured tympanic membrane (40% of cases), or less commonly, a dull erythematous tympanic membrane (20% of cases) is seen. Posterior auricular swelling caused by occlusion of the mastoid emissary vein should be sought. This finding, named Gresinger sign, has been described in nearly half the previous cases.

Eye and Neurologic Examination Bilateral prominent papilledema, a manifestation of raised intracranial pressure, is found in over half the cases. Papilledema may also be associated with retinal hemorrhage. Loss of visual acuity is noted in approximately 15% of cases with papilledema. Unilateral sixth nerve palsy, causing a lateral gaze palsy and diplopia, is reported in over a third of patients. This symptom may be preceded by lateral gaze nystagmus. Sixth nerve dysfunction is thought to be caused by compression of the nerve by swelling of the inferior petrosal sinus in the closed space of Dorello's canal (100). Otitis media and sixth nerve paralysis, combined with symptoms of fifth nerve irritation (temporoparietal and retroorbital pain), is known as Gradenigo's syndrome. When present this symptom complex provides strong evidence for lateral sinus thrombosis or inflammation of the petrous ridge of the temporal bone (100). Other focal neurologic deficits are rare. Approximately 2% of all cases develop contralateral hemiparesis. Another physical finding noted in nearly one third of patients is mild nucchal rigidity, a likely reflection of meningeal irritation. This finding may be accompanied by depression of mental status (approximately 14% of all cases).

Laboratory Findings

As observed in cavernous sinus infection, peripheral leukocytosis is the rule (80% of cases), suggesting an acute inflammatory process.

Bacteriology The principal organisms associated with septic lateral sinus thrombosis reflect the bacteriology of chronic otitis media. In order of frequency *Proteus* species, *S. aureus*, *Escherichia coli*, and anaerobes (*Bacteroides fragilis* and anaerobic streptococci) are the major pathogens reported. Cultures of the material draining from the external meatus do not accurately reflect the etiology of otitis media and mastoiditis; therefore, whenever possible, intraoperative, blood, and CSF cultures should be obtained.

Cerebrospinal Fluid Analysis After excluding the diagnosis of brain abscess by performing an MRI or CT scan, lumbar puncture should be performed in all cases of suspected septic lateral sinus thrombosis. CSF pressure is frequently markedly elevated (75% of cases), pressures being in the range of 450 to 500 mm H_2O. Elevation of CSF pressure is likely to be due to interference with CSF resorption by the arachnoid villi, which drain into the superior sagittal sinus. If the lateral sinus responsible for drainage of the superior sagittal sinus is occluded, CSF resorption is blocked and a communicating hydrocephalus (sometimes called otitic hydrocephalus) develops. The Queckenstedt or Tobey-Ayer maneuver has proven to be unreliable and may precipitate brain stem herniation (105,139) and, therefore, is no longer recommended. Two thirds of CSF samples demonstrate normal cellular and biochemical composition. The other one third contains a mixture of PMN and mononuclear cells, suggesting a parameningeal focus of infection. One half of patients with increased white blood cells in their CSF have been found to harbor a brain or epidural abscess (81).

Radiology   Mastoid radiographs should be performed in all patients with suspected lateral sinus thrombosis. Findings consistent with mastoid infection are found in nearly all cases. Abnormalities may include increased density with loss of mastoid air cell trabeculae, bony sclerosis of the mastoid region, and lytic lesions of the temporal or parietal bones. Although venous phase angiography and dynamic brain scan were once used for diagnosis, MRI is now the diagnostic study of choice (136,137). Techniques to assess venous flow using MRI angiography are now available (Figure 8.7A). In addition, T1-weighted images can readily detect methemoglobin in thrombosed vessels which results in a marked increase in signal intensity (Figure 8.7B). CT scan is helpful for assessing bony erosion in the regions of the mastoid air cells (Figure 8.7C), but cannot specifically demonstrate thrombus formation or detect reduced venous flow of the lateral sinuses. Chest x-ray should also be performed to look for septic emboli that can pass via the jugular veins into the pulmonary vasculature.

Treatment

High-dose broad-spectrum intravenous antibiotics should be initiated immediately. Nafcillin or oxacillin should be administered until *S. aureus* has been definitely excluded. A third-generation cephalosporin such as ceftriaxone or cefotaxime, as well as metronidazole, should also be initiated pending culture results (for doses see treatment of septic cavernous sinus thrombosis). Although *Pseudomonas* is frequently cultured from the external ear, this organism has not been isolated from intraoperative culture in any antibiotic era cases.

Surgical drainage and debridement are also generally required (75% of patients). If the patient remains febrile and toxic after 12 to 24 hours of antibiotic treatment, radical mastoidectomy should be performed. During surgery the area overlying the lateral sinus should be explored. Infected granulation tissue or purulent collections requiring drainage are often found. Removal of thrombus from the lateral sinus is not recommended because recanalization as well as development of collateral venous circulation and normalization of CSF pressure generally occur once the overlying inflammatory focus is removed. If papilledema and increased CSF pressure persist, serial lumbar punctures every 48 hours may be necessary. If communicating hydrocephalus and increased CSF pressure fail to resolve, particularly if there is progressive loss of visual acuity, placement of a ventricular shunt may have to be considered. Although once commonly performed, ligation of the jugular vein to prevent septic pulmonary emboli is no longer recommended because septic emboli are rare in the antibiotic era. Anticoagulation is not recommended because cortical venous occlusion may occur in the region overlying the infected mastoid and result in

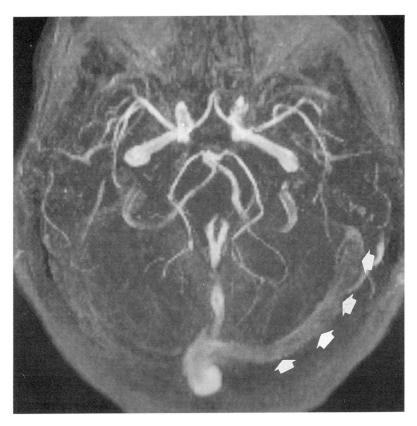

Figure 8.7A. MRI angiogram, coronal section shows normal flow in the right lateral sinus (*thick white arrows*) and absence of flow in the left lateral sinus.

small venous hemorrhagic infarcts. Such infarcts are likely to increase the risk of anticoagulant-induced intracerebral hemorrhage. In addition, the majority of patients completely recover without systemic anticoagulation.

Outcome

Complications reported in the earlier decades of the antibiotic era included meningitis (109), cerebellar abscess (97,101,107,109), septic pulmonary emboli (100,102,106,129), superior vena cava syndrome (122), and uncontrollable sepsis (115). With the development of a more aggressive surgical approach to this disease, these complications are now uncommon and mortality is low. The majority of patients fully recover, although 10 to 15% suffer with chronic sequelae including otitic hydrocephalus, decreased visual acuity, chronic eighth nerve dysfunction, and residual hemiparesis.

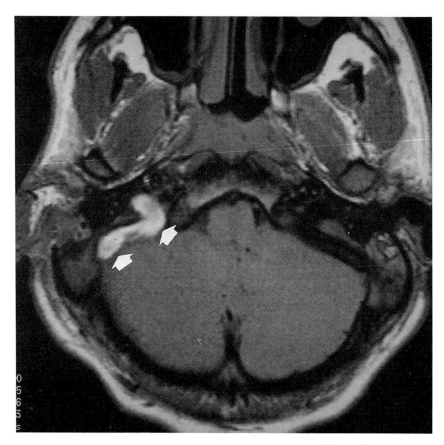

Figure 8.7B. MRI coronal section, T1 image without contrast shows a marked increase in signal intensity at the junction of the left sigmoid and internal jugular vein indicative of thrombus formation (*thick white arrows*). Note the thickened soft tissue in the region of the left middle ear and mastoid.

SEPTIC THROMBOSIS OF THE SUPERIOR SAGITTAL SINUS

The superior sagittal sinus, the largest of the intracerebral venous sinuses, becomes obstructed by septic thrombosis less commonly than the cavernous do and lateral sinuses (1,81,140–148).

Primary Sites of Infection

Bacterial meningitis is the most common infection that predisposes to septic superior sagittal sinus thrombosis (81,146). Infection probably spreads from the meninges via the diploic veins, which drain into the superior sagittal sinus. Air

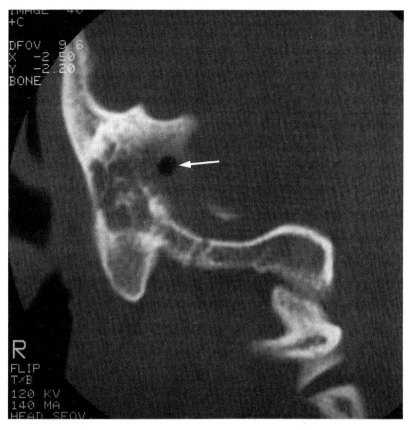

Figure 8.7C.   CT scan, coronal section shows the bony detail of the left mastoid region. Note the marked erosion of the bone in this region as well as gas in the sigmoid sinus (*white arrow*).

sinus infection is the second most common primary site. Ethmoid and maxillary sinus infection can spread to this venous sinus via ethmoidal veins. Frontal sinusitis associated with epidural abscess can induce cortical vein thrombosis, which in turn may extend into the superior sagittal sinus. Septic lateral sinus thrombus can on occasion spread retrograde into the superior sagittal sinus. Pulmonary infection, tonsillitis, tooth infection, and pelvic infection have also preceded septic superior sagittal sinus thrombosis.

Symptoms and History of Predisposing Illness

The onset of this illness is generally acute, over a period of 1 to 3 days. The most common presentation is that of fulminant bacterial meningitis. Severe generalized headache, nausea, and vomiting are rapidly followed by the onset of confusion. Change in mental status is also usually associated with the onset of focal or grand mal seizures, which are often refractory to antiseizure medications. Within hours confusion progresses to coma. A milder form of the illness, one in which patients complain of frontal headaches for several weeks prior to the onset of seizures or motor deficits, has been associated with frontal sinusitis. Approximately one third of patients have a predisposing illness. Sickle cell anemia, osteopetrosis, Down syndrome, breast cancer, and malignant lymphoma have been reported in association with septic superior sagittal sinus thrombosis. Two cases developed in women during the peripartum period (1,140).

Physical Findings

High fever is generally present (70% of cases). An abnormal mental status is usually apparent at the time of admission (65% of cases), the majority of patients being unresponsive to voice or painful stimuli. Nuchal rigidity resulting from meningitis is present in most cases. Hemiparesis, caused by cortical vein thrombosis and associated venous cerebral infarction, is evident in nearly half of cases. Signs of brain stem compression (lack of eye movements with caloric stimulation, dilated unreactive pupils, and generalized flaccid motor paralysis) may develop within hours of admission. Papilledema may be seen on funduscopic examination. However, many patients do not survive long enough to develop this manifestation of increased CSF pressure. Septic thrombosis of only the anterior segment of the superior sagittal sinus is generally associated with frontal sinusitis. The neurologic deficits are generally milder in these patients.

Differential Diagnosis

Many of the symptoms and signs of septic superior sagittal sinus thrombosis are not specific. Similar findings can be associated with lateral sinus thrombosis; brain, epidural, or subdural abscess; or bacterial meningitis complicated by septic arteritis, extensive cortical vein thrombosis, or severe cerebritis.

Laboratory Findings

As observed in the other forms of septic dural sinus thrombosis, most patients have a peripheral leukocytosis suggesting a bacterial infection.

Bacteriology The pathogens associated with this disorder reflect the causes of community-acquired and nosocomial meningitis as well as brain abscess and include. *S. pneumoniae.* Other aerobic and anaerobic streptococci, *Klebsiella* species, *S. aureus*, *Listeria monocytogenes*, and *Pseudomonas* species are less commonly isolated. Rarer etiologic agents have included *Trichinella spiralis* (141) and *Treponema pallidum* (148).

Cerebrospinal Fluid The CSF pressure is often elevated, occlusion of the superior sagittal preventing normal CSF resorption by the arachnoid villi. In patients with meningitis the CSF contains increased numbers of PMN, a low glucose concentration, and an elevated protein level.

Radiology A CT scan with contrast may demonstrate an "empty delta sign," a triangular area of decreased density surrounded by a region of enhancement. This darkened area represents thrombus within the sinus with contrast material being taken up by the surrounding collateral veins and sinus wall. This finding is relatively specific for superior sagittal sinus thrombosis (149) but may disappear when recanalization of the venous sinus begins (150). A pseudo "empty delta sign" may also be seen following head trauma (151). This sign may also be seen on occasion in CT scans of lateral sinus thrombosis (134). Gyral enhancement secondary to increased venous collateral circulation and focal areas of cerebral edema may also be seen. Conventional angiography and dynamic brain scan are no longer necessary. MRI is now the diagnostic study of choice in this disorder. As described in the septic lateral sinus thrombosis section, MRI can readily demonstrate decreased flow and thrombus in the superior sagittal sinus (147,152–154).

Treatment and Outcome

The consequences of complete thrombosis of the superior sagittal sinus are profound. Cerebral edema immediately ensues. The many cortical veins that drain into the sinus also thrombose, leading to multiple hemorrhagic venous infarcts. The arachnoid villi, which drain into this sinus, no longer are capable of resorbing CSF and the patient also develops communicating hydrocephalus. The marked increase in cerebral cortical volume often results in transtentorial brain stem herniation. A fatal outcome is the rule (nearly 80% of cases). Treatment with broad-spectrum antibiotics should be initiated. In cases of meningitis, ceftriaxone or cefotaxime is recommended. This antibiotic should be combined with intravenous ampicillin (10 to 12 g/d in q6h doses) in immunocompromised patients. If the primary focus of infection is an air sinus or brain abscess, nafcillin and metronidazole should be added to this regimen. If pseudomonas is known to be the primary pathogen, treatment with intravenous ceftazidime (2 g q6h iv) and an aminoglycoside such as tobramycin (5 mg/kg/d divided into three doses given q8h) should be instituted. Intravenous mannitol may decrease cerebral edema and reduce the risk of brain stem herniation (155). Mannitol, however, should be used with caution because this agent can produce severe dehydration, a condition that may predispose to further dural sinus thrombosis. In cases of pediatric meningitis, steroids in high doses have been found to reduce the CSF pressure and neurologic sequelae and may help to prevent septic superior sagittal sinus thrombosis (156, 157). Once this complication has developed, they may help to reduce cerebral edema.

The role of anticoagulants remains controversial. Mortality is presently extremely high in this disease. Therefore, any therapy that might improve outcome needs to be considered. The presence of multiple hemorrhagic venous infarcts increases the risk of intracerebral hemorrhage. Use of constant infusion heparin in cases of aseptic superior sagittal sinus thrombosis with intracerebral hemorrhage, however, was associated with a significantly improved outcome without an increase in intracerebral hemorrhage as compared to controls (158). Animal studies suggest that early institution of heparin therapy may prevent thrombosis of the bridging veins and the cortical veins and prevent the development of cortical infarcts and communicating hydrocephalus (159). In several cases of aseptic superior sagittal sinus thrombosis, urokinase has also been used without complication (160,161). Ideally controlled studies should be performed to determine the relative risks and benefits of anticoagulation in septic dural sinus thrombosis.

Patients with partial subacute thrombosis, particularly of the anterior segment of the superior sagittal sinus (usually associated with frontal or ethmoid sinusitis), have much milder clinical manifestations and may recover fully. With time, an extensive collateral venous circulation develops and communicating hydrocephalus resolves.

CONCLUSIONS

Infections of the facial area, air sinuses, middle ear, and meninges can be complicated by septic dural sinus thrombosis. Physicians need to recognize and treat these primary infections early in their course to prevent this very serious complication. With the advent of MRI and CT scanning, dural sinus thrombosis can be readily diagnosed and appropriately treated. Broad-spectrum, high-dose antibiotic therapy and surgical drainage of the infected air sinuses or middle ear are the mainstays of therapy. The role of anticoagulation is in transition. Constant infusion heparin may be considered in early cases of septic cavernous sinus thrombosis. Patients with septic lateral sinus thrombosis usually fully recover without receiving anticoagulants. The role of heparin therapy in septic superior sagittal sinus thrombosis remains controversial.

ACKNOWLEDGMENTS

I would like to thank Dr. Anthony Mancuso for providing the CT scan and MRI images and Ms. Leanne Williams for her secretarial assistance.

REFERENCES

1 **Kalbag RM, Woolf AL.** Cerebral venous thrombosis: with special reference to primary aseptic thrombosis. New York: Oxford University Press, 1967:23.

2 **Bedford MA.** The "cavernous sinus." Br J Ophthalmol 1966;50:41–46.

3 **Harris FS, Rhoton AL.** Anatomy of the cavernous sinus. J Neurosurg 1976;45:169–180.

4 **Bisaria KK.** Anatomic variations of venous sinuses in the region of the torcula Herophili. J Neurosurg 1985;62:90–95.

5 **Woodhall B.** Variations of the cranial venous sinuses in the region of the torcula Herophili. Arch Surg 1936;33:297–314.

6 **Ershler IL, Blaisdell IH.** Massive hematuria following use of heparin in cavernous sinus thrombosis. JAMA 1941;117:927.

7 **Eagleton W.** Cavernous sinus thrombophlebitis and allied septic traumatic lesions of the basal venous sinuses. New York: Macmillan, 1926:1.

8 **Grove WE.** Septic and aseptic types of thrombosis of the cavernous sinus. Arch Otolaryngol 1936;24:29–50.

9 **Bassey OO, Elebute EA.** Septic thrombosis of the cavernous sinus. West Afr Med J 1968;17:39–41.

10 **Bell RW.** Orbital cellulitis and cavernous sinus thrombosis caused by rhabdomyosarcoma of the middle ear. Ann Ophthalmol 1972;4:1090–1092.

11 **Brown P.** Septic cavernous sinus thrombosis. Bull Johns Hopkins Hosp 1961;109:68–75.

12 **Bucky TL, Lahey WJ, Kunkel P.** Bilateral cavernous sinus thrombophlebitis. Conn State Med J 1948;12:996–999.

13 **Casaubon JN, Dion MA, Larbrissea US.** Septic cavernous sinus thrombosis after rhinoplasty. Plast Reconstruct Surg 1977;59:119–123.

14 **Childress RC, Bitzer W.** Cavernous sinus thrombosis. J Fla Med Assoc 1964;51:94–95.

15 **Clune JP.** Septic thrombosis within the cavernous chamber. Am J Ophthalmol 1963;56:33–39.

16 **D'Arbela PG.** Cavernous sinus thrombosis. East Afr Med J 1964;41:551–559.

17 **Doorly ARC.** Thrombophlebitis of the cavernous sinus with recovery. Br Med J 1942;1:42.

18 **Elfman LK.** Thrombosis of the cavernous sinus. Arch Otolaryngol 1950;51:188–195.

19 **Evans HW.** Cavernous sinus thrombosis. J Lancet 1965;85:109–111.

20 **Fairclough WA.** Drainage in infected cavernous sinus thrombosis. Aust N Z J Surg 1947;16:194–196.

21 **Feinfeld DA, Al-Acjlar G, Lipner HI, Chirayil SJ, Hakim J, Avram MM.** Syndrome of inappropriate secretion of antidiuretic hormone. JAMA 1978;240:856–857.

22 **Fox SL, West GB.** Thrombosis of the cavernous sinus. JAMA 1947;134:1452–1456.

23 **Friberg TR, Sogg RL.** Ischemic optic neuropathy in cavernous sinus thrombosis. Arch Ophthalmol 1978;96:453–456.

24 **Gallagher JP.** Septic thrombosis of the cavernous sinus. Med Ann Distr Columbia 1960;29:278–283.

25 **Gialldrenzi AF, Weiss WW, Furman DJ, Greenwald AM.** Septic cavernous sinus thrombosis in a diabetic after dental extraction. J Oral Surg 1974;32:924–930.

26 **Goodhill V.** Cavernous sinus thrombosis. JAMA 1944;125:28–31.

27 **Greenish BVI.** Cavernous sinus thrombosis. Br Med J 1945;1:876–877.

28 **Harvey JE.** Streptokinase therapy and cavernous sinus thrombosis. Br Med J 1974;4:46.

29 **Henner R, Ridall EG.** Thrombosis of cavernous sinus treated with penicillin and heparin. Arch Otolaryngol 1945;41:295–297.

30 **Ivey KJ, Smith H.** Hypopituitarism associated with cavernous sinus thrombosis. J Neurol Neurosurg Psychiatry 1968;31:187–189.

31 **Johnston DF.** Cavernous sinus thrombosis treated with penicillin. Lancet 1945;1:9–10.

32 **Karlin FJ, Robinson WA.** Septic cavernous sinus thrombosis. Ann Emerg Med 1984;13:449–455.

33 **Khare BB.** Pyrrolidinomethyltetracycline in cavernous sinus thrombosis. Br J Ophthalmol 1967;51:712–713.

34 **Lawton C, Hobin M.** Cavernous sinus thrombosis. Can Nurse 1956;52:120–121.

35 **Lillie HL.** Prognosis of septic thrombophlebitis of the cavernous sinus. J Int Coll Surg 1951;15:754–759.

36 **Malik SRK, Gupta AK, Singh G, Choudhry S.** Pyrrolidinomethyltetracycline in cavernous sinus thrombosis. Br J Ophthalmol 1970;54:113–116.

37 **Mathew NY, Abraham J, Toari GM, Lyer GV.** Internal carotid artery occlusion in cavernous sinus thrombosis. Arch Neurol 1971;24:11–16.

38 **McAllen PM, Shaw RE.** Cavernous sinus thrombophlebitis. Br J Surg 1952;40:49–52.

39 **Mehra KS, Somani PN.** Multiple emboli in central retinal artery following cavernous sinus thrombosis. J All-India Ophthalmol Soc 1967;15:71–72.

40 **Miklos A.** The cure of cavernous sinus thrombosis phlebitis. Br J Ophthalmol 1950;34:234.

41 **Morrison LF, Schindler M.** Cavernous sinus thrombosis. Arch Otolaryngol 1940; 31:948–954.

42 **Nicholson WM, Anderson WB.** Penicillin in the treatment of cavernous sinus thrombophlebitis. JAMA 1944;126:12–15.

43 **Oliver KS, Diab AE, Abu-Jaudeh CN.** Thrombophlebitis of the cavernous sinus originating from acute dental infection. Arch Otolaryngol 1948;48:36–40.

44 **Pace E.** Thrombosis of the cavernous sinus. Arch Otolaryngol 1941;33:216–230.

45 **Palmersheim LA, Hamilton MK.** Fatal cavernous sinus thrombosis following 3rd molar removal. J Oral Maxillofac Surg 1982;40:371–376.

46 **Pascarelli E, Lemlich A.** Diplopia and photophobia as premonitory symptoms in cavernous sinus thrombosis. Ann Otol 1964;73:210–217.

47 **Pirkey WP.** Thrombosis of the cavernous sinus. Arch Otolaryngol 1950;51:917–924.

48 **Pratt LW.** Cavernous sinus thrombosis. J Maine Med Assoc 1959;50:817–822.

49 **Price CD, Hameroff SB, Richards RD.** Cavernous sinus thrombosis and orbital cellulitis. South Med J 1971;64:1243–1247.

50 **Russel A, Fearing SJ.** Cavernous sinus thrombosis in a diabetic. Oral Surg 1955; 8:372–377.

51 **Sears TP, Wilson FL.** Recovery from cavernous sinus thrombosis and staphylococcal pneumonia by combined use of penicillin, sulfadiazine and antistaphylococcus serum. Rocky Mt Med 1945;42: 838–841.

52 **Shaw RE.** Cavernous sinus thrombophlebitis: a review. Br J Surg 1952;40: 40–48.

53 **Solomon OD, Moses L, Volk M.** Steroid therapy in cavernous sinus thrombosis. Am J Ophthalmol 1962;54:1122–1124.

54 **Stevens J, Robinson K.** Chronic cavernous sinus thrombosis: discussion and report of case. J Oral Surg 1977;35:136–139.

55 **Stool JA, Lomas RD.** Thrombophlebitis of cavernous sinus with recovery. Texas State J Med 1948;44:372–373.

56 **Taylor PJ.** Cavernous sinus thrombosis. Br J Ophthalmol 1957;41:228–237.

57 **Tempae V, Dorun G.** Cavernous sinus thrombosis. Arch Otolaryngol 1959;69: 220–223.

58 **Weisman AD.** Cavernous sinus thrombophlebitis. N Engl J Med 1944;231: 118–122.

59 **Welty RF.** Bacterial thrombophlebitis of a cavernous sinus with recovery. Arch Otolaryngol 1946;43:70–72.

60 **Wiesenfeld IH, Phillips E.** Thrombophlebitis of a cavernous sinus following extraction of teeth. Arch Otolaryngol 1944;40:497–500.

61 **Williams E.** Hypopituitarism following sinusitis and cavernous sinus thrombosis. Proc R Soc Med 1956;49:827–828.

62 **Wolf JW.** Thrombosis of the cavernous sinus with hemolytic streptococcal bacteremia. Arch Otolaryngol 1944;40:33–37.

63 **Wolfe WC, Gain JF.** Thrombosis of the cavernous sinuses. Arch Otolaryngol 1944;40:79–84.

64 **Yarington CT.** Septic thrombosis of the cavernous sinus. JAMA 1960;173:506–508.

65 **Yarington CT.** The prognosis and treatment of cavernous sinus thrombosis. Ann Rhinol Laryngol Otol 1961;70:263–267.

66 **Yarington CT.** Thrombosis of the cavernous sinus. Otorhinolaryng Surg 1963;40: 66–71.

67 **Zahller M, Spector RH, Skoglund R, Digby D, Nyhan WL.** Cavernous sinus thrombosis. West J Med 1980;133:44–48.

68 **Ellie E, Houang B, Louail C, et al.** CT and high field MRI in septic thrombosis of the cavernous sinuses. Neuroradiology 1992; 34:22–24.

69 **Yun MW, Hwang CF, Lui CC.** Cavernous sinus thrombosis following odontogenic and cervicofacial infection. Eur Arch Otorhinolaryngol 1991;248:422–424.

70 **Todo T, Inoya H.** Sudden appearance of a mycotic aneurysm of the intracavernous carotid artery after symptoms resembling cluster headache: case report. Neurosurgery 1991;29:594–599.

71 Jones TH, Bergvall V, Bradshaw JP. Carotid artery stenoses and thrombosis secondary to cavernous sinus thromboses in *Fusobacterium necrophorum* meningitis. Postgrad Med J 1990;66:747–750.

72 Ben-Uri R, Palma L, Kaveh Z. Septic thrombosis of the cavernous sinus: diagnosis with the aid of computed tomography. Clin Radiol 1989;40:520–522.

73 Endo S, Ohtsuji T, Fukuda O, Oka N, Takaku A. A case of septic cavernous sinus thrombosis with sequential dynamic angiographic changes. A case report. Surg Neurol 1989;32:59–63.

74 Levine SR, Twyman RE, Gilman S. The role of anticoagulation in cavernous sinus thrombosis. Neurology 1988;38:517–522.

75 MacDonald RL, Findlay JM, Tator CH. Sphenoethmoidal sinusitis complicated by cavernous sinus thrombosis and pontocerebellar infarction. Can J Neurol Sci 1988;15:310–313.

76 Hartmann B, Kremer K, Gutman I, Krakowski D, Kam J. Cavernous sinus infection manifested by Horner's syndrome and ipsilateral sixth nerve palsy. J Clin Neuroophthalmol 1987;7:223–226.

77 Harbour RC, Trobe JD, Ballinger WE. Septic cavernous sinus thrombosis associated with gingivitis and parapharyngeal abscess. Arch Ophthalmol 1984;102:94–97.

78 Silver HS, Morris LR. Hypopituitarism secondary to cavernous sinus thrombosis. South Med J 1983;76:642–646.

79 Hladky JP, Leys D, Vantyghem MC, et al. Early hypopituitarism following cavernous sinus thrombosis: total recovery within one year. Clin Neurol Neurosurg 1991;93:249–252.

80 Gupta A, Jalali S, Bansal RK, Grewal SP. Anterior ischemic optic neuropathy and branch retinal artery occlusion in cavernous sinus thrombosis. J Clin Neuroophthalmol 1990;10:193–196.

81 Southwick FS, Richardson EP Jr, Swartz MN. Septic thrombosis of the dural venous sinuses. Medicine 1986;65:82–106.

82 Lew PD, Southwick FS, Montgomery WW, Weber AL, Baker AS. Sphenoid sinusitis: a review of 30 cases. N Engl J Med 1983;309:1149–1154.

83 DiNubile MJ. Septic thrombosis of the cavernous sinuses. Arch Neurol 1988;45:567–572.

84 Palmer BW. Unilateral exophthalmos. Arch Otolaryngol 1965;62:415–424.

85 Hunt WE. Tolosa-Hunt syndrome: one cause of painful ophthalmoplegia. J Neurosurg 1976;44:544–549.

86 Hunt WE, Meagher JN, LeFever HE, Zeman W. Painful ophthalmoplegia. Neurology 1961;11:56–62.

87 Yousem DM, Atlas SW, Grossman RI, Sergott RC, Savino PH, Bosley TM. MR imaging of Tolosa-Hunt syndrome. Am J Roentgenol 1990;154:167–170.

88 Gilbert WS, Talbot FJ. Cogan's syndrome. Arch Ophthalmol 1969;82:633–636.

89 Chung JW, Chang KH, Han MH, Kim BH, Song CS. Computed tomography of cavernous sinus diseases. Neuroradiology 1988;30:319–328.

90 Komiyama M. Magnetic resonance imaging of the cavernous sinus. Radiat Med 1990;8:136–144.

91 Ata M. Cerebral infarction due to intracranial sinus thrombosis. J Clin Pathol 1965;18:636–640.

92 Bronson SR, Dunbar HS. Thrombosis of the dural venous sinuses as a cause of "pseudotumor cerebri." Ann Surg 1951;134:376–385.

93 Davidson AS. Otogenic pulmonary infection. J Laryngol 1960;74:877.

94 Foley J. Benign forms of intracranial hypertension. Toxic and otitic hydrocephalus. Brain 1955;78:1–41.

95 Gagnon NB, Sierra-Dupont S, Huot LA, Larochelle D. Thrombosis of the lateral sinus. J Otolaryngol 1977;6:257–261.

96 Greer M. Benign intracranial hypertension. Neurology 1962;12:472–476.

97 Harpman JA. On the management of otorhinogenic intracranial infections. J Laryngol Otol 1955;69:180–194.

98 Hitchcock ER, Cowie RA. Sino-jugular venous graft in otitic hydrocephalus. Acta Neurochir 1981;59:187–193.

99 Horowitz S. Otogenic intracranial hypertension. J Laryngol Otol 1949;63:363–381.

100 Jahrsdoerfer RA, Fitz-Huge GS. Lateral sinus thrombosis. South Med J 1968;61:1271–1275.

101 Jensen AM. Sinus thrombosis and otogenic sepsis. Acta Otolaryngol 1962;55:237–243.

102 Kimmick H, Myers D. Lateral sinus thrombosis. Arch Otolaryngol 1958;68:156–159.

103 Kinal ME, Jaeger RM. Thrombophlebitis of dural venous sinuses following otitis media. J Neurosurg 1960;17:81–89.

104 **Lund WS.** A review of 50 cases of intracranial complications from otogenic infection between 1961 and 1971. Clin Otolaryngol 1978;3:495–501.

105 **Meltzer PE.** Treatment of thrombosis of the lateral sinus. Arch Otolaryngol 1935; 22:131–142.

106 **Merei L.** Necrosis of the wall of the sigmoid sinus and the jugular vein. Acta Oto-Laryngol 1950;38:78–81.

107 **Miglets AW, Harrington JW.** Complications of chronic mastoiditis. R I Med J 1970;53:152–159.

108 **Morantz RA, Lansky L, Batnitzky S.** Non-operative management of pseudotumor cerebri caused by lateral sinus thrombosis. J Kansas Med Soc 1980;465–466.

109 **Morse HR.** Intracranial complications of chronic mastoiditis. Arch Otolaryngol 1956;63:142–145.

110 **Nail BM.** Otitic hydrocephalus. South Med J 1966;5:1168–1169.

111 **Neffson AH.** Occult thrombosis of sigmoid and lateral sinuses. Arch Otolaryngol 1945;41:77–78.

112 **O'Connor AEF, Moffat DA.** Otogenic intracranial hypertension: otitic hydrocephalus. J Laryngol Otol 1978;92:767–775.

113 **Pang LQ.** Intracranial complications of otitis media in this antibiotic era. Hawaii Med J 1967;5:426–430.

114 **Proctor CA.** Intracranial complications of otitic origin. Laryngoscope 1966;76:288–308.

115 **Seid AB, Sellars AL.** The management of otogenic lateral sinus disease at Groote Shuur Hospital. Laryngoscope 1973;83:397–403.

116 **Sindou M, Mercier P, Boker J, Brunon J.** Bilateral thrombosis of the transverse sinuses: microsurgical revascularization with venous bypass. Surg Neurol 1979;13:215–220.

117 **Symonds CP.** Otitic hydrocephalus. Neurology 1956;6:681–685.

118 **Venezio FR, Naidich TP, Shulman ST.** Complications of mastoiditis with special emphasis on venous sinus thrombosis. J Pediatr 1982;101:509–513.

119 **Wright JLW, Grimaldi PMGB.** Otogenic intracranial complications. J Laryngol Otol 1973;87:1085–1095.

120 **Yu WK, Shimo G.** Otitic hydrocephalus. Can J Otolaryngol 1975;4:712–719.

121 **Tveteras K, Kristensen S, Dommerby H.** Septic cavernous and lateral sinus thrombosis: modern diagnostic and therapeutic principles. J Laryngol Otol 1988; 102:877–882.

122 **Tovi F, Hirsch M, Gatot A.** Superior vena cava syndrome: presenting symptom of silent otitis media. J Laryngol Otol 1988; 102:623–625.

123 **Habib RG, Girgis NI, Abu-el-Ella AH, Faird Z, Woody J.** The treatment and outcome of intracranial infections of otogenic origin. J Trop Med Hyg 1988;91:83–86.

124 **Mathews TJ.** Lateral sinus pathology (22 cases managed at Groote Schuur Hospital). J Laryngol Otol 1988; 102:118–120.

125 **Samuel J, Fernandes CM.** Lateral sinus thrombosis (a review of 45 cases). J Laryngol Otol 1987;101:1227–1229.

126 **Rizer FM, Amiri CA, Schroeder WW, Brackmann DE.** Lateral sinus thrombosis: diagnosis and treatment—a case report. J Otolaryngol 1987;16:77–79.

127 **Samuel J, Fernandes CM, Steinberg JL.** Intracranial otogenic complications: a persisting problem. Laryngoscope 1986;96: 272–278.

128 **Samuel J, Fernandes CM.** Otogenic complications with an intact tympanic membrane. Laryngoscope 1985;95:1387–1390.

129 **Hawkins DB.** Lateral sinus thrombosis: a sometimes unexpected diagnosis. Laryngoscope 1985;95:674–677.

130 **Gower DJ, McGuirt WF, Kelly DL Jr.** Intracranial complications of ear disease in a pediatric population with special emphasis on subdural effusion and empyema. South Med J 1985;78:429–434.

131 **Debruyne F.** Lateral sinus thrombosis in the eighties. J Laryngol Otol 1985;99:91–93.

132 **Kraus M, Tovi F.** Central nervous system complications secondary to otorhinologic infections. An analysis of 39 pediatric cases. Int J Pediatr Otorhinolaryngol 1992;24:217–226.

133 **Podoshin L, Fradis M, Gertner R.** Late development of lateral sinus vein thrombosis. Ear Nose Throat J 1992;71: 243–245.

134 **Goh DW, Hamilton JG.** Lateral sinus abscess: the empty delta sign. Br J Hosp Med 1991;46:401–402.

135 **Kraus M, Tovi F.** CNS complications of ear, nose and throat infections: an analysis of 50 consecutive cases. J Otolaryngol 1991;20:329–335.

136 Irving RM, Jones NS, Hall-Craggs MA, Kendall B. CT and MR imaging in lateral sinus thrombosis. J Laryngol Otol 1991; 105:693–695.

137 Mas JL, Meder JF, Meary E, Bousser MG. Magnetic resonance imaging in lateral sinus hypoplasia and thrombosis. Stroke 1990;21:1350–1356.

138 Oyarzabal MF, Patel KS, Tolley NS. Bilateral acute mastoiditis complicated by lateral sinus thrombosis. J Laryngol Otol 1992;106:535–537.

139 Albert DM, Williams SR. Clinical and anatomic considerations of the Tobey-Ayer test in lateral sinus thrombosis. J Laryngol Otol 1986;100:1311–1313.

140 Askenasy HM, Kosary IZ, Braham J. Thrombosis of the longitudinal sinus. Neurology 1962;12:288–292.

141 Evans RW, Patten BM. Trichinosis associated with superior sagittal sinus thrombosis. Ann Neurol 1982;11:216–217.

142 Krayenbuhl H. Cerebral venous thrombosis. Clin Neurosurg 1967;14:1–24.

143 Polters AA, Jones AW. Intracranial venous thrombosis in Uganda. East Afr Med J 1973;50:634–643.

144 Strauss SI, Stern NS, Mendelow H, Spatz SS. Septic superior sagittal sinus thrombosis after oral surgery. J Oral Surg 1973;31:560–565.

145 Stuart EA, O'Brien FH, McNally WJ. Cerebral venous thrombosis. Ann Otol Rhinol Laryngol 1951;60:406–438.

146 Pfister HW, Borasio GD, Dirnagl U, Bauer M, Einhaupl KM. Cerebovascular complications of bacterial meningitis in adults. Neurology 1992;42:1497–1504.

147 Thron A, Wessel K, Linden D, Schroth G, Dichgans J. Superior sagittal sinus thrombosis: neuroradiological evaluation and clinical findings. J Neurol 1986;233:283–288.

148 el Alaoui-Faris M, Birouk N, Slassi I, Jiddane M, Chkili T. Thrombosis of the upper longitudinal sinus and syphilitic cranial osteitis. Rev Neurol Paris 1992;148:783–785.

149 Rao KCVG, Knipp HC, Wagner EJ. Computer tomographic findings in cerebral sinus and venous thrombosis. Radiology 1981;140:391–398.

150 Shinohara Y, Yoshitoshi M, Yoshii F. Appearance and disappearance of empty sign in superior sagittal sinus thrombosis. Stroke 1986;17:1282–1284.

151 Yeakley JW, Mayer JS, Patchell LL, Lee KF, Miner ME. The pseudodelta sign in acute head trauma. J Neurosurg 1988;69:867–868.

152 Nadel L, Braun IF, Kraft KA, Fatouros PP, Laine FJ. Intracranial vascular abnormalities: value of MR phase imaging to distinguish thrombus from flowing blood. Am J Roentgenol 1991;156:373–380.

153 Nadel L, Braun IF, Kraft KA, Jensen ME, Laine FJ. MRI of intracranial sinovenous thrombosis: the role of phase imaging. Magn Reson Imaging 1990;8:315–320.

154 Diaz JM, Schiffman JS, Urban ES, Maccario M. Superior sagittal sinus thrombosis and pulmonary embolism: a syndrome rediscovered. Acta Neurol Scand 1992;86:390–396.

155 Ravussin P, Abou-Madi M, Archer D, et al. Changes in CSF pressure after mannitol in patients with and without elevated CSF pressure. J Neurosurg 1988;69:869–876.

156 Lebel MH, Freij BJ, Syrogiannopoulos GA, et al. Dexamethasone therapy for bacterial meningitis. Results of two double-blind, placebo-controlled trials. N Engl J Med 1988;319:964–971.

157 Odio CM, Faingezicht I, Paris M, et al. The beneficial effects of early dexamethasone administration in infants and children with bacterial meningitis. N Engl J Med 1991;324:1525–1531.

158 Einhaupl KM, Villringer A, Meister W, et al. Heparin treatment in sinus venous thrombosis. Lancet 1991;388:597–600.

159 Fries G, Wallenfang T, Hennen J, et al. Occlusion of the pig superior sagittal sinus, bridging and cortical veins: multistep evolution of sinus-vein thrombosis. J Neurosurg 1992;77:127–133.

160 Tsai FY, Higashida RT, Matovich V, Alfieri K. Acute thrombosis of the intracranial dural sinus: direct thrombolytic treatment. Am J Neuroradiol 1992;13:1137–1141.

161 Manthous CA, Chen H. Case report: treatment of superior sagittal sinus thrombosis with urokinase. Conn Med 1992;56:529–530.

Acute and Chronic Mastoiditis: Clinical Presentation, Diagnosis, and Management

JOSEPH B. NADOL, JR.
ROLAND D. EAVEY

Acute and chronic infections of the mastoid are still relatively common despite the introduction of antimicrobials in the 1930s. However, the incidence of acute mastoiditis has diminished substantially coincident with the introduction of sulfonamides and antibiotics. For example, in 1936, before the use of sulfonamides, 45.9% of patients admitted to Los Angeles County Hospital with acute suppurative otitis media eventually required mastoidectomy. However, by 1943, only 17.6% of cases treated with sulfonamide compounds required surgery (1). The need for simple mastoidectomy at one institution in Pennsylvania dropped from 119 in 1937 to only 6 from 1951 to 1954 (2). By 1959, the incidence of acute mastoiditis was 0.4% in a series of 12,000 cases of acute suppurative otitis media reported by Palva and Pulkkinen (3). In a review of the effectiveness of antimicrobial therapy for acute otitis media in 1954, Rudberg found that 9.3 to 69.5% of patients eventually required mastoid surgery prior to the introduction of antibiotics, whereas thereafter the need for mastoidectomy dropped to 1.5 to 28% of cases (4). The incidence of secondary complications due to acute mastoiditis, including brain abscess and meningitis, has also declined substantially (5).

Despite the success of antibiotic treatment of acute otitis media in preventing mastoiditis and other complications, acute mastoiditis still occurs, and the incidence of chronic otitis media has probably been little changed.

ANATOMY OF THE MIDDLE EAR AND MASTOID

The pneumatized regions of the temporal bone include the middle ear, mastoid, perilabyrinthine cells, petrous apex, and accessory pneumatized areas including the squamous, occipital, and styloid bones (6) (Figure 9.1). The degree of pneumatization of the temporal bone is highly variable. Pneumatization of the mastoid and petrous apex regions progress rapidly in the neonatal and adoles-

204

cent periods and may continue slowly throughout life (7). The principal communication between the mastoid and middle ear compartments is the aditus ad antrum (see Figure 9.1), which may easily become blocked by an inflammatory process, which in turn leads to sequestration and poor drainage of the mastoid compartment (8,9).

ACUTE MASTOIDITIS

Although every case of acute suppurative otitis media demonstrates an inflammatory process in the communicating mastoid compartment, acute mastoiditis will be defined as an acute infection that results in pyogenic granulation in the mastoid and middle ear (Figure 9.2) and osteolysis of its bony trabeculae, as shown by computerized tomography (CT) imaging.

Pathophysiology

Infrequently, acute mastoiditis can be a complication of leukemia, mononucleosis, sarcoma of the temporal bone, and Kawasaki disease (10). More commonly, acute mastoiditis follows an episode of acute suppurative otitis media. As the mucoperiosteum becomes inflamed, obstruction and sequestration of the infection may occur at the aditus ad antrum or in smaller air cell tracts. As the infection intensifies, active bone remodeling with osteoclastic bone resorption occurs. Much of the calcified trabecular network and periosteal bone may be

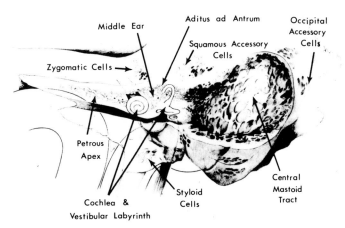

Figure 9.1. Pneumatized compartments of the temporal bone. The middle ear communicates with the mastoid air cell system primarily through the aditus ad antrum. In addition to the middle ear and mastoid, the petrous apex may be pneumatized in some individuals. In particularly well-pneumatized temporal bone, accessory air cells may be found in the root of the zygoma, squamous, occipital, and styloid bones.

replaced by noncalcified, soft woven bone. This is referred to as the coalescent stage of acute mastoiditis. Such bony changes involve not only the trabeculae within the mastoid, but also the plates of bone that separate the mastoid air cells from the external auditory canal, postauricular soft tissues, middle cranial fossa superiorly, and the sigmoid sinus posteriorly.

Diagnosis

Acute mastoiditis is most commonly preceded by acute otitis media. However, the absence of a history of acute otitis media does not rule out acute mastoiditis. Approximately 80% of cases of acute mastoiditis occur in chidren and adolescents. Pain in the ear and postauricular area is universal in chidren and adults. In infants, fussiness and ear pulling are common.

   On physical examination, an anterior, lateral, and inferior displacement of the auricle is common, but not universally present (Figure 9.3). Almost all patients will have postauricular or supra-auricular tenderness. Fever, erythema, and edema in the postauricular area are common. The external auditory canal may be narrowed by "sagging" of the skin of the posterosuperior canal due to a subperiosteal abscess or cellulitis.

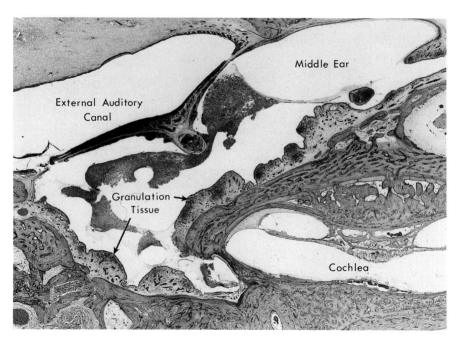

Figure 9.2.   Acute suppurative otitis media and mastoiditis secondary to *Haemophilus influenzae* in a 7-month-old girl who died of meningitis five days after the onset of fever and ear pain. There was no evidence of bacterial labyrinthitis (original magnification ×8.5).

The tympanic membrane may be difficult to visualize if the canal is narrowed. In about 10% of cases of acute mastoiditis, the tympanic membrane may be normal because the infection of the middle ear has resolved and the aditus ad antrum has become blocked by pyogenic granulation tissue. It is even possible to have a significant sequela of acute mastoiditis, such as sigmoid sinus thrombophlebitis, without significant postauricular or tympanic membrane findings (11). Conversely, some conditions can mimic acute mastoiditis such as retroauricular lymphadenitis or external otitis with postauricular extension of cellulitis.

Ancillary Studies

Leukocytosis is common. A blood culture may be positive, particularly in thrombophlebitis of the lateral venous sinus.

Plain radiographs of the mastoid have been superceded by CT, which is the single most useful radiographic technique and will demonstrate a fluid-filled middle ear and mastoid, demineralization of the bony trabeculae of the mastoid (Figure 9.4) and may demonstrate intracranial complications (Figure 9.5). Thrombophlebitis of the lateral venous sinus is best demonstrated by magnetic resonance imaging (MRI), digital subtraction angiography, or radionucleotide scanning (Figures 9.6 and 9.7). An audiogram can be performed although this may prove uncomfortable in a patient with a tender mastoid. Audiology should

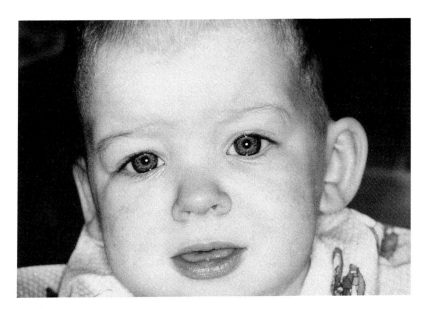

Figure 9.3. The left auricle is displaced anteriorly and laterally by a subperiosteal abscess in this infant with acute mastoiditis.

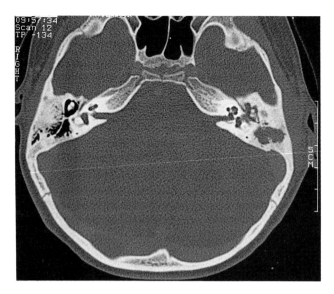

Figure 9.4.   Axial CT scan with bone technique demonstrates acute left mastoiditis in a 7-year-old boy. In addition to opacification of the middle ear and mastoid air cells, there has been loss of the trabecular pattern of the mastoid air cell system on the left, secondary to the acute osteolytic process.

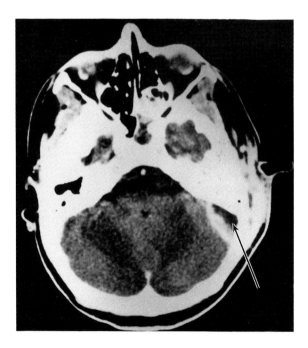

Figure 9.5.   Soft tissue windows and axial CT scan in a patient with acute mastoiditis demonstrate an epidural abscess of the left posterior fossa (*arrow*).

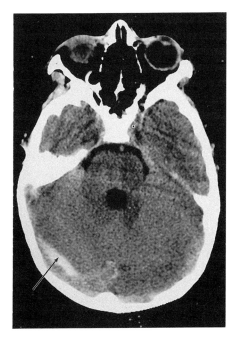 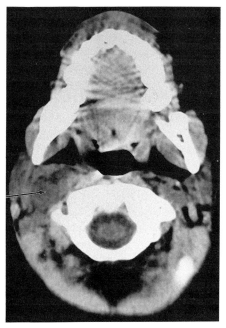

Figure 9.6. A (Left). Acute mastoiditis of the right ear, complicated by thrombosis of the right transverse sinus in a 6-year-old boy with a temperature of 103°F and headache. Soft tissue CT scan without contrast demonstrates thrombus in the right transverse sinus (*arrow*). B (Right). Soft tissue CT scan of the upper neck demonstrates edema around the internal jugular vein (*arrow*).

also be deferred if the patient has a serious complication requiring immediate surgical management.

Microbiology

The most common pathogens in acute suppurative otitis media are *Haemophilus influenzae*, *Streptococcus pneumoniae*, and *Moraxella catarrhalis*. However, mixed cultures of aerobes and anaerobes are common in acute mastoiditis. Occasionally, anaerobes are the sole organism isolated, including gram-positive cocci, gram-positive bacilli, and gram-negative bacilli. The most common aerobes are group A β-hemolytic streptococci, *Staphylococcus aureus*, *Proteus mirabilis*, *Staphylococcus epidermidis*, and *Pseudomonas aeruginosa*.

In some studies there has been less disparity between cultures in acute otitis media and acute mastoiditis. In a study of 30 children with acute mastoiditis between 1973 and 1984, cultures were positive for *S. pneumoniae* in seven, *S.*

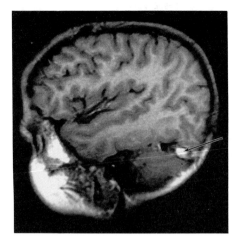
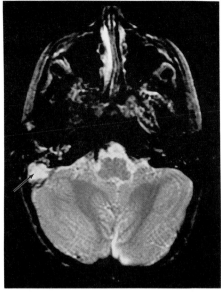

Figure 9.6. C (Top Left). Sagittal MRI with T1-weighted image demonstrates thrombus in the right transverse sinus (*arrow*). D (Top Right). T2-weighted axial MRI image demonstrates thrombus in the right sigmoid sinus (*arrow*).

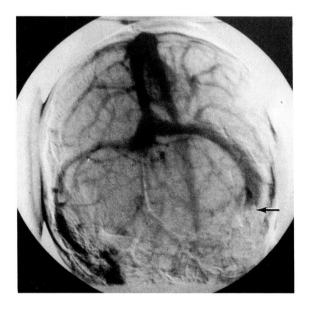

Figure 9.7. Occlusion of the sigmoid sinus (*arrow*) demonstrated by digital subtraction angiography in a child with acute mastoiditis.

epidermidis in five, *H. influenzae* in three, group A β-hemolytic streptococci in three, anaerobes in three, *S. aureus* in three, *P. aeruginosa* in one (12). Although Prellner and Rydell found a predominance of *S. pneumoniae*, the other organisms were almost evenly divided between *H. influenzae*, β-hemolytic streptococci, *S. aureus*, *P. mirabilis*, *Pseudomonas* and *Bacteroides* species (13).

The bacterial spectrum of acute otitis media has changed in the last half of this century. Before 1940, almost half the cases of acute mastoiditis were caused by group A β-hemolytic streptococci compared to a 0 to 10% incidence during the years 1970 to 1983. In addition, evidence suggests that the serotypes of pneumococcus isolated from patients with acute otitis media have changed over time (14). Although the overall incidence of acute mastoiditis caused by *Mycobacterium tuberculosis* has declined, there has been an increase in acute otitis media and mastoiditis caused by *Mycobacterium fortuitum* and *Mycobacterium chelonae* (15). It is uncertain whether the changes in the bacteriology of acute mastoiditis are in part responsible for the decline in incidence and the severity of this infection.

Management of Uncomplicated Acute Mastoiditis

Medical Management   Ideally, the choice of antibiotics should be based on the results of Gram stain and bacterial culture and susceptibility testing. However, culture results are not be available for 1 to 3 days, and in approximately one third of cultures, no growth occurs.

Selection of initial parenteral antibiotics should be based on the prevalence of common organisms. For example, a logical choice would be a combination of a semisynthetic penicillin and chloramphenicol. This combination provides broad-spectrum coverage for gram-positive organisms such as *Streptococcus* and *Staphylococcus* in addition to such organisms as *H. influenzae* and gram-negative bacteria. These antibiotics also penetrate the blood–brain barrier. Should *Pseudomonas* be suspected, treatment is best achieved by using two agents, including an aminoglycoside such as gentamicin or tobramycin and a third-generation cephalosporin such as ceftazidime. Should the tympanic membrane be open from either a spontaneous perforation or a myringotomy, antibiotic ear drops should also be used. In uncomplicated cases, clinical improvement should occur within 24 to 48 hours. Proof of efficacy of newer antibiotics is hampered by the decreased incidence of mastoiditis, which makes clinical trials difficult.

Intravenous antibiotics should be continued until acute signs and symptoms have resolved, usually about one week (16,17). However, the period of resolution can range from 3 days to 3 weeks. Because the pathology of acute mastoiditis involves osteitis and not osteomyelitis, a longer course of intravenous antibiotics is almost never required. After cessation of intravenous antibiotics, an oral antibiotic should be continued for approximately 2 additional weeks. In the case of a mastoiditis due to *Pseudomonas*, outpatient therapy may not be possible in children because ciprofloxin is not approved for this age group, and home intravenous therapy may not be practical.

Surgery   Should the patient not be making obvious progress with intravenous antibiotics, surgery is indicated. Mastoid surgery is required in approximately one half of the patients admitted with acute mastoiditis (16,17). The goals of surgery include drainage of an abscess if present, procurement of representative material for Gram stain, culture and susceptibility testing; debridement of infected bone and granulation tissue to reestablish communication between the middle ear and mastoid; and placement of a ventilation tube in the tympanic membrane to provide drainage.

When urgent surgery is indicated, antibiotics should be withheld until purulent material has been obtained. Surgery for complicated acute mastoiditis depends on the location and extent of the complication.

Complications

Although the mortality rate has dropped to 0%, the frequency of complications of acute mastoiditis is still in the range of 20 to 30% (16).

Subperiosteal Abscess The most common extracranial complication of acute mastoiditis is subperiosteal abscess (14). This occurs most frequently in the postauricular region or in the posterior-superior aspect of the external canal. Occasionally, an abscess may occur in the root of the zygomatic bone or in the neck as a Bezold's abscess. Surgical drainage via postauricular incision and simple mastoidectomy is indicated.

Paralysis of Facial Nerve Facial paralysis should raise the suspicion of a virulent organism or an immunocompromised patient. A higher incidence of gram-negative organisms, especially *P. aeruginosa*, has been reported in association with this complication (18). Failure to respond to intravenous antibiotic therapy requires surgical drainage and exploration of the facial nerve.

Intracranial Abscess, Meningitis, and Thrombophlebitis of a Venous Sinus An intracranial abscess is generally evacuated prior to mastoidectomy although the two procedures may be performed under the same anesthesia. For intracranial septic complications without abscess formation, such as meningitis, otitic hydrocephalus, and thrombophlebitis of the sigmoid sinus, mastoidectomy is almost always indicated although it may be delayed until the patient has been stabilized on intravenous antibiotics. The mortality rate for thrombosis of the lateral venous sinus in the preantibiotic era was 24% (19) despite surgical intervention. With a combination of intravenous antibiotics and timely surgical intervention, this rate has been reduced to nearly 0%.

Future Considerations and Prevention

Strategies to reduce the incidence of acute otitis media should correlate with the further diminution of the incidence of acute mastoiditis. A high index of suspicion and rapid diagnosis and treatment of these patients would also help to minimize complications and shorten length of hospital stay. It is ironic that the diagnosis of acute otitis media has increased about 200% in the last 20 years in the younger age groups (20). This has been ascribed to increased use of day care for children and improved instruments for otoscopy. Vaccines for *S. pneumoniae,* nontypeable *H. influenzae* and *Moraxella catarrhalis* may reduce the incidence of otitis media and hence acute mastoiditis. Recognition of the common and atypical presentations of acute mastoiditis will reduce the morbidity of this disease.

CHRONIC MASTOIDITIS

Definition and Categories

Chronic mastoiditis or chronic otitis media is best understood by defining several subcategories (Table 9.1). Chronic active otitis media implies a chronic progressive inflammatory process in the middle ear and mastoid but not always with suppuration. In chronic active otitis media with cholesteatoma, an epidermal cyst in the middle ear or mastoid may cause progressive resorption of bone with or without infection. Chronic active otitis media without cholesteatoma implies a chronic perforation and suppurative drainage from the tympanomastoid compartment.

Chronic inactive otitis media may occur with and without frequent reactivation. By definition, in neither category is cholesteatoma present. The typical presentation of chronic inactive otitis media with frequent reactivation is intermittent otorrhea, which promptly responds to medical management but recurs soon after cessation of treatment. Chronic inactive otitis media without frequent reactivation implies the presence of the residua of previous suppuration and inflammation, but without active or progressive disease. Thus, chronic perforation (without suppuration), ossicular fixation or resorption, or deposition of fibrous tissue in the mucosa and around ossicles (chronic adhesive otitis media or tympanosclerosis) are common findings. These subcategories of chronic otitis media have significant therapeutic implications, as will be discussed.

Table 9.1. Categories of Chronic Otitis Media (COM)

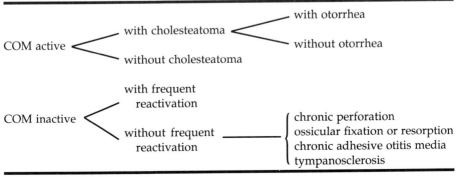

Pathogenesis

Chronic active otitis media without cholesteatoma generally begins as acute suppurative otitis media and mastoiditis. The mechanisms by which chronic suppurative otitis media progresses to chronic otitis media are unknown. However, it is generally believed that obstruction within the tympanomastoid compartment is an important factor in sequestration and chronicity of the suppurative process. Thus, poor function of the eustachian tube leading to middle ear effusion and subsequent infection plays a role in the pathogenesis of chronic suppurative otitis media. Likewise, inflammatory obstruction at the small communication between the middle ear compartment and the mastoid compartment called the aditus ad antrum may result in sequestration and poor drainage of the mastoid compartment (8,9).

The pathogenesis of cholesteatoma remains controversial. A cholesteatoma is an epithelial inclusion cyst in the tympanic or mastoid compartment, which may become secondarily infected. Clinically, these lesions are divided into congenital and acquired forms. Congenital cholesteatoma is rare and is thought to result from an epithelial rest in the middle ear during development. Acquired cholesteatoma is further subdivided into primary and secondary types. Secondary acquired cholesteatoma results from epithelial migration through a perforation into the tympanomastoid compartment and the subsequent development of an epithelial inclusion cyst. A primary acquired cholesteatoma develops without true perforation of the tympanic membrane. The usual mechanism involves progressive medial retraction of the tympanic membrane, usually in its superior portion (pars flaccida). Such retractions are thought to be secondary to chronic negative pressure within the middle ear, in turn due to dysfunction of the eustachian tube. Thus, progressive retraction of the tympanic membrane results in trapping of squamous epithelium of the lateral surface of the tympanic membrane in a "retraction pocket" that then invades the middle ear and mastoid compartments. Other mechanisms of cholesteatoma formation have also been proposed, including squamous metaplasia of the respiratory mucosa of the middle ear (21,22) or hyperplasia of basal cells of the tympanic membrane resulting in epithelial invasion of the middle ear (23,24).

Prevalence

There is little information concerning the prevalence of the various forms of chronic otitis media. It is generally believed that chronic active otitis media without cholesteatoma is three to four times more common than chronic otitis media with cholesteatoma (25). In 1978, it was estimated that there were approximately 4.2 and 13.8 hospital discharges per 100,000 population with chronic otitis media with and without cholesteatoma, respectively (26).

Bacteriology

The most common aerobic organisms cultured from ears with chronic otitis media are *Pseudomonas*, *Proteus*, *Streptococcus*, *Staphylococcus* species, and *Escherichia coli*. Compared to earlier reports in which anerobic organisms comprised only 1 to 5% of isolated organisms, more current reports suggest that the incidence of anerobic organisms is between 30 and 60% of all cases of chronic otitis media. Most commonly anaerobes are found as mixed flora along with an aerobic organism (27–29). It is assumed that this change in prevalence of anerobic organisms is related to better microbiologic technique rather than a true change in prevalence.

Histopathology

A review of the histopathology of chronic otitis media will provide a basis for better understanding of the options for treatment of chronic suppuration and reconstruction of the middle ear to achieve improvement in hearing.

Rarefying Osteitis and Fibrocystic Sclerosis   Osteoclastic resorption of bone is a common finding in chronic otitis media (Figure 9.8). This process results in

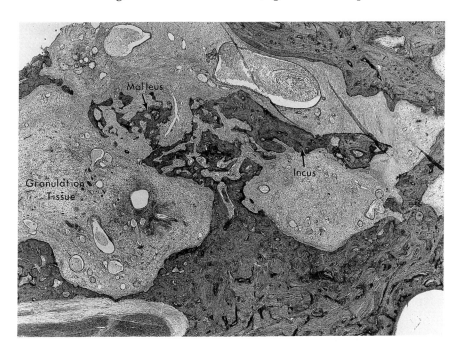

Figure 9.8.   Rarifying osteitis of malleus and incus. This horizontal section is taken through the attic, or epitympanum, of a 44-year-old man with chronic active otitis media without cholesteatoma. The epitympanum is filled with granulation tissue and there is active resorption of the head of the malleus and body of the incus (original magnification ×23).

loss of the normal trabecular architecture of the mastoid, which can be recognized on CT scan, dehiscences between the mastoid and the dura of the middle or posterior fossa, dehiscences in the otic capsule resulting in labyrinthine fistulas, and resorption and discontinuity of the ossicular chain. It is important to differentiate this process from osteomyelitis of the temporal bone, which is most frequently seen as a complication of malignant or invasive external otitis. In osteomyelitis of the temporal bone, the resorptive and suppurative process spreads along vascular and fascial planes and creates microabscesses, often in noncontinuous foci (30). In contrast, in uncomplicated chronic otitis media, rarefying osteitis occurs along the interface with either cholesteatoma or granulation tissue in the tympanomastoid compartment.

As granulation tissue matures, fibrous tissue is deposited in the submucosal region of the previous air space of the tympanomasoid compartment. This fibrocystic sclerosis may cause further obstruction of the mastoid compartment, producing aditus block and may produce a conductive hearing loss by interfering with the motion of the ossicular chain and round window membrane (Figure 9.9).

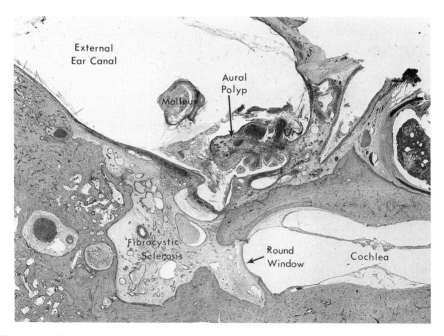

Figure 9.9.   Fibrocystic sclerosis of the middle ear. This 83-year-old woman had bilateral chronic active otitis media for many years. This horizontal section through the left temporal bone demonstrates a large perforation and an aural polyp eminating from the middle ear mucosa. In the round window niche, the normally aerated middle ear is replaced by a subepithelial deposition of fibrous tissue termed "fibrocystic sclerosis" (original magnification ×7.6).

Cholesteatoma   Cholesteatoma is best understood as an epidermal inclusion cyst within the tympanomastoid compartment (Figure 9.10). In such a closed space, it has an osteolytic potential, resulting in resorption of bone of the mastoid, dural plates, otic capsule, or ossicular chain. This bone resorption is thought to be secondary to both enzymatic and cell-mediated processes (31,32). Both superinfection and presumed increased pressure, caused by cholesteatoma formation in a closed space, may potentiate the osteolytic process (Figure 9.11). Despite experimental evidence that enzymatic processes are involved in the osteolytic potential of cholesteatoma, clinically it is clear that entrapment and superinfection play dominant roles. Thus, during a surgical procedure, if cholesteatoma is left in situ and only decompressed by exteriorization, reparative bone formation may occur subjacent to cholesteatoma, resulting in closure of a previous fistula.

Tympanosclerosis   Hyalin may be deposited in a submucosal plane as a consequence of chronic otitis media. This may occur within the tympanic membrane (Figure 9.12) around ligaments of the ossicular chain (Figure 9.13), resulting in conductive hearing loss or in further obstruction of the tympanomastoid compartment. Occasionally, new bone formation may be seen within a tympanosclerotic focus (see Figure 9.12).

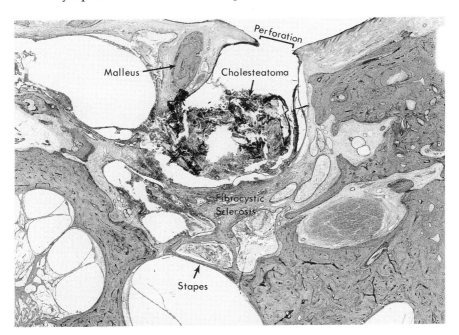

Figure 9.10.   Posterior perforation with cholesteatoma in a 64-year-old man with mixed hearing loss. There was also resorption of the long process of incus and head of stapes and fibrocystic sclerosis of the posterior middle ear space (original magnification ×13).

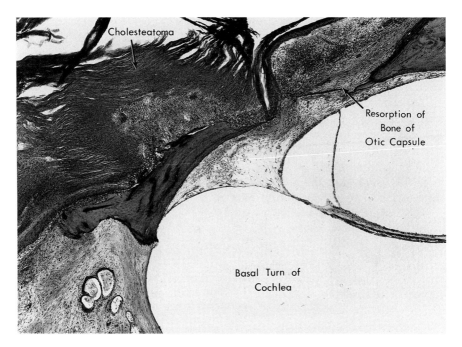

Figure 9.11. Cholesteatoma with resorption of bone of the otic capsule. This 71-year-old man had a lifelong history of bilateral chronic active otitis media. Subjacent to cholesteatoma there was bone resorption overlying the otic capsule of the basal turn of the cochlea (original magnification ×60).

Cholesterol Granuloma   Poor eustachian tube function and subsequent inflammation of the tympanomastoid compartment results in decreased aeration of the air spaces of the petrous bone and microhemorrhages. A cholesterol granuloma is considered to be a foreign body reaction to cholesterol from such exudates (Figure 9.14). A cholesterol granuloma, or cholesterol cyst, may contain blue-brown fluid with cholesterol crystals and may present clinically as an effusion behind an intact tympanic membrane (idiopathic hemotympanum). In chronic otitis media a cholesterol granuloma may be diagnosed on the basis of pathognomonic signs on imaging (Figure 9.15) or as a blue-domed cyst in a postoperative mastoid cavity (33). Cholesterol granuloma may also occur in the petrous apex region of the temporal bone without a clear history of previous otitis media (34). A cholesterol granuloma may cause localized destruction of bone (35).

Diagnosis

The presenting symptoms and signs of chronic otitis media without cholesteatoma include hearing loss and painless and malodorous, intermittent or chronic otorrhea, and perforation of the tympanic membrane. In chronic

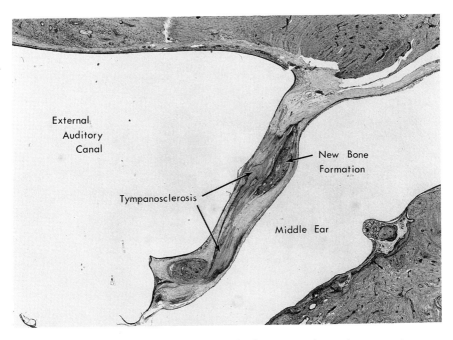

Figure 9.12. Histologic section through the external canal, tympanic membrane, and middle ear of a 73-year-old woman with chronic inactive otitis media of the left ear. The tympanic membrane is thickened by subepithelial deposition of tympanosclerosis with new bone formation (original magnification ×28).

active otitis media with cholesteatoma, otorrhea may not be present. The most common location for cholesteatoma is in the pars flaccida area of the tympanic membrane. Conductive hearing loss may be caused by interference with the motion of the ossicular chain by cholesteatoma, granulation tissue, perforation of the tympanic membrane, or ossicular discontinuity. In chronic inactive otitis media there may be a perforation or retraction of the tympanic membrane and usually significant scarring or tympanosclerosis. The presenting signs and symptoms of complications of chronic mastoiditis are presented later in this chapter. Vertigo, facial paresis, and pain are not part of the presenting symptoms of uncomplicated chronic otitis media. The differential diagnosis of purulent otorrhea with granulomatous material in the middle ear compartment include tuberculous otitis media (36), chronic granulomatous disease, including Wegener's granulomatosis (37), or neoplastic processes, including squamous cell carcinoma. The incidence of tuberculosis of the middle ear seems to be increasing in immunocompromised patients (38). In general, in a patient with otorrhea and granulomatous material in the middle ear, a transcanal biopsy is indicated if the presenting signs and symptoms are atypical for uncomplicated chronic otitis media, including pain, vertigo, sensorineural

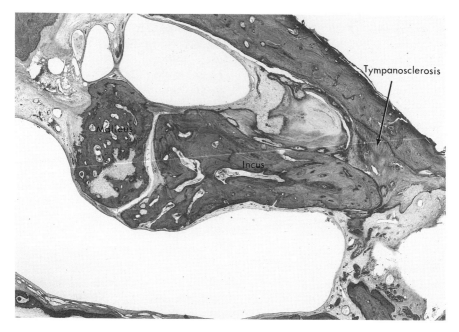

Figure 9.13. Tympanosclerosis fixing the short process of the incus in the epitympanum in a 69-year-old man with chronic inactive otitis media of the right ear (original magnification ×20).

hearing loss, and facial nerve or lower cranial nerve deficits. Malignant external otitis may also present with otorrhea and granulation tissue within the external auditory canal. However, in most cases, the tympanic membrane is intact and severe pain and tenderness are hallmarks of malignant external otitis and not of chronic otitis media.

Role of Bacterial Culture and Radiographic Imaging of the Temporal Bone

Bacterial culture of otorrhea is helpful in management decisions and is absolutely indicated in the presence of complications of chronic otitis media or in the immunocompromised host. Previous treatment with oral antibiotics or topical antibiotic drops will clearly interfere with culture. To avoid skin contaminants, the technique of culture should include suction cleansing of the external ear canal and the use of a microswab placed directly through the perforation into the middle ear space for both aerobic and anaerobic cultures. Imaging of the temporal bone is seldom necessary for the diagnosis of chronic otitis media, but may be extremely helpful in determining the extent of disease in recurrent chronic otitis media, or to evaluate complications of chronic otitis media, such as vertigo, facial paresis, pain, headache, sensorineural hearing

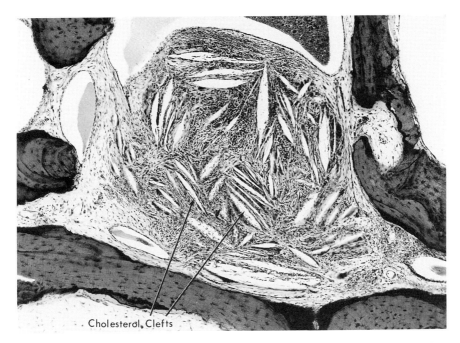

Cholesterol Clefts

Figure 9.14. Cholesterol granuloma in mastoid air cells of a 75-year-old woman with chronic otitis media. Cholesterol clefts are surrounded by fibrous tissue with multinucleated giant cells (original magnification ×105).

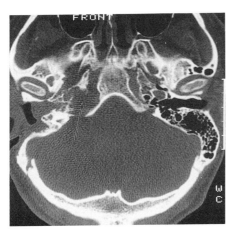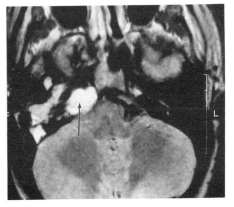

Figure 9.15. Cholesterol granuloma of the right petrous apex in a 32-year-old man with recurrent right ear symptoms following previous mastoidectomy. Left. Bone window axial CT scan demonstrates a lytic lesion of the right petrous apex (*arrow*). Right. T2-weighted axial MRI demonstrates a bright lesion (*arrow*) corresponding to the lytic area on CT scan.

loss, or suspected abscess formation. In general, CT scanning is the preferred method of imaging. MRI is particularly suited to cases of suspected intracranial complications of chronic otitis media, such as lateral venous sinus thrombosis or abscess formation.

Treatment

Medical Management In cases of chronic active otitis media without cholesteatoma, medical management may result in resolution of otorrhea. Medical management includes local hygiene, topical and oral antibiotics, and occasionally parenteral antibiotic administration (39,40).

Instructing the patient to observe water precautions is an essential element of management. Topical administration of antibiotics such as Cortisporin® may result in resolution of the edema and subsequent obstruction. Generally, oral antibiotics are selected on the basis of culture results and are continued for a minimum of two weeks, and otic drops may be necessary for three or more weeks. If the infection responds, a waiting period must be instituted to determine whether the process has been rendered inactive (chronic inactive otitis media) or whether the infection will promptly recur due to a subclinical nidus within the tympanomastoid compartment or the presence of aditus block (chronic inactive otitis media with frequent reactivation). If, after three months, there has been no recurrence of infection, no further treatment may be necessary or, alternatively, the patient may be considered for elective reconstructive surgery to repair the perforation and to treat conductive hearing loss due to ossicular discontinuity or fixation. On the other hand, if the infection promply recurs, a diagnosis of chronic inactive otitis media with frequent reactivation has been established. In such cases, CT imaging of the temporal bone, particularly during the quiescent phase, may be useful. In general, a surgical procedure is indicated to prevent recurrence.

In chronic active otitis media with cholesteatoma, surgical removal of the cholesteatoma and reconstruction of the middle ear are indicated in most situations unless contraindicated by other medical conditions of the patient.

Surgery The objectives of surgery for chronic otitis media include extirpation of the disease, alteration of the anatomy of the tympanomastoid compartment to prevent recurrence and, finally, reconstruction of the hearing mechanism (40). The proper surgical approach depends on the subcategory of chronic active otitis media. Thus, for example, in chronic active otitis media with cholesteatoma limited to the attic region and with no history of otorrhea, a limited transcanal procedure (tympanoplasty and atticotomy) may be sufficient. In all cases in which there has been recalcitrant otorrhea (chronic active otitis media with or without cholesteatoma; chronic inactive otitis media with frequent reactivation) mastoidectomy is a necessary component of the surgical approach. In the otologic literature, there is still controversy concerning the relative indications for "canal wall up" versus "canal wall down" tympanomastoidectomy. In both procedures, a mastoidectomy is done. However, in the canal wall down approach the bony canal between the external auditory canal and the mastoid is removed, effectively resulting in exteriorization of the mastoid to the external ear canal. The principle rationale of the canal wall up approach is to preserve the normal anatomy of the external auditory canal and obviate the need for periodic cleaning of a mastoid bowl. However, the incidence of recurrent or residual cholesteatoma in the canal up approach is higher than that for canal wall down surgery and approaches 30% (41,42). In general, the canal wall down approach may be preferable in cases of large cholesteatoma, recurrent chronic otitis media after previous surgery, in the presence of complications of chronic otitis media, or in individuals in whom possible revision surgery is medically contraindicated. On the other hand, the canal wall up approach is ideal in cases of chronic inactive otitis media with frequent reactivation.

Reconstruction   Reconstruction of the tympanic membrane and ossicular chain may be done in conjunction with either a canal up or canal down approach, as a secondary and staged procedure following mastoid surgery, or as a primary procedure in chronic inactive otitis media. In general, the limiting factor in successful reconstruction is the function of the eustachian tube. There is no reliable clinical means of assessing eustachian tube function in the face of chronic ear disease. However, the presence of bilateral chronic otitis media, chronic adhesive otitis media, or previous surgical failure in reconstruction of the middle ear or ossicles are relative contraindications to reconstructive tympanoplasty. Details of tympanoplastic surgery are beyond the scope of this review, and the reader is referred elsewhere for this discussion (43,44).

Expected Surgical Confinement, Success Rates, Complications of Surgery
Mastoidectomy and tympanoplasty are now done on an ambulatory basis in most centers. General anesthesia for two to five hours is usually necessary. Complete healing of the surgical site including tympanic graft and external auditory canal may take from one to four months. Complications of tympanomastoid surgery include failure to control the disease process resulting in the need for revision surgery (45,46), sensorineural hearing loss, vertigo, facial nerve injury, and rarely intracranial complications. The success rate of tympanomastoid surgery for control of otorrhea approaches 85% (45), whereas the results of tympanoplastic surgery are highly variable and depend in large measure on residual eustachian tube function.

Complications

Because the only symptoms of chronic otitis media may be hearing loss and painless otorrhea, many patients still present only when complications of this disease process have occurred.

Fistulization of the Vestibular or Auditory Labyrinth Cholesteatoma or the rarefying osteitis of chronic otitis media may result in resorption of bone covering the semicircular canals or cochlea, resulting in a fistula between the inner ear and mastoid or middle ear, labyrinthitis, vertigo, and sensorineural hearing loss or meningitis (Figures 9.16 and 9.17). Fortunately, in most cases dehiscence of the bone overlying the inner ear results in clinical symptoms, such as unsteadiness, prior to an overt fistula, labyrinthitis, or meningitis. The suspicion of dehiscence or fistulization requires urgent surgical intervention, ideally with culture identification of pathogens and proper antibiotic coverage.

Paresis of the Facial Nerve Chronic otitis media with or without cholesteatoma may cause a progressive paresis of the facial nerve over hours or weeks. Differential diagnosis between facial paresis due to chronic otitis media or concomitant Bell's palsy is often difficult to make with certainty. Therefore, facial paresis in the face of chronic active otitis media should be treated as a complication of chronic otitis media and deserves emergent surgical drainage and decompression of the facial nerve. Delay of mastoid surgery for facial paralysis until degeneration of the facial nerve has occurred generally does not result in satisfactory recovery of facial nerve function.

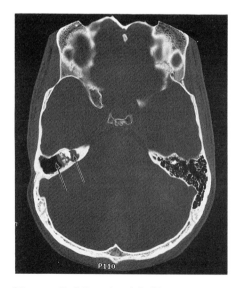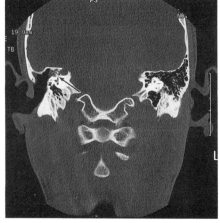

Figure 9.16. Axial (left) and coronal (right) sections demonstrate recurrent cholesteatoma in a previously operated right mastoid. In the axial section, a soft tissue mass (*arrows*), verified as cholesteatoma by subsequent surgery, is demonstrated lateral and medial to the otic capsule. In coronal section, a fistula of the superior semicircular canal is demonstrated (*arrow*).

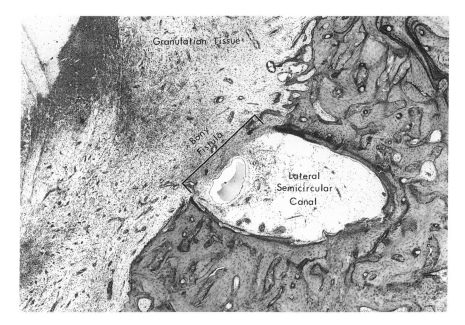

Figure 9.17. Bony fistula of the lateral semicircular canal in a 15-year-old boy with chronic active otitis media (original magnification ×45).

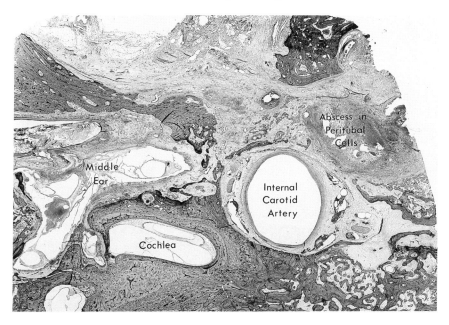

Figure 9.18. Petrous apicitis complicating chronic active otitis media of the left ear in a 76-year-old man. There was a history of recurring left otorrhea for many years. Approximately 2 months prior to death there was onset of left-sided headache and increased otorrhea. Palsy of the left sixth and tenth nerves was noted on the day of death, and bacterial culture revealed *S. aureus*. A microabscess was found in the peritubal air cells near the carotid artery (original magnification ×7.3).

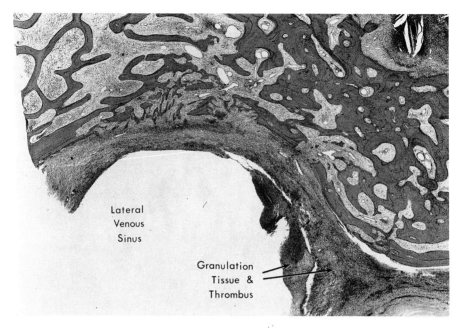

Figure 9.19. Thrombophlebitis of the lateral venous sinus in a 16-year-old boy with chronic active otitis media with cholesteatoma. Two weeks prior to death he complained of headache. On admission he was febrile, and culture of the spinal fluid revealed meningococcus. He died several hours following emergency craniotomy for left temporal lobe abscess. Histologic examination of the left mastoid showed chronic suppurative otitis media with cholesteatoma extending to the lateral venous sinus. An active thrombophlebitis with polymorphonuclear leukocytes is seen within the lumen of the lateral venous sinus (original magnification ×16).

Petrous Apicitis Ear pain or headache in the setting of chronic active otitis media is an ominous sign, suggesting either the presence of concurrent neoplasm or impending intracranial complication, including petrous apicitis. Petrous apicitis may present with sudden onset in the classically described Gradenigo's syndrome or may present as relatively slowly progressive signs and symptoms including sensorineural hearing loss and facial paresis over months to years before a precipitous and decompensating event such as meningitis, brain abscess, or thrombosis of the internal carotid artery (Figure 9.18).

Thrombophlebitis of the Lateral Venous Sinus Ear pain, headache, and a febrile response, especially the classical "picket fence" pyrexia in the presence of chronic otitis media, should suggest intracranial complication including thrombosis of the lateral venous sinus (Figure 9.19). Suspicion of this complication should be evaluated by CT or MRI of the temporal bone on an emergency

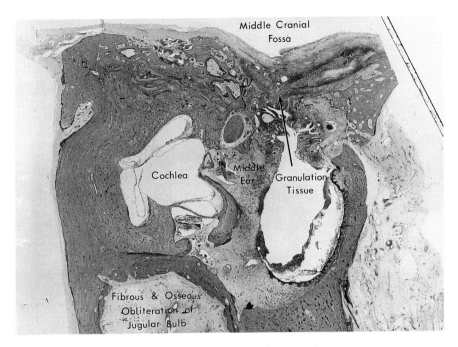

Figure 9.20. Temporal lobe abscess secondary to chronic suppurative otitis media in a 58-year-old man. He died 2 weeks following a left canal wall down mastoidectomy and one day following temporal craniotomy for drainage of a temporal lobe abscess. In this vertical section of the temporal bone, granulation tissue is seen within the middle ear, extending through a defect in the bony tegmen and into the middle cranial fossa. A long-standing fibrous obliteration and new bone formation within the jugular bulb were presumably secondary to previous thrombophlebitis from chronic otitis media (original magnification ×7.5).

basis. In the preantibiotic era, the diagnosis of suspected thrombophlebitis of the lateral venous sinus was managed by ligation of the jugular vein in the neck and emergency mastoidectomy and venotomy. Current therapy depends on the response to intravenous antibiotic therapy based on culture results. In cases in which there has been a prompt response to antibiotic therapy, surgery is delayed until the patient has become afebrile and is done only if strong evidence suggests the possibility of recurrent disease, such as the presence of cholesteatoma or chronic active otitis media. In general, opening of the lateral venous sinus is done only to drain an empyema and thrombectomy only is usually not indicated.

Meningitis and Brain Abscess Meningitis as a complication of chronic otitis media (Figure 9.20) should be treated initially with intravenous antibiotics. Surgery is delayed until the patient is stable and preferably afebrile. In cases of brain abscess complicating chronic otitis media, primary treatment should be directed toward the management of the brain abscess. Intraparenchymal abscess, in selected cases, is treated with intravenous antibiotics alone and without drainage. Tympanomastoid surgery is delayed until the patient is stable and definitive management of the abscess has been achieved. In some cases where the abscess is juxtaposed to the mastoid compartment, tympanomastoid surgery may be done to eliminate the source of the infection and simultaneously to effect drainage of the intracranial abscess.

REFERENCES

1 **House HP.** Otitis media. A comparative study of the results obtained in therapy before and after the introduction of the sulfonamide compounds. Arch Otolaryngol 1946;43:371–378.

2 **Davison FW.** Otitis media—then and now. Laryngoscope 1955;65:142–151.

3 **Palva T, Pulkkinen K.** Mastoiditis. J Laryngol Otol 1959;73:573–588.

4 **Rudberg RD.** Acute otitis media: comparative therapeutic results of sulfonamide and penicillin administered in various forms. Acta Otolaryngol (Stockh) 1954;(suppl 113):9–79.

5 **Proctor CA.** Intracranial complications of otitic origin. Laryngoscope 1966;76:288–308.

6 **Allam A.** Pneumatization of the temporal bone. Ann Otol Rhinol Laryngol 1969;78:49–64.

7 **Eby TL, Nadol JB Jr.** Postnatal growth of the human temporal bone; implications for cochlear implants in children. Ann Otol Rhinol Laryngol 1986;95:356–364.

8 **Proctor B.** Attic-aditus block and the tympanic diaphragm. Ann Otol Rhinol Laryngol 1971;80:371–375.

9 **Richardson GS.** Aditus block. Ann Otol 1963;72:223–236.

10 **McKenna M, Eavey R.** Acute mastoiditis. In: Nadol JB, Schuknecht HF, eds. Surgery of the ear and temporal bone. New York: Raven Press, 1993:145–154.

11 Case records of the Massachusetts General Hospital. Sigmoid sinus thrombosis. N Engl J Med 1988;318:1322–1328.

12 **Ogle JW, Lauer BA.** Acute mastoiditis: diagnosis and complications. Am J Dis Child 1986:1178–1182.

13 **Prellner K, Rydell R.** Acute mastoiditis: influence of antibiotic treatment on the bacterial spectrum. Acta Otolaryngol (Stockh) 1986;102:52–56.

14 **Hansman D.** Serotypes of pneumococci in pneumonia, meningitis and other pneumococcal infections. Aust N Z J Med 1977;7:267–270.

15 **Neitch SM, Sydnor JB, Schleupner CJ.** *Mycobacterium fortunitum* as a cause of mastoiditis and wound infection. Arch Otolaryngol 1982;108:11–14.

16 **Gliklich RE, Eavey RD, Iannuzzi RA, Camacho A.** A contemporary analysis of acute mastoiditis. Otolaryngol Head Neck Surg (in press).

17 **Hawkins DB, Dru D, House JW, Clark RW.** Acute mastoiditis in children: a review of 54 cases. Laryngoscope 1983;98:568–572.

18 **Ostfeld E, Rubinstein E.** Acute gram-negative bacillary infections of the middle ear and mastoid. Ann Otol Rhinol Laryngol 1980;89:33–36.

19 **Meltzer PE.** Treatment of thrombosis of the lateral sinus: a summary of the results obtained during 12 years at the Massachusetts Eye and Ear Infirmary. Arch Otolaryngol 1935;22:131–142.

20 **Schappert SM.** Office visits for otitis media: United States 1975–90. Advance data from Vital and Health Statistics of the Centers for Disease Control/National Center for Health Statistics, U.S. Department of Health and Human Services, no. 214. September 8, 1992.

21 **Sade J.** Cellular differentiation in the middle ear lining. Ann Otol Rhinol Laryngol 1971;80:376.

22 **Chole RA, Fruch DP.** Quantitative studies of eustachian tube epithelium during experimental vitamin A deprivation and reversal. In: Sade J, ed. Cholesteatoma and mastoid surgery. Amsterdam: Kugler Publications, 1982.

23 **Ruedi L.** Cholesteatoma formation in the middle ear in animal experiments. Acta Otolaryngol 1959;50:233.

24 **Huang CC, Shi GS, Yi ZX.** Experimental induction of middle ear cholesteatoma in rats. Am J Otolaryngol 1988;9:165–172.

25 **Papparella MM, Kim CS.** Mastoidectomy update. Laryngoscope 1977;87:1977–1988.

26 **Rubin RJ.** The disease in society: evaluation of chronic otitis media in general and cholesteatoma in particular. In: Sade J, ed. Cholesteatoma and mastoid surgery. Amsterdam. Kugler Publications, 1982.

27 **Harker LA, Koontz FP.** Bacteriology of cholesteatoma: clinical significance. Transactions of the American Academy of Ophthalmology and Otolaryngology-Otolaryngology Series. 1977:683–686.

28 **Jokipii AMM, Karma P, Ojala K, Jokipii L.** Anaerobic bacteria in chronic otitis media. Arch Otolaryngol 1977;103:273–280.

29 **Brooke I.** Aerobic and anaerobic bacteriology of cholesteatoma. Laryngoscope 1981; 91:250–253.

30 **Nadol JB Jr.** Histopathology of pseudomonas osteomyelitis of the temporal bone starting as malignant external otitis. Am J Otolaryngol 1980;1:359–371.

31 **Chole RA.** Cellular and subcellular events of bone resorption in human and experimental cholesteatoma: the role of osteoclasts. Laryngoscope 1984;94:76–95.

32 **Morigama H, Huang CC, Abramson M, Kato M.** Bone resorption factors in chronic otitis media. Otolaryngol Head Neck Surg 1984;92:322–328.

33 **Palva T, Lehto VP, Johnsson L-G, Virtinen, I, Makinen J.** Large cholesterol granuloma cysts in the mastoid. Clinical and histopathologic findings. Arch Otolaryngol 1985;111:786–791.

34 **Thedinger BA, Nadol JB Jr, Montgomery WW, Thedinger BS, Greenberg JJ.** Radiographic diagnosis, surgical treatment and long term follow-up of cholesterol granulomas of the petrous apex. Laryngoscope 1989;99:896–907.

35 **Nager GT, Vanderveen TS.** Cholesterol granuloma involving the temporal bone.

Ann Otol Rhinol Laryngol 1976;85: 204–209.

36 **Turner AL, Fraser JS.** Tuberculosis of the middle ear cleft in children. A clinical and pathological study. J Laryngol Rhinol Otol 1915;30:209–247.

37 **Karmody CS.** Wegener's granulomatosis: Presentation as an otologic problem. Otolaryngology 1978;86:573–584.

38 **Ognibene FP.** Upper and lower airway manifestations of human immunodeficiency virus infection. Ear Nose Throat J 1990;69:424–431.

39 **Kenna MA, Bluestone CD, Reilly JS, Lusk RP.** Medical management of chronic suppurative otitis media without cholesteatoma in children. Laryngoscope 1986; 96:146–151.

40 **Nadol JB Jr.** The chronic draining ear. In: Gates GA, ed. Current therapy in otolaryngology head and neck surgery. Philadelphia: BC Decker, 1987:18–22.

41 **Smyth GD.** Postoperative cholesteatoma in combined approach tympanoplasty. J Laryngol Otolaryngol 1976;90:597–621.

42 **Sheehy J, Brackmann DE, Graham MD.** Cholesteatoma Surgery: Residual and Recurrent Disease. A review of 1024 cases. Ann Otol 1977;86:451–462.

43 **Montandon P.** Ossiculoplasty and tympanoplasty combined with surgery for active chronic otitis media. In: Nadol JB Jr, Schuknecht HF, eds. Surgery of the Ear and Temporal Bone. New York: Raven Press, 1993:245–253.

44 **Arrigg FG Jr, Arrigg FG Sr.** Ossicular reconstruction in chronic inactive otitis media. In: Nadol JB Jr, Schuknecht HF, eds. Surgery of the ear and temporal bone. New York: Raven Press, 1993:255–262.

45 **Nadol JB Jr.** Causes of failure of mastoidectomy for chronic otitis media. Laryngoscope 1985;95:410–493.

46 **Nadol JB Jr, Krouse JH.** The hypotympanum and infralabyrinthine cells in chronic otitis media. Laryngoscope 1991;101: 137–141.

Enteropathogenic and Enteroaggregative Strains of *Escherichia coli*: Clinical Features of Infection, Epidemiology, and Pathogenesis

CHRISTINE A. WANKE

Escherichia coli are nearly ubiquitous organisms, distributed throughout the soil and plant and animal kingdoms. These organisms were originally described by Theodore Escherich in 1885 as *Bacterium coli commune*, a name that suggests their common presence in the colon of mammalian species (1). *E. coli* are present in virtually all animal and human intestinal tracts although they may not be the predominant species. *E. coli* capable of causing disease in human or animal hosts are not morphologically or generally biochemically distinct from those that exist as normal, commensal flora. In some parts of the world, diarrheal illnesses remain a leading cause of morbidity and mortality and *E. coli* may be the etiologic agent responsible for the majority of these (2).

The ability to distinguish pathogenic *E. coli* has relied on a variety of identification techniques from associations of specific serogroups of organisms with specific diseases, bioassays for various virulence factors, and recently, recognition of homologous genetic material by DNA probes. Five groups of *E. coli* have emerged in the last 50 years as etiologic agents in diarrheal disease. The five groups include the enterotoxigenic *E. coli* (ETEC), the enterohemorrhagic *E. coli* (EHEC), the enteroinvasive *E. coli* (EIEC), the enteropathogenic *E. coli* (EPEC), and the most recently described and still controversial enteroaggregative *E. coli* (EAggEc). ETEC organisms produce a variety of secretory enterotoxins that are recognized by animal or cell culture bioassays or by DNA probes. The EHEC produce a cytotoxin similar to that of *Shigella* and are recognized by cytopathic changes in cell culture or by DNA probe; the EIEC possess the same ability to invade as *Shigella* organisms and may be recognized by the ability to cause an inflammatory conjunctivitis in guinea pigs (Sereny test) as well as by DNA probe for invasion genes. Until recently the EPEC were identified by exclusion criteria: EPEC were organisms capable of causing intestinal disease, belonged to several common serogroups, produced no enterotoxins and no cytotoxins, and were not invasive (3). Recently, more definitive means of identifying EPEC, including tissue culture adherence assays and DNA probes for adhesins, have more clearly defined these organisms (4–7). These techniques have also allowed the identification of additional groups of *E. coli* that are associated with diarrheal disease. The EAggEc also have a distinctive aggregative adherence phenotype and appear to be associated with persistent diarrheal disease in children in the developing world (2,8,9). The role of other groups of epithelial cell-adherent *E. coli*, such as those that exhibit diffuse adherence to tissue culture cells in the production of diarrheal disease, has remained more speculative (10,11).

Recent advances in the understanding of the pathogenesis of diarrheal disease by the EPEC organisms has added an exciting dimension to the understanding of intestinal cell physiology as well. Recognition that the process of adherence of bacterial cells to intestinal cells can initiate a series of host cell signal transduction pathways and can itself be responsible for the production of diarrheal disease has occurred only within the last several years (12). The widely held belief that adherence factors of enteric organisms occurred simply to reduce the clearance of organisms from the intestine or to hold an organism in the proper position to deliver a toxin to the epithelial cell has been called into question with this recognition. That adherence is an active process that can stimulate a variety of intestinal cell responses including phosphorylation of intestinal cell proteins, actin accumulation, and intracellular calcium transport has dramatically advanced the understanding of the pathogenesis of diarrheal disease by EPEC and other adherent organisms.

ENTEROPATHOGENIC *Escherichia coli*

Historical Perspective

Outbreaks of severe diarrheal disease in children have been noted since the late 1700s (1). Cholera infantum was first described in the United States by Benjamin Rush in 1789 and shortly thereafter in the United Kingdom. Epidemiologic work revealed that this disease occurred in community and hospital outbreaks, was more common in warm weather, and appeared to be associated with poorer economic status and weaning; all of these factors suggested an infectious etiology. *E. coli* were proposed as possible etiologic agents by various investigators beginning in 1889. Veterinarians had convincingly demonstrated that *E. coli* were capable of producing severe diarrhea in calves (calf scours) before 1920 by feeding strains of *E. coli* to calves and demonstrating that some organisms produced diarrhea and other *E. coli* did not (1). In the 1920s, distinct groups of *E. coli*, identified as *dyspepsiekoli*, were felt to be associated with childhood diarrhea in Germany and still other *E. coli* were identified in diarrheal outbreaks in the United States (13,14).

In 1945 in the United Kingdom, John Bray investigated an outbreak of infantile diarrhea in Uxbridge and identified an antigenically homogenous strain of *E. coli* in children with disease (1,15). This discovery led to the recognition of antigenically similar *E. coli* in other outbreaks of infantile or summer diarrhea in Scotland, London, and the United States. Simultaneously, a serotyping scheme for *E. coli* was developed by Kauffmann (16). This scheme classified *E. coli* into 160 serogroups based on somatic O antigens and was used to characterize the *E. coli* from diarrheal outbreaks. Serogroups 55 and 111 were the first to be associated with infantile diarrhea. Retrospective analysis identified these as the serogroups of the organisms first known as the *dyspepsiekoli* as well as the organisms isolated by John Bray (17,18).

Serogrouping of *E. coli* remained the standard for identification of diarrheagenic strains until the discovery of the secretory enterotoxins in the 1950s and 1960s. These toxins were detectable by bioassay with fluid production in rabbit ileal loop or suckling mouse models (2,19). The separation of diarrheagenic *E. coli* into toxin or nontoxin producing led to confusion about the role of the nontoxin-producing EPEC strains in diarrheal disease. The nontoxin-producing EPEC remained categorized by serogroup and their epidemiologic association with diarrheal disease seemed secure (Table 10.1). In retrospect, this association has held up well because studies that have determined the adherence phenotype and presence of the genetic material responsible for the recognized EPEC adherence factor have confirmed that the original outbreaks were associated with EPEC organisms. Studies in which volunteers ingested 1×10^6 to 1×10^{10} colony-forming units (CFU) of organisms of traditional EPEC serogroups also demonstrated that in adults these organisms were fully capable of causing diarrheal disease, which in some cases was severe and dehydrating (21,22).

Epidemiology

Diarrheal disease caused by EPEC organisms occurs in endemic and epidemic patterns, as does diarrheal disease caused by the majority of enteric pathogens.

Table 10.1. Classic Enteropathogenic *Escherichia coli* Serogroups

026
055*
086
0111*
0119*
0125
0126
0127*
0128*
0142*

*Signifies type 1 EPEC: serogroups that are EPEC adherence factor positive and exhibit localized adherence.

The prevalence of endemic disease varies with geographical location and season of the year. However, as with all studies examining the prevalence of diarrheal pathogens, it is difficult to exclude the possibility that study design, problems with collection of samples, or adequacy of evaluation of the samples influences the results.

Endemic Disease   Endemic EPEC disease occurs most frequently in very young infants. In urban southern Brazil, EPEC caused 26% of the diarrheal illnesses in children less than six months of age (23). In Canada, 10% of the children under one year of age hospitalized for diarrheal disease had EPEC organisms in the stool, and 6% of children of the same age with diarrhea in the community harbored EPEC in the stool (3). In the same population, EPEC were isolated from only 0.5% of children of the same age without diarrhea. EPEC were isolated from the stools of 6% of the children, aged one to three years, with diarrhea in the community and in none of the controls. *Shigella* and *Salmonella* species were the two most frequently isolated pathogens in this age group, EPEC was the third most common, and *Campylobacter* was fourth.

The rate of endemic disease caused by EPEC is higher in the summer or warm months. This has been true in studies in temperate climates from Europe and the United States and in warmer climates such as South Africa where the rate of endemic EPEC disease in blacks is increased in the hot summer months (24).

Although data strongly suggest that there has been a dramatic decrease in disease morbidity in the developed world in the last century, data from the United Kingdom suggest that there has not been a change in the incidence of sporadic or endemic disease in the last 15 to 20 years (3). Studies from around the world have demonstrated that endemic disease associated with EPEC exists as well in Israel, Egypt, Ethiopia, the Central African Republic, China, South Africa, Thailand, India, Bangladesh, Australia, and throughout Latin America (3,24–27). The proportion of endemic diarrheal disease caused by EPEC varies widely, however, from 1.8% of all acute childhood diarrhea in a study from an urban area in Peru to 3% in Bangkok and Israel to 8% in Australia and the nearly 30% in São Paulo, Brazil. In another community study from a slum in northeastern Brazil, the rate of isolation of EPEC from stools of children with acute diarrhea was no greater than the rate of isolation of EPEC from control children in the same community (28). Some of these apparent differences in prevalence may be due to detection technique. The study from São Paulo reported only serogroups of *E. coli* isolated from stools of children with diarrhea (which may overrepresent the role of EPEC), and the study from the community in northeastern Brazil reported only adherence phenotype of *E. coli* isolated from stool (and may underrepresent the contribution of EPEC). Others document EPEC adherence factor (EAF) DNA probe homology data or probe data in conjunction with adherence assay data and serogroup. Even with differences in technique taken into account, probably true geographical variation exists in the prevalence of EPEC disease, depending on environmental conditions, duration of breast-feeding in the community, and sanitation, among other factors. Because the tools to distinguish EPEC from *E. coli* that are normal flora are available only in research laboratories, it is likely that a large proportion of sporadic EPEC disease is unrecognized.

Epidemic Disease   Outbreaks or miniepidemics of EPEC-associated disease also occur. These are best documented in the developed world and occur in day care settings as well as hospital settings such as neonatal nurseries (1,3,29,30). In contrast to endemic disease, outbreaks in temperate climates occur in colder, winter months. As recently as the 1930s, the mortality rate for outbreaks in the United States was as high as 47% (1). Six to 10 outbreaks per year are documented in the United Kingdom. In the United States, the number of EPEC outbreaks has decreased since 1972, with a corresponding increase in number of outbreaks of ETEC disease in older children and adults (3). The mortality rate in these outbreaks has also significantly decreased over time. However, in a retrospective evaluation of *E. coli* collected by the Centers for Disease Control and Prevention (CDC) from 50 outbreaks of diarrheal disease between 1934 and 1987, it was possible to demonstrate an EPEC serogroup in association with 56% of the outbreaks and the EPEC adherence phenotype and homology with the EAF DNA probe in 46% of the outbreaks (3,31).

Recently, increasing epidemiologic data have linked EPEC to persistent (duration > 14 days) wasting diarrheal diseases that occur in 3% to 27% of children in the developing world (32). EPEC strains were isolated from 3.4% of children with persistent diarrhea in Peru and from 13% of children under age 5 with persistent diarrhea in an urban slum in northeastern Brazil (33,34).

Awareness of persistent diarrhea as a major health problem in the developing world has increased with the rise of the acquired immunodeficiency syndrome (AIDS) epidemic. In the human immunodeficiency virus (HIV)-infected population, persistent diarrheal disease occurs in adults as well as children (2). Few data are available about the prevalence of EPEC in diarrheal disease in either children or adults with HIV disease, but these organisms may play a role in diarrheal disease in this compromised population, as do the other enteric bacterial pathogens. Diarrheal disease was the cause of hospitalization for 70% of the children with HIV infection in São Paolo in one study and EPEC were isolated from 28% of those children. No data were available for non–HIV-infected children in this study (35). Persistent diarrheal disease was a predictor of mortality for children with AIDS in Zaire, but EPEC were isolated no more frequently from children with HIV and diarrhea than from children with HIV and no diarrhea or children without diarrhea who were not infected with the HIV virus (36). In an adult AIDS patient with persistent diarrheal disease in New York, organisms consistent with *E. coli* were visualized on fixed colonic biopsy specimens. Whether these organisms were EPEC or EAggEc or some unrelated organism requires further study (37).

An additional group at risk for EPEC diarrheal disease is travelers. ETEC cause the majority of diarrhea in travelers to the less developed world, but EPEC organisms contribute to the disease burden as well. Some authors estimate the EPEC may cause as much as 10% of diarrheal disease in travelers to some areas (38,39).

Clinical Disease

The spectrum of diarrheal disease caused by EPEC is broad, from mild diarrhea to fulminant, prolonged, and ultimately fatal disease (1,3,22,29). Many of the published series of EPEC diarrhea report outbreaks in which the morbidity and mortality were high, but milder outbreaks may not be investigated. Watery, greenish stool is described in children with EPEC diarrhea; dehydration is reported as a complication in up to 70% of children (40). Children with protracted disease may present with poor growth and a metabolic acidosis as well as dehydration. The mean duration of hospitalization of children with uncomplicated EPEC disease was 4.6 days in one study, compared with 2.4 days for children with nonbacterial gastroenteritis, 2.5 days for children with *Shigella sonnei* diarrhea, and 5.1 days for children with *Shigella flexneri* infection. Fever was reported to last a mean of 2.7 days (3). Vomiting was present during illness in 80% of children (23).

In children hospitalized with persistent and severe diarrheal disease, EPEC organisms may be recovered from stool and jejunal fluid and seen on biopsies taken throughout the length of the intestine, including the colon and rectum (40). The histologic hallmark of EPEC infection is the attaching and effacing lesion seen on the mucosal surface, with a cuplike pedestal underlying the organisms (Figure 10.1). Jejunal biopsies may also exhibit moderate to severe atrophy with disordered enterocytes. Adherent bacteria may be identified on these enterocytes and immunohistochemical staining has confirmed that these organisms belong to EPEC serogroups. Serogroup 0119 has often been associated with outbreaks of increased severity. Functionally, these children have severe malabsorption and often require parenteral nutrition. Further evidence of the severity of disease in these children, who were between the ages of 3 and 28 weeks in one study and 4 to 10 months in a second, is that even with the proper diagnosis and treatment, the younger children were hospitalized for a mean of 21 to 120 days and the older children for a mean of 7 to 28 days (41–43).

Treatment

There have been no controlled trials of treatment of EPEC disease. Reports of the efficacy of oral gentamicin or neomycin in children hospitalized with severe EPEC diarrhea have been published. Treatment for 5 to 7 days resulted in clearance of the organisms from stool during the course of treatment, but diarrhea resolved more gradually in these severely ill children and abated entirely only when nutrition had been reestablished, often parenterally (41,42). More recently, trials of oral gentamicin for 6 days in children with persistent diarrhea in Guatemala and India did not provide any benefit in resolution of disease or in increased weight gain over placebo (44,45). Forty-six percent of the

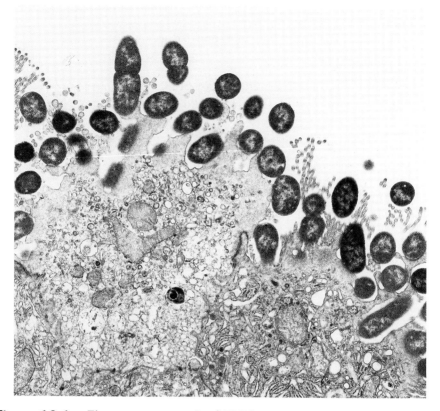

Figure 10.1.   Electron micrograph of EPEC organisms adherent to intestinal mucosa. The classic cuplike pedestals, loss of microvilli, and effacement and disorganization of the involved enterocytes can be seen. (Micrograph courtesy of Dr. Saul Tzipori.)

children in the study from Guatemala had EPEC isolated from stool, but these children were not distinguished from other children with persistent diarrhea in the evaluation of the response rate to treatment. EPEC identification was not attempted in the Indian study. These studies did not report any concomitant nutritional interventions in these children and did not report whether EPEC organisms were cleared in the treated children.

The case report of the adult AIDS patient with chronic diarrhea who had *E. coli*-like organisms seen on biopsy suggested that 2 weeks of therapy with an oral quinolone was completely successful in aborting the prolonged diarrheal illness in this patient. This anecdotal report is not accompanied by any culture data (37).

The EPEC organisms have been reported to be resistant to commonly used antibiotics (23,31). Eleven percent of organisms studied retrospectively from EPEC outbreaks in the United States from 1934 to 1987 were resistant to one antibiotic, 7% were resistant to two antibiotics, and 57% were resistant to three antibiotics (31). In Brazil, nearly all EPEC isolates were resistant to trimethoprim-sulfamethoxazole, ampicillin, and tetracycline. Sixty-five percent of organisms were susceptible only to broad-spectrum cephalosporins, colistin, naladixic acid, and norfloxacin (23). In vitro studies suggest that the macrolide antibiotic azithromycin is effective against EPEC, but clinical trials have not been performed (46).

Alternative or nonantibiotic therapy may also be useful. EPEC organisms are recognized antigenically by sIgA in breast milk, and breast-feeding has long been considered to be fairly effective prophylaxis against disease (47). Recently, oligosaccharides purified from breast milk have been shown to inhibit attachment of EPEC organisms in the tissue culture assay. Pentasaccharide and difucosyl-lactose were the most successful in inhibiting adherence. This inhibition was specific for EPEC strains and did not inhibit adherence of other *E. coli* strains (47). In Guatemala, more than 480 plants are used in herbal or folk remedies for diarrheal illness. Sixteen of these were tested for antibacterial effects and three of the plant extracts tested were documented to have significant inhibitory activity against EPEC growth (48). These kinds of nonantibiotic approaches may provide new strategies for therapy against EPEC disease in the future.

Diagnosis

In the routine clinical microbiology laboratory work-up for enteric pathogens, lactose-fermenting colonies on MacConkey plates are not evaluated, and the presence of EPEC organisms, along with other *E. coli* that cause enteric disease, such as ETEC, are not detected. Serogrouping of *E. coli*, which previously was done fairly routinely in the clinical microbiology laboratory, has not been done in the majority of laboratories for the last 20 years. At present, the group-specific antisera necessary to identify the major EPEC serogroups are no longer commercially available (3,31). In research laboratories three methods for identifying EPEC have existed since the mid-1980s.

In 1985, a 1.0-kb DNA probe prepared from the large plasmid of EPEC strain 2348/69 was first reported (7). This probe identified a portion of the plasmid that, when interrupted, caused the EPEC strain to lose its ability to adhere to HEp-2 tissue culture cells and was presumed to encode for at least a portion of the genetic material responsible for the ability of EPEC to adhere. This EAF probe consistently hybridized with EPEC strains that adhere to tissue culture cells and has been widely used since for the identification of EPEC strains. Neither the ability to adhere to tissue culture cells nor homology with the EAF probe is present in all organisms that fall into the classic EPEC serogroups (see Table 10.1). Only 24 of 109 EPEC strains identified by serogroup demonstrated homology with the adherence probe (7). Additional strains within the same serogroups of EPEC that exhibit adherence to tissue culture cells and homology with the EAF probe may be adherence and probe negative. Since the development of the EAF probe, research probes have been constructed from additional genetic fragments associated with other virulence factors, such as *eae*, which do not invariably correlate with EAF (49). All of the probes remain research surveillance tools and are not commercially available.

The tissue culture adherence factor that distinguishes EPEC strains was originally described in 1979 (4). In 1987, modifications were made in the interpretation of the tissue culture adherence assay and a specific pattern of adherence was ascribed to EPEC strains (5). The distinctive phenotype for the EAF-positive strains was termed "localized adherence" (LA). LA is characterized by clusters or microcolonies of *E. coli* adhering only to the surface of the tissue culture cells. In this first report, 97% of 95 LA EPEC were recognized by the EAF probe as compared to none of the strains with other patterns of adherence to tissue culture cells. The recognition of LA in tissue culture was proposed as an alternative screening assay for EPEC in centers particularly in the developing world, where access to genetic techniques or the use of radiolabeled DNA probes might be problematic. In practical terms, the ability to perform tissue culture is also problematic because of the need for specialized facilities and the expense of the reagents. The amount of time required to perform and read the adherence assays also limits their usefulness.

Other investigators have developed an assay using fluorescent staining of actin as an alternative means to identify the attaching and effacing lesions caused by EPEC (50–52). Actin accumulates under the site of the localized adherence of the EPEC organism and can be stained by fluorescein isothiocyanate (FITC)-conjugated phalloidin for visualization under a fluorescent microscope. Thirty-nine percent of *E. coli* strains that fell into classic EPEC serogroups were positive in the fluorescent-actin (f-actin) stain. Forty-three percent of the strains that were positive with the f-actin stain demonstrated LA and were positive by the EAF probe. However, the strains that were f-actin stain positive and LA/EAF negative did attach to human duodenal mucosal tissue obtained by biopsy and maintained in culture. This raises the possibility that the f-actin stain might be more sensitive than the LA/EAF probe for detecting EPEC strains that do adhere to intestine. The f-actin stain, however, also requires access to a fluorescent microscope and specialized reagents, which limit its usefulness in the developing world.

The f-actin test, the EAF probe, the LA tissue culture assay, and specific serotyping to identify clonality are all useful in epidemiologic studies but are of little use in the diagnosis or management of diarrheal illness in the clinical setting. Physicians should, however, consider EPEC as a potential pathogen in a prolonged diarrheal illness that escapes diagnosis on routine examination in an infant, a traveler with high-risk exposures, or an AIDS patient. EPEC should also be considered as a potential etiology for an outbreak of diarrheal illness, which is not caused by a routine pathogen, in a preschool, day care setting, or in hospitals. In this setting the physician could consider sending *E. coli* specimens to a research center for more specific examination for virulence factors.

Pathogenesis

The mechanism by which EPEC organisms cause diarrheal disease is unclear. Because these organisms have been defined as those *E. coli* that did not produce secretory toxins or cytotoxins and were negative in the Sereny test, there was no clear virulence factor to implicate in the production of disease. It has been presumed that the attachment of EPEC to the intestine caused sufficient disruption of the brush border to produce a malabsorptive diarrhea; it has also been postulated that some as yet undetected toxin was delivered directly to the intestinal epithelium after the organisms attached. In the late 1970s, one study reported that organisms of a classic EPEC serogroup did produce a secretory toxin that was able to cause fluid secretion in an animal model, but this finding was not confirmed (53). The above theories do not recognize the intriguing possibility that it is the act of adherence itself that signals cell secretory processes and leads to diarrheal disease. Current evidence suggests that this may be so although it has not been proven definitively (12,54).

A three-stage model that potentially explains EPEC pathogenesis has been put forth recently by Donnenberg and Kaper on the basis of unique genetic determinants of EPEC that encode a variety of adhesins (12). This model proposes that bacteria adhere initially to the intestinal microvilli and to each other by fimbrial adhesins (stage 1). This self-aggregation may explain the microcolony formation that appears as LA in the tissue culture assays. LA is consistently associated with a 60-MDa plasmid (pMAR); the 1.0-kb EAF probe developed from a region of this plasmid is quite specific for LA, and EPEC strains that are cured of this 60-MDa plasmid are less pathogenic (22,55–58). However, the molecular nature of LA is still not understood (12,59). Recently, a bundle-forming pilus has been described on an EPEC strain and has been visualized on other strains although not on strains cured of the pMAR plasmid (60,61). This pilus may be responsible for this initialized LA.

In stage 2, additional adherence factors come into play and pull the bacteria into closer contact with the epithelium and initiate cell signal transduction pathways that lead to increased intracellular calcium levels and protein phosphorylation and ultimately the cytoskeletal changes that lead to effacement of the microvilli (12). Although LA does not occur in EPEC strains that have been cured of the pMAR plasmid, attachment and effacement persist at a lower level in EPEC strains that have been cured of this plasmid. Investigators have not been able to detect induced alterations in host cell cyclic nucleotide levels after infections with EPEC, but two groups of investigators have found that EPEC attachment induces elevations in intracellular calcium, another cellular second messenger (62–64). There is additional speculation that protein kinase C might be involved in phosphorylation of two distinct proteins in host cells after infection with EPEC in vitro (65). Other proteins have been reported to be phosphorylated after EPEC infection, including three large proteins of 90, 100, and 130 kDa (66,67). One hypothesis generated from these observations is that EPEC infection might activate phospholipase C, resulting in the cleavage of phosphatidyl inositol to inositol triphosphate and diacyl glycerol. Inositol triphosphate could release intracellular calcium and diacyl glycerol could then activate protein kinase C resulting in protein phosphorylation (12). The elevated intracellular calcium and phosphorylated proteins could produce many of the cytoskeletal changes seen with EPEC infection. In addition, the adherence of EPEC organisms to intestinal cells in tissue culture deceases electrical resistance across cellular monolayers, suggesting a potential mechanism for the induction of secretory processes (68). These hypotheses are attractive but evidence to date is insufficient to implicate them as the sole explanation for EPEC diarrheal disease.

Finally, in the third stage of pathogenesis, an additional adherence factor may be activated; the latter may then pull the bacterium into intimate contact with the epithelium and permit the accumulation of actin and other cytoskeletal proteins such as myosin, talin, and ezrin under the bacterium with the formation of the cuplike pedestal that is so characteristic of the EPEC organisms (69) (see Figure 10.1). This intimate adherence under these circumstances permits some EPEC organisms to be taken up by epithelial cells; whether this is active invasion of the cell by the bacterium or activation of the cell leading to the engulfing or phagocytosis of the bacteria is not clear (70–73). The intimate adherence factor appears to be the gene product of a nonplasmid gene cluster termed *eae* (49). One recognized product of this gene cluster is a 94-kDa outer membrane protein, which has been called intimin, and is similar to the invasins of the *Yersinia* species (74,75). Although *eae* is not plasmid associated, a regulatory factor or factors on the LA/EAF 60-MDa plasmid appear to enhance the expression of the *eae* gene (76). The *eaeA* gene appears to be necessary for intimate attachment of EPEC but does not appear to be sufficient to totally explain the intimate attachment and effacement that is ultimately recognized with EPEC disease (77). When the entire *eae* gene cluster is cloned into non-EPEC *E. coli*, these mutants do not induce actin accumulation in epithelial cells (78). Mutants in which the *eae* gene cluster is disrupted are also still able to phosphorylate proteins, alter the cytoskeleton, and damage microvilli (79). EPEC mutants with disruption at chromosomal sites other than the *eae* gene cluster are able to adhere tightly but do not alter the cytoskeleton or phosphorylate proteins (80,81). It is likely, therefore, that additional genetic material is also necessary for the disease ultimately caused by EPEC organisms.

The virulence of many of the bacterial products defined by this molecular methodology have been confirmed in animal models using rabbits or piglets. Not only did the presence of the EAF plasmid and the *eae* gene cluster permit the attaching and effacing lesions in the intestine of these animal models, the absence of one or the other altered the distribution of lesions along the gut, suggesting that these gene products do mediate specific interactions with intestinal mucosal receptors (78,82). Alterations in enterocyte function with loss of microvillus membrane enzymes have been noted in both animal models and in biopsy specimens taken from children with disease (83,84). Interestingly, in a rabbit model, inhibition of bacterial replication by the use of bacteriostatic antibiotics did not alter the course of the intestinal damage done by EPEC strains (85). This suggests that the bacterial-mucosal interaction becomes committed early in the course of infection, once the initial adherence occurs with fully pathogenic organisms.

Although EPEC pathogenesis is incompletely understood, the elucidation of the interaction of the potential virulence factors in the recent past has been remarkable. EPEC organisms have served as the means to identify mechanisms by which bacterial adherence may well participate in the production of diarrheal disease by activating cell signal transduction pathways. The use of molecular methodology in studying these organisms has provided insights into the multiplicity of mechanisms that appear to be necessary for these organisms to produce disease and to begin to sort out the role that each of the postulated virulence factors may play.

ENTEROAGGREGATIVE *Escherichia coli*

The recognition of the specific pattern of LA of EPEC to epithelial cells in culture was accompanied by the recognition of alternative patterns of adherence such as that exhibited by the EAggEc (5,6). The EAggEc are defined by their ability to adhere to tissue culture cells in a stacked brick pattern; they also palisade over the glass between the tissue culture cells in a distinctive fashion (Figure 10.2). An additional pattern of adherence, termed diffuse adherence, in which isolated bacteria appear scattered across the surface of the epithelial cells, was recognized at the same time, but the association of organisms with this adherence pattern with diarrheal disease is less secure (5). The tissue culture adherence assay became used relatively widely in epidemiologic studies of diarrheal disease in children in the developing world in the mid-1980s, particularly in studies attempting to identify potential infectious agents in children with persistent diarrheal disease from whom no other pathogen could be identified. The association of EAggEc with diarrheal disease has been recognized only since the late 1980s and little is known about these organisms and the diarrheal disease with which they are associated. Certainly, the mechanism by which these organisms cause diarrheal disease is not known. Whether they, with their distinctive adherence phenotype, like EPEC, have the potential to use adherence as an active process to initiate cell signal transduction pathways is not known.

Epidemiology

Data extracted from retrospective studies in Asia and South America suggest that from 3 to 27% of all childhood diarrhea is prolonged beyond 14 days, the accepted definition of persistent diarrhea (32). In prospective studies done more recently 5 to 23% of all diarrheal illness in children appeared to be prolonged and appeared to be most common in children between the ages of 6 and 18 months. In these prospective studies of persistent diarrhea in Mexico,

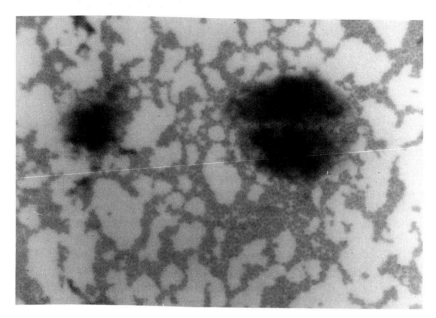

Figure 10.2. High power (oil immersion lens) of the distinctive cascading appearance of EAggEc in the HeLa tissue culture cell assay. The adherence of organisms to and around cells as well as to the glass can be seen.

Brazil, India, and Bangladesh, EAggEc were identified by tissue culture adherence assay more frequently than any other enteric pathogen in 19 to 53% of stools of children with persistent diarrhea (8,9,86–90). In these same studies, EAggEc were isolated from the stools of 8 to 24% of the children with acute diarrhea but only from 5 to 19% of the stools of children who served as nondiarrheal controls. The first prospective study reporting the presence of EAggEc did not document the duration of diarrheal illness but found EAggEc were present in the stools of 36% of the children with diarrhea in Santiago, Chile, as compared to 23% of children without diarrhea (5).

Unexpectedly, when organisms isolated from stools of children under age 3 years in the United Kingdom since 1985 (which were classified as EPEC by serogroup) were examined for adherence phenotype, 55% were reclassified as EAggEc (91). Only 2 of 32 E. coli isolated from children in the United Kingdom selected as age-matched controls demonstrated the EAggEc phenotype. Although E. coli diarrheal illnesses are more common in children, E. coli strains isolated from elderly patients (over age 65 years) with diarrhea were also noted to be aggregative (91). Adults also proved to be susceptible to EAggEc diarrheal disease in a study done of acute diarrheal illnesses in U.S. servicemen stationed overseas. EAggEc were the only pathogens isolated from 4% of the servicemen with acute diarrhea stationed in West Africa and 6% of the servicemen stationed in South America (92).

Additional studies done in Peru, Bangladesh, and Thailand and in Australian aboriginal children with diarrheal disease demonstrated no association between the isolation of EAggEc organisms and diarrheal disease (33,93–95).

Enteroaggregative *E. coli* disease appears to cause mostly endemic disease because outbreaks of diarrhea have rarely been examined for EAggEc organisms. Three small outbreaks of diarrhea in elderly individuals hospitalized in the United Kingdom were associated with EAggEc and one small day care outbreak in the United Kingdom in 1980 was associated with EAggEc. In this outbreak, EAggEc were isolated from three children with diarrheal disease, some asymptomatic children in the same day care facility, and in four adult staff members with diarrhea (91). To date no seasonal variation has been noted, but there does appear to be geographical variation with servicemen stationed in South America more likely to acquire diarrheal disease due to EAggEc than servicemen in Africa (92).

The HIV epidemic has increased awareness of the role that diarrhea may play in morbidity and mortality in these compromised patients. The one study that has investigated the pathogens in persistent diarrhea in children with HIV disease in Zaire documented EAggEc in 41% of children with HIV infection and diarrhea and in 30% of children uninfected with HIV with diarrhea. In this population, 28% of HIV-uninfected children without diarrhea also had EAggEc isolated from stool. The level of recovery of EAggEc was higher in this population than any other reported to date. EAggEc were detected in this study by an EAggEc probe, which has not consistently identified all EAggEc strains that are detectable by tissue culture assay (36). *E. coli* consistent with EAggEc have been identified by biopsy in AIDS patients with chronic diarrhea (37). We have demonstrated aggregative *E. coli* by tissue culture adherence assay in the stools of HIV patients with chronic, pathogen-negative diarrhea. The one patient who was treated with two weeks of quinolone antibiotic responded dramatically to therapy with cessation of diarrhea and weight gain (personal data). The role of EAggEc in otherwise pathogen-negative diarrhea of AIDS patients requires additional study.

Because travelers are immunologically the equivalent of children, it is also possible that EAggEc could be a cause of travelers' diarrhea. EAggEc were recognized in the stools of 27 to 33% of travelers with and without diarrhea and no other recognized pathogen (96). Although this study did not demonstrate an association between colonization of adult travelers with EAggEc and diarrhea, it did demonstrate that EAggEc organisms may be acquired during the course of travel because before travel only 2.5% of individuals had EAggEc isolated from stool. The data from U.S. servicemen stationed abroad also suggest that EAggEc may be a cause of diarrhea in travelers (92).

Volunteer studies in which adults ingested 1×10^{10} CFU of an EAggEc strain (with aggregative adherence fimbriae I) orally in bicarbonate buffer caused disease in only one of 19 volunteers (97,98). Twelve volunteers, however, developed antibody responses that appeared to be to the fimbrial adhesion. Whether children, hosts with some underlying mucosal deficit due to immunocompromise or malnutrition, or individuals who are repeatedly exposed to organisms are at greater risk for developing EAggEc diarrheal disease needs to be clarified further.

Clinical Disease

Little is written about the clinical disease associated with EAggEc, and though inferences about clinical disease may be drawn from some of the animal work done with EAggEc, any correlation of the animal data with human disease is not clear. The only study that characterized the clinical disease of children with persistent diarrhea from whom EAggEc were isolated was done in Mexico. One third of the children with EAggEC in that study had diarrhea that was bloody, albeit not frankly dysenteric, as well as prolonged (84).

The findings in these children may be consistent with the fact that inflammatory intestinal lesions were seen in gnotobiotic piglets, rats, and rabbits when these animals were inoculated with EAggEc organisms (9,99,100). In the rabbit ileal loop model, EAggEc strains tested produced villus shortening, hemorrhagic necrosis of the villus tips, inflammation with edema, and elongated microvilli (101). Alternatively, two proteins of 108 and 116 kDa purified from EAggEc culture media induced similar histologic changes in rat intestine (102). In the reversible ileal tie rabbit model using 1.0-kg rabbits, EAggEc strains isolated from children with diarrhea reproducibly produced diarrheal illnesses that persisted for 3 to 10 days and caused systemic illness in the rabbit, whereas an EAggEc strain isolated from a child without diarrhea did not produce diarrhea (9). Six of 12 neonatal gnotobiotic piglets fed EAggEc developed diarrhea. Mucosal changes were seen in these animals as well, with hyperemia of the distal small bowel and cecum and swelling of the villi in the small intestine. Aggregation of bacteria was seen in the intestines of the gnotobiotic piglets; the aggregates of bacteria coated the surface epithelium and formed a continuous coat over villus tips (99). Aggregates of bacteria were also seen on rabbit and human mucosal explants used in adherence assays with EAggEc strains (101). These observations suggest that the aggregative adherence phenotype is more than an epiphenomena, although the phenotype may still represent a group of organisms that cause diarrheal disease by a heterogeneous group of mechanisms.

In additional in vitro studies done with EAggEc, the organisms also appeared to adhere more to the mucous coat of formalin-fixed human intestine rather than the absorptive surface (99,101). The EAggEc also appeared to adhere more to the lymphoid cells of the gut, particularly M cells, than did other intestinal pathogens such as ETEC (103). In this study, adherence assays done with biopsies taken from the length of human and animal intestine demonstrated more adherence of EAggEc organisms to the colonic mucosa than to ileal or jejunal mucosa. Confirmation of these histologic observations exist in data that demonstrate that EAggEc have a strong specific avidity for binding purified intestinal mucin (104).

The spectrum of clinical disease associated with EAggEc is poorly defined and no treatment trials have been performed. Short trials of oral gentamicin alone did not change the course of persistent diarrhea in children. However, these studies did not examine the stools of children for the presence of EAggEc organisms (44,45). EAggEc strains isolated from U.S. servicemen in South America and West Africa and from children in Brazil, Mexico, Chile, and Thailand have exhibited multiple antibiotic resistance (28,92,105). Resistance is routinely present to penicillin, tetracycline, chloramphenicol, streptomycin, kanamycin, and trimethoprim/sulfamethoxazole. This resistance may be encoded on the same plasmid that encodes for aggregative adherence (105). Susceptibility is generally preserved to date for carbapenems, broad-spectrum cephalosporins, quinolones, and gentamicin. The expense of these agents and the inability to safely and routinely use quinolone antibiotics in children limit the prospect of treatment trials.

The diagnosis of EAggEc is also cumbersome. Screening strains in the tissue culture adherence assay is probably the most reliable method to identify EAggEc organisms. A DNA probe has been constructed from sequential restriction fragments of purified plasmid DNA from an EAggEc strain from a child with diarrhea in Chile. This probe has been remarkably specific in the identification of EAggEc strains also identified by adherence assay (106,107). The sensitivity of the strain for identification of EAggEc strains from a variety of geographical locations has varied widely (38 to 89%) when compared to the tissue culture assay.

A more rapid method of detection of EAggEc strains has been described recently. In liquid broth media, all EAggEc strains from a variety of geographical areas formed a thick scum at the surface of the broth (108). This clump formation was specific for EAggEc and appeared to be plasmid mediated (103,108). The ultimate usefulness of this technique needs to be validated.

The Organism

Unlike the EPEC, serogrouping of EAggEc organisms has not been a useful means of categorizing strains. In one study, 68% of strains were O nontypable. When these nontypable strains were screened with rough specific phages, only 18% were attacked by the phages, implying that the majority did produce smooth lipopolysaccharide and that the aggregative phenotype interfered with serogrouping. Strains have also been shown to have type I fimbriae, to hemagglutinate human, rat, or bovine red blood cells, and to be hydrophobic (9,90,98). The O antigen polysaccharide of one EAggEc strain has recently been characterized as repetitive pentasaccharide units (109).

Pathogenesis

The aggregative phenotype is presumed to be a marker for the virulence factor responsible for the diarrheal disease associated with the EAggEc organisms.

Transposon mutagenesis has been used to generate nonadherent mutants that have been characterized to identify the genetic material responsible for aggregative adherence. Aggregative adherence has been consistently associated with the 60-MDa plasmid, which encodes a bundle-forming fimbria that has been called the aggregative adherence fimbriae I (AAF/I) and appears to be responsible by complementation for the aggregative phenotype. AAF/I also appears to mediate hemagglutination to human red blood cells. Expression of the fimbriae requires two separate plasmid regions with 9 kb of DNA between the two regions that is not associated with fimbrial expression (98,110). Four morphologically distinct fimbriae have been visualized on EAggEc by electron microscopy (111).

A secretory toxin has also been identified in select EAggEc strains. Although EAggEc strains do not have any of the recognized secretory toxins of the ETEC group by bioassay and DNA homology studies, culture filtrates of EAggEc strains were noted to have enterotoxigenic activity on rabbit ileal mucosa mounted in Ussing chambers. The genetic material that encodes this toxin has been localized to the large plasmid of the EAggEc, in the 9-kb fragment of DNA between the two AAF/I loci (112,113). An early report suggested that this secretory toxin activated cyclic glucose monophosphate (GMP), and cloned toxin has been shown to elevate tissue cyclic GMP. In addition, DNA sequence homology to *E. coli* heat-stable toxin A (STa) and to guanylin have been noted, suggesting that cyclic GMP may well be involved (113,114). The role of this toxin in the clinical disease associated with EAggEc is not known.

Other investigators have found that EAggEc and culture filtrates of EAggEc elevated levels of intracellular calcium in epithelial cells (102). Gel electrophoresis of protein precipitates prepared from broth cultures of EAggEc revealed a 120- to 140-kDa protein, which by immunoblot was cross-reactive with previously described hemolysins (115). Hemolysins may form ion-specific pores in cell membranes and allow the influx of calcium. In contrast to EPEC infection, in which intracellular calcium is mobilized by activation of signal transduction pathways, calcium elevations were not abolished in EAggEc infection when epithelial cells were treated to prevent the mobilization of intracellular calcium. Culture filtrates of EAggEc were also able to induce protein phosphorylation in epithelial cells, again in distinction to EPEC infection, in which close contact of the bacteria and the epithelial cell is necessary. EAggEc strains are not clinically hemolytic, however, and what role these phenomena play in EAggEc virulence is not known.

In addition, some EAggEc strains may be taken up by epithelial cells in the gentamicin invasion assay (116). It is possible that this process is not an active bacterial process but represents the epithelial cell actively engulfing the bacteria. This process is inhibited by cytochalasin D, staurosporine, and genisten, which suggests that actin filaments and signal transduction by protein kinase and tyrosine kinase may be important for this process (116). Whether this phenomenon is mediated by the same protein that appears to phosphorylate proteins is not known.

It is not clear if all of the putative virulence factors and mechanisms discussed above occur consistently in EAggEc from various geographical areas. It is equally likely that the EAggEc phenotype represents a heterogeneous group of organisms. It is also possible that a concert of virulence factors may be working together as in EPEC, and the associations of these factors remain to be elucidated.

Much remains to be learned about the epidemiology and mechanisms by which the EAggEc cause diarrheal disease. Although the pathogenesis of EPEC infections is better understood, prior to this decade, these organisms were not defined by any consistent criteria other than serogroup and exclusion from any of the other diarrheagenic group of *E. coli*. Both EPEC and EAggEc organisms can potentially serve as probes to provide better understanding of both normal intestinal physiology and pathogenesis of diarrheal disease. The EPEC have opened the door on the exciting possibility that bacterial adherence is an active process that can subvert host cell physiology by initiating signal transduction pathways. What further physiologic processes will be linked to bacterial adherence in the gut are still to be defined.

REFERENCES

1   Robins-Browne RM. Traditional entero-pathogenic *Escherichia coli* of infantile diarrhea. Rev Infect Dis 1987;9:28–53.

2   Guerrant RL, Bobak DA. Bacterial and protozoal gastroenteritis. N Engl J Med 1991;325:327–340.

3   National Institute of Allergy and Infectious Disease. Summary of a workshop on enteropathogenic *Escherichia coli*. J Infect Dis 1983;147:1108–1118.

4   Cravioto A, Gross RJ, Scotland S, et al. An adhesive factor found in strains of *Escherichia coli* belonging to the traditional infantile enteropathogenic serotypes. Curr Microbiol 1979;3:95–99.

5   Nataro JP, Kaper JB, Robins-Browne R, Prado V, Vial P, Levine MM. Patterns of adherence of diarrheagenic *Escherichia coli* to HEp-2 cells. Pediatr Infect Dis J 1987;6:829–831.

6   Vial PA, Mathewson JJ, DuPont HL, Guers L, Levine MM. Comparison of two assay methods for patterns of adherence to HEp-2 cells of *Escherichia coli* from patients with diarrhea. J Clin Microbiol 1990;28:882–885.

7   Nataro JP, Baldini MM, Kaper JB, Black RE, Bravo N, Levine MM. Detection of an adherence factor of enteropathogenic *Escherichia coli* with a DNA probe. J Clin Infect Dis 1985;152:560–565.

8   Bhan MK, Khoshoo V, Sommerfelt H, Raj P, Sazawal S, Srivastava R. Enteroaggregative *Escherichia coli* and *Salmonella* associated with nondysenteric persistent diarrhea. Pediatr Infect Dis J 1989;8:499–502.

9   Wanke CA, Schorling JB, Barrett JL, Desouza MA, Guerrant RL. Potential role of adherence traits of *Escherichia coli* in persistent diarrhea in an urban Brazilian slum. Pediatr Infect Dis J 1991;10:746–751.

10 Giron JA, Jones T, Millan-Velasco F, et al. Diffuse-adhering *Escherichia coli* (DAEC) as a putative cause of diarrhea in Mayan children in Mexico. J Infect Dis 1991;163:507–513.

11 Tacket CO, Moseley SL, Kay B, Losonsky G, Levine MM. Challenge studies in volunteers using *Escherichia coli* strains with diffuse adherence to HEp-2 cells. J Infect Dis 1990;162:550–552.

12 Donnenberg MS, Kaper JB. Enteropathogenic *Escherichia coli*. Infect Immun 1992;60:3953–3961.

13 Davison WC. Duodenal contents of infants in health and during and following diarrhea. Am J Dis Child 1925;29:743–756.

14 **Dulaney AD, Michelson ID.** A strain of *E. coli* mutabile from an outbreak of diarrhea in the newborn. Am J Public Health 1935;25:1241–1251.

15 **Anonymous.** Bray's discovery of pathogenic *E. coli* as a cause of infantile gastroenteritis. Arch Dis Child 1973;48:923–926.

16 **Kauffmann F.** The serology of the coli group. J Immunol 1947;57:71–100.

17 **Kauffmann F, Dupont A.** *Escherichia* strains from infantile epidemic gastroenteritis. Acta Pathol Microbiol Scand 1950;27:552–564.

18 **Neter E, Korns RF, Trussell RE.** Association of *Escherichia coli* serogroup 0111 with two hospital outbreaks of epidemic diarrhea of the newborn infant in New York State during 1947. Pediatrics 1953;12:377–383.

19 **De SN.** Enterotoxicity of bacteria-free culture-filtrates of *Vibrio cholera*. Nature 1959;183:1533–1534.

20 **Beutin L, Orskov I, Orskov F, et al.** Clonal diversity and virulence factors in strains of *Escherichia coli* of the classic enteropathogenic serogroup 0114. J Infect Dis 1990;162:1329–1334.

21 **Levine MM, Bergquist EJ, Nalin DR, et al.** *Escherichia coli* strains that cause diarrhoea but do not produce heat-labile or heat-stable enterotoxins and are noninvasive. Lancet 1978;I:1119–1122.

22 **Levine MM, Nataro JP, Karch H, et al.** The diarrheal response of humans to some classic serotypes of enteropathogenic *Escherichia coli* is dependent on a plasmid encoding an enteroadhesiveness factor. J Infect Dis 1985;152:550–559.

23 **Gomes TAT, Rassi V, MacDonald KL, et al.** Enteropathogens associated with acute diarrheal disease in urban infants in Sao Paulo, Brazil. J Infect Dis 1991;164:331–337.

24 **Robins-Browne R, Still CS, Miliotis MD, et al.** Summer diarrhoea in African infants and children. Arch Dis Child 1980;55:923–928.

25 **Kain KC, Barteluk RL, Kelly MT, et al.** Etiology of childhood diarrhea in Beijing, China. J Clin Microbiol 1991;29:90–95.

26 **Echeverria P, Orskov F, Orskov I, et al.** Attaching and effacing enteropathogenic *Escherichia coli* as a cause of infantile diarrhea in Bangkok. J Infect Dis 1991;164:550–554.

27 **Gunzburg ST, Chang BJ, Burke V, Gracey M.** Virulence factors of enteric

Escherichia coli in young Aboriginal children in north-west Australia. Epidemiol Infect 1992;109:283–289.

28 **Schorling JB, Wanke CA, Schorling SK, et al.** A prospective study of persistent diarrhea among children in an urban Brazilian slum: patterns of occurrence and etiologic agents. Am J Epidemiol 1990;132:144–155.

29 **Bower JR, Congeni BL, Cleary TG, et al.** *Escherichia coli* 0114: nonmotile as a pathogen in an outbreak of severe diarrhea associated with a day care center. J Infect Dis 1989;160:243–247.

30 **Paulozzi LJ, Johnson KE, Kamahele LM, Clausen CR, Riley LW, Helgerson SD.** Diarrhea associated with adherent enteropathogenic *Escherichia coli* in an infant and toddler center, Seattle, Washington. Pediatrics 1986;77:296–300.

31 **Moyenuddin M, Wachsmuth IK, Moseley SL, Bopp CA, Blake PA.** Serotype, antimicrobial resistance, and adherence properties of *Escherichia coli* strains associated with outbreaks of diarrheal illness in children in the United States. J Clin Microbiol 1989;27:2234–2239.

32 **Wanke CA.** Infectious causes of prolonged diarrhoea. In: Guerrant RL, ed. Clinical Tropical Medicine and Communicable Disease, vol. 3. England: Balliere & Tindall, 1988:567–590.

33 **Lanata CF, Black RE, Maurtua D, et al.** Etiologic agents in acute vs. persistent diarrhea in children under three years of age in peri-urban Lima, Peru. Acta Pediatr 1992;381(suppl):32–38.

34 **Lima AAM, Fang G, Schorling JB, et al.** Persistent diarrhea in northeast Brazil: Etiologies and interactions with malnutrition. Acta Pediatr 1992;381(suppl):39–44.

35 **Ito H, Della Negra M, Queiroz W, Janini M, Rodriguez C.** Diarrheal illness among pediatric AIDS patients. Abstracts of the Sixth International Conference on AIDS, San Francisco, California, 1990. Abstract no. S.B.29.

36 **Thea DM, St. Louis ME, Atido U, et al.** A prospective study of diarrhea and HIV-1 infection among 429 Zairian infants. N Engl J Med 1993;329:1696–1702.

37 **Kotler DP, Orenstein JM.** Chronic diarrhea and malabsorption associated with enteropathogenic bacterial infection in a patient with AIDS. Ann Intern Med 1993;119:127–128.

38 **DuPont HL, Ericsson CD.** Prevention and treatment of traveler's diarrhea. N Engl J Med 1993;328:1821–1827.

39 Mathewson JJ, Johnson PC, DuPont HL, et al. A newly recognized cause of travelers' diarrhea: enteroadherent *Escherichia coli*. J Infect Dis 1985;151:471–475.

40 Levine MM. *Escherichia coli* that cause diarrhea: enterotoxigenic, enteropathogenic, enteroinvasive, enterohemorrhagic, enteroadherent. J Infect Dis 1987;155:377–389.

41 Rothbaum R, McAdams AJ, Giannella R, Partin JC. A clinicopathologic study of enterocyte-adherent *Escherichia coli*: a cause of protracted diarrhea in infants. Gastroenterology 1982;83:441–454.

42 Clausen CR, Christie DL. Chronic diarrhea in infants caused by adherent enteropathogenic *Escherichia coli*. J Pediatr 1982;100:358–361.

43 Ulshen MH, Rollo JL. Pathogenesis of *Escherichia coli* gastroenteritis in man: another mechanism. N Engl J Med 1980; 302:99–101.

44 Bartlett AV, Turun B, Morales C, Cano F, Cruz JR. Oral gentamicin is not effective treatment for persistent diarrhea. Acta Pediatr 1992;381(suppl):149–154.

45 Bhatnagar S, Bhan MK, Sazawal S, et al. Efficacy of massive dose oral gentamicin therapy in nonbloody persistent diarrhea with associated malnutrition. J Pediatr Gastroenterol Nutr 1992;12:1117–1124.

46 Gordillo ME, Singh KV, Murray BE. In vitro activity of azithromycin against bacterial enteric pathogens. Antimicrob Agents Chemother 1993;37:1203–1205.

47 Cravioto A, Tello A, Villafan H, Ruiz J, del Vedovo S, Neeser JR. Inhibition of localized adhesin of enteropathogenic *Escherichia coli* to HEp-2 cells by immunoglobulin and oligosaccharide fractions of human colostrum and breast milk. J Infect Dis 1991;163:1247–1255.

48 Caceres A, Fletes L, Aguilar L, et al. Plants used in Guatemala for treatment of gastrointestinal disorders. J Ethnopharmacol 1993;38:31–38.

49 Jerse AE, Yu J, Tall BD, Kaper JB. A genetic locus of enteropathogenic *Escherichia coli* necessary for the production of attaching and effacing lesions on tissue culture cells. Proc Natl Acad Sci USA 1990;87: 7839–7843.

50 Knulton S, Baldwin T, Williams PH, McNeish AS. Actin accumulation at sites of bacterial adhesion to tissue culture cells: basis of a new diagnostic test for enteropathogenic and enterohemorrhagic *Escherichia coli*. Infect Immun 1989;57: 1290–1298.

51 Knutton S, Phillips AD, Smith HR, et al. Screening for enteropathogenic *Escherichia coli* in infants with diarrhea by fluorescent-actin staining test. Infect Immun 1991;59:365–371.

52 Shariff M, Bhan MK, Knutton S, Das BK, Saini S, Kumar R. Evaluation of the fluorescence actin staining test for detection of enteropathogenic *Escherichia coli*. J Clin Microbiol 1993;31:386–389.

53 Klipstein FA, Rowe B, Engert RF, Short HB, Gross RJ. Enterotoxigenicity of enteropathogenic serotypes of *Escherichia coli* isolated from infants with epidemic diarrhea. Infect Immun 1978;21:171–178.

54 Hoepelman AIM, Tuomanen EI. Consequences of microbial attachment: directing host cell functions with adhesins. Infect Immun 1992;60:1729–1733.

55 Baldini MM, Kaper JB, Levine MM, Candy DCA, Moon HW. Plasmid-mediated adhesion in enteropathogenic *Escherichia coli*. J Pediatr Gastroenterol Nutr 1983;2:534–538.

56 Nataro JP, Scaletsky ICA, Kaper JB, Levine MM, Trabulsi LR. Plasmid-mediated factors conferring diffuse and localized adherence of enteropathogenic *Escherichia coli*. Infect Immun 1985;48:378–383.

57 Baldini MM, Nataro JP, Kaper JB. Localization of a determinant for HEp-2 adherence by enteropathogenic *Escherichia coli*. Infect Immun 1986;52:334–336.

58 Laporta MZ, Silva MLM, Scaletsky ICA, Trabulsi LR. Plasmids coding for drug resistance and localized adherence to HeLa cells in enteropathogenic *Escherichia coli* O55:H⁻ and O55:H6. Infect Immun 1986;51:715–717.

59 Scaletsky ICA, Milani SR, Trabulsi LR, Travassos LR. Isolation and characterization of the localized adherence factor of enteropathogenic *Escherichia coli*. Infect Immun 1988;56:2979–2983.

60 Giron JA, Donnenberg MS, Martin WC, Jarvis KG, Kaper JB. Distribution of bundle-forming pilus structural gene (*bfpA*) among enteropathogenic *Escherichia coli*. J Infect Dis 1993;168:1037–1041.

61 Giron JA, Ho ASY, Schoolnik GK. Characterization of fimbriae produced by enteropathogenic *Escherichia coli*. J Bacteriol 1993;175:7391–7403.

62 Baldwin TJ, Ward W, Aitken A, Knutton S, Williams PH. Elevation of intracellular free calcium levels in HEp-2 cells infected

with enteropathogenic *Escherichia coli*. Infect Immun 1991;59:1599–1604.

63 **Baldwin TJ, Lee-Delaunay MB, Knutton S, Williams PH.** Calcium-calmodulin dependence of actin accretion and lethality in cultured HEp-2 cells infected with enteropathogenic *Escherichia coli*. Infect Immun 1993;61:760–763.

64 **Dytoc M, Fedorko L, Sherman P.** Changes in cytosolic free calcium in HEp-2 cells infected with attaching and effacing *Escherichia coli*. Abstracts of the 91st General Meeting of the American Society of Microbiology, Washington, DC, 1991. Abstract no. B-108.

65 **Baldwin TJ, Brooks SF, Knutton S, Manjarrez Hernandez HA, Aitken A, Williams PH.** Protein phosphorylation by protein kinase C in HEp-2 cells infected with enteropathogenic *Escherichia coli*. Infect Immun 1990;58:761–765.

66 **Rosenshine I, Donnenberg MS, Kaper JB, Finaly BB.** Signal transduction between enteropathogenic *Escherichia coli* (EPEC) and epithelial cells: EPEC-induced tyrosine phosphorylation of host cell proteins to initiate cytoskeletal rearrangement and bacterial uptake. EMBO J 1992; 11:3551–3560.

67 **Manjarrez-Hernandez HA, Baldwin TJ, Aitken A, Knutton S, Williams PH.** Intestinal epithelial cell protein phosphorylation in enteropathogenic *Escherichia coli* diarrhea. Lancet 1992;339:521–524.

68 **Canil C, Rosenshine I, Ruschkowski S, Donnenberg MS, Kaper JB, Finlay BB.** Enteropathogenic *E. coli* decreases the transepithelial electrical resistance of polarized epithelial monolayers. Infect Immun 1993;61:2755–2762.

69 **Finlay BB, Rosenshine I, Donnenberg MS, Kaper JB.** Cytoskeletal composition of attaching and effacing lesions associated with enteropathogenic *Escherichia coli* adherence to HeLa cells. Infect Immun 1992;60:2541–2543.

70 **Donnenberg MS, Donohue-Rolfe A, Keusch GT.** Epithelial cell invasion: an overlooked property of enteropathogenic *Escherichia coli* (EPEC) associated with the EPEC adherence factor. J Infect Dis 1989; 160:452–459.

71 **Fletcher JN, Embaye HE, Getty B, Batt RM, Hart CA, Saunders JR.** Novel invasion determinant of enteropathogenic *Escherichia coli* plasmid pLV501: the ability to invade intestinal epithelial cells and

HEp-2 cells. Infect Immun 1992;60:2229–2236.

72 **Miliotis MD, Koornhof HJ, Phillips JI.** Invasive potential of noncytotoxic enteropathogenic *Escherichia coli* in an in vitro Henle 407 cell model. Infect Immun 1989; 57:1928–1935.

73 **Donnenberg MS, Calderwood SB, Donohue-Rolfe A, Keusch GT, Kaper JB.** Construction and analysis of Tn*phoA* mutants of enteropathogenic *Escherichia coli* unable to invade HEp-2 cells. Infect Immun 1990;58:1565–1571.

74 **Jerse AE, Yu J, Tau BD, Kaper JB.** A genetic locus of EPEC necessary for the production of attaching and effacing lesions on tissue culture cells. Proc Natl Acad Sci USA 1990;87:7839–7843.

75 **Jerse AE, Kaper JB.** The *eae* gene of enteropathogenic *Escherichia coli* encodes a 94-kilodalton membrane protein, the expression of which is influenced by the EAF plasmid. Infect Immun 1991;59:4302–4309.

76 **Donnenberg MS, Kaper JB.** Construction of an *eae* deletion mutant of enteropathogenic *Escherichia coli* by using a positive-selection suicide vector. Infect Immun 1991;59:4310–4317.

77 **Donnenberg MS, Tacket CO, James SP, et al.** Role of *eaeA* gene in experimental enteropathogenic *Escherichia coli* infection. J Clin Invest 1993;92:1412–1417.

78 **Donnenberg MS, Tzipori S, McKee ML, O'Brien AD, Alroy J, Kaper JB.** The role of *eae* gene of enterohemorrhagic *Escherichia coli* in intimate attachment in vitro and in a porcine model. J Clin Invest 1993; 92:1418–1424.

79 **Donnenberg MS, Yu J, Kaper JB.** A second chromosomal gene necessary for intimate attachment of enteropathogenic *Escherichia coli* to epithelial cells. J Bacteriol 1993;175:4670–4680.

80 **Rosenshine I, Duronio V, Finaly BB.** Tyrosine protein kinase inhibitors block invasin-promoted bacterial uptake by epithelial cells. Infect Immun 1992;60:2211–2217.

81 **Cantey JR, Moseley SL.** HeLa cell adherence, actin aggregation, and invasion by nonenteropathogenic *Escherichia coli* possessing the *eae* gene. Infect Immun 1991;59:3924–3929.

82 **Tzipori S, Gibson R, Montanaro J.** Nature and distribution of mucosal lesions associated with enteropathogenic and enterohemorrhagic *E. coli* in piglets and

the role of plasmid mediated factors. Infect Immun 1989;57:1142–1150.

83 Taylor CJ, Hart CA, Batt RM, McDougall C, McLean L. Ultrastructural and biochemical changes in human jejunal mucosa associated with EPEC 0111 infection. J Pediatr Gastroenterol Nutr 1986;5:70–73.

84 Embaye H, Hart CA, Getty B, Fletcher JN, Saunders JR, Batt RM. Effects of enteropathogenic *Escherichia coli* on microvillar membrane proteins during organ culture of rabbit intestinal mucosa. Gut 1992;33:1184–1189.

85 Embaye H, Batt RM, Saunders JR, Getty B, Hart CA. Interaction of enteropathogenic *Escherichia coli* 0111 with rabbit intestinal mucosa in vitro. Gastroenterology 1989;96:1079–1086.

86 Cravioto A, Tello A, Navarro A, et al. Association of *Escherichia coli* HEp-2 adherence patterns with type and duration of diarrhoea. Lancet 1991;337:262–264.

87 Henry FJ, Udoy AS, Wanke CA, Aziz KMA. Epidemiology of persistent diarrhea and etiologic agents in Mirzapur, Bangladesh. Acta Pediatr 1992;381(suppl): 27–31.

88 Bhatnagar S, Bhan MK, Sommerflet H, Sazawal S, Kumar R, Saini S. Enteroaggregative *Escherichia coli* may be a new pathogen causing acute and persistent diarrhea. Scand J Infect Dis 1993;25:579–583.

89 Bhan MK, Raj P, Levine MM, et al. Enteroaggregative *Escherichia coli* associated with persistent diarrhea in a cohort of rural children in India. J Infect Dis 1989;159:1061–1064.

90 Levine MM, Ferreccio C, Prado V, et al. Epidemiologic studies of *Escherichia coli* diarrheal illness in a low socio-economic level peri-urban community in Santiago, Chile. Am J Epidemiol 1993;138:849–869.

91 Scotland SM, Smith HR, Said B, Willshaw GA, Cheasty T, Rowe B. Identification of EPEC isolated in Britain as EAgg or as members of A/E *Escherichia coli* not hybridizing with EPEC probe. J Med Microbiol 1991;35:278–283.

92 Bourgeois AL, Gardiner CH, Thornton SA, et al. Etiology of acute diarrhea among United States military personnel deployed to South America and West Africa. Am J Trop Med Hyg 1993;48:243–248.

93 Baqui AH, Sack RB, Black RE, et al. Enteropathogens associated with acute and persistent diarrhea in Bangladeshi children less than 5 years of age. J Infect Dis 1992;166:792–796.

94 Gunzburg ST, Chang BJ, Elliott SJ, Burke V, Gracey M. Diffuse and enteroaggregative patterns of adherence of enteric *Escherichia coli* isolated from Aboriginal children from the Kimberley Region of Western Australia. J Infect Dis 1993;167:755–758.

95 Echeverria P, Serichantalerg O, Changchawalit S, et al. Tissue culture-adherent *Escherichia coli* in infantile diarrhea. J Infect Dis 1992;165:141–143.

96 Cohen MB, Hawkins JA, Weckbach LA, Staneck JL, Levine MM, Heck JE. Colonization by enteroaggregative *Escherichia coli* in travelers with and without diarrhea. J Clin Microbiol 1993;31:351–353.

97 Levine MM, Savarino S, Losonsky G, Guers L, Tacket CO. Volunteer studies of enteroaggregative *Escherichia coli*. Abstracts of the 93rd General Meeting of the American Society for Microbiology, Las Vegas, Nevada, April 1994. Abstract no. B-315.

98 Nataro JP, Deng Y, Maneval DR, German AL, Martin WC, Levine MM. Aggregative adherence fimbriae I of enteroaggregative *Escherichia coli* mediate adherence to HEp-2 cells and hemagglutination of human erythrocytes. Infect Immun 1992;60:2297–2304.

99 Tzipori S, Montanaro J, Robins-Browne RM, Vial P, Gibson R, Levine MM. Studies with enteroaggregative *Escherichia coli* in the gnotobiotic piglet gastroenteritis model. Infect Immun 1992;60:5302–5306.

100 Vial PA, Robins-Browne R, Lior H, et al. Characterization of enteroadherence-aggregative *Escherichia coli*, a putative agent of diarrheal disease. J Infect Dis 1988;158:70–79.

101 Yamamoto T, Koyana Y, Matsumoto M, et al. Localized, aggregative, and diffuse adherence to HeLa cells, plastic, and human small intestines by *Escherichia coli* isolated from patients with diarrhea. J Infect Dis 1992;166:1295–1310.

102 Baldwin TJ, Knutton S, Sellers L, Manjarrez-Hernandez A, Aitken A, Williams PH. Enteroaggregative *Escherichia coli* strains secrete a heat-labile toxin antigenically related to *Escherichia coli* hemolysin. Infect Immun 1992;60:2092–2095.

103 Yamamoto T, Endo S, Yokota T, Echeverria P. Characteristics of adherence of enteroaggregative *Escherichia coli* to hu-

man and animal mucosa. Infect Immun 1991;59:3722–3739.

104 **Wanke CA, Cronan S, Goss C, Chadee K, Guerrant RL.** Characterization of binding of *Escherichia coli* strains which are enteropathogens to small-bowel mucin. Infect Immun 1990;58:794–800.

105 **Yamamoto T, Echeverria P, Yokota T.** Drug resistance and adherence to human intestines of enteroaggregative *Escherichia coli*. J Infect Dis 1992;165:744–749.

106 **Levine MM, Prado V, Robins-Browne R, et al.** Use of DNA probes and HEp-2 cell adherence assay to detect diarrheagenic *Escherichia coli*. J Infect Dis 1988;158:224–228.

107 **Baudry B, Savarino SJ, Vial P, Kaper JB, Levine MM.** A sensitive and specific DNA probe to identify enteroaggregative *Escherichia coli*, a recently discovered diarrheal pathogen. J Infect Dis 1990;161:1249–1251.

108 **Albert MJ, Qadri F, Haque A, Bhuiyan NA.** Bacterial clump formation at the surface of liquid culture as a rapid test for identification of enteroaggregative *Escherichia coli*. J Clin Microbiol 1993;31:1397–1399.

109 **Weintraub A, Leontein K, Widmalm G, Vial P, Levine MM, Lindberg AA.** Structural studies of the O-antigenic polysaccharide of an EAggEC strain. Eur J Biochem 1993;213:859–864.

110 **Nataro JP, Yikang D, Giron JA, Savarino SJ, Kothary MH, Hall R.** Aggregative adherence fimbria I expression in enteroaggregative *Escherichia coli* requires two unlinked plasmid regions. Infect Immun 1993;61:1126–1131.

111 **Knutton S, Shaw RK, Bhan MK, et al.** Ability of EAggEC strains to adhere in vitro to human intestinal mucosa. Infect Immun 1992;60:2083–2091.

112 **Savarino SJ, Fasano A, Robertson DC, Levine MM.** Enteroaggregative *Escherichia coli* elaborate a heat-stable enterotoxin demonstrable in an in vitro rabbit intestinal model. J Clin Invest 1991;87:1450–1455.

113 **Savarino SJ, Fasano A, Watson J, et al.** Enteroaggregative *Escherichia coli* heat-stable enterotoxin 1 represents another subfamily of *Escherichia coli* heat-stable toxin. Proc Natl Acad Sci USA 1993;90:3093–3097.

114 **Fang GD, Savarino SJ, Fasano A, Levine MM, Guerrant RL.** Cyclic GMP is increased in intestinal epithelial cells by enteroaggregative *Escherichia coli*. Abstracts of the 31st Interscience Conference on Antimicrobial Agents and Chemotherapy, Chicago, Illinois, October 1991. Abstract no. 1322.

115 **Eslava C, Villaseca J, Morales R, Navarro A, Cravioto A.** Identification of a protein with toxigenic activity produced by enteroaggregative *Escherichia coli*. Abstracts of the 93rd General Meeting of the American Society for Microbiology, Las Vegas, Nevada, April 1994. Abstract no. 88.

116 **Benjamin P, Cronan S, Miller SI, Wanke CA.** Characterization of an invasive genetic locus in enteroaggregative *Escherichia coli*. Abstracts of 93rd General Meeting of the American Society for Microbiology, Las Vegas, Nevada, May 1994. Abstract.

BCG Immunization: Review of Past Experience, Current Use, and Future Prospects

TIMOTHY F. BREWER
MARY E. WILSON
EDWARD A. NARDELL

The resurgence of tuberculosis in late twentieth century America has rekindled interest in all aspects of this long-neglected disease—its history, pathogenesis, transmission, diagnosis, treatment, and prevention. The alarming emergence of multiple drug-resistant (MDR) tuberculosis in a number of urban areas and its predictable transmission to health care workers have spawned new urgency in finding alternatives to isoniazid (INH) chemoprophylaxis—the only drug proven effective in preventing disease in large clinical trials. Unfortunately, when neither isoniazid nor rifampin can be used, the remaining antibiotics for the treatment of either infection or disease are both more toxic and much less effective. Combinations of pyrazinamide, ethambutol, and ofloxacin (or ciprofloxacin) have been recommended empirically as prophylaxis for the contacts of known MDR cases, but evidence of efficacy, tolerance, and acceptability is lacking, and the quinolones are not approved for use in children due to concerns about their safety (1). Indeed, even for drug-susceptible tuberculous infection, where the efficacy of INH has been proven in preventing disease, patient acceptance, adherence to treatment, and drug toxicity have been barriers limiting the impact of chemoprophylaxis as a tuberculosis control strategy (2).

Another highly controversial approach to preventing exposure and transmission in high-risk settings has been the strict application of administrative and environmental engineering controls and the use of personal respirators where exposure cannot be eliminated (3). However, because environmental controls and respirators cannot protect completely, especially against infection from unsuspected tuberculosis cases, immunization with bacille Calmette-Guérin (BCG) has been suggested as an additional control strategy (4,5). This chapter reviews previous experience with BCG among populations with high and low prevalence rates of tuberculosis, its present usage, its potential impact on the current skin testing and chemoprophylaxis strategy in this country, and the prospects for using BCG, or future tuberculosis vaccines, in the United States.

THE TUBERCULOSIS RESURGENCE IN PERSPECTIVE— IMPLICATIONS FOR BCG USAGE

Since 1985, when the long-standing nationwide decline in tuberculosis ceased and the resurgence began, the factors responsible for this unanticipated reversal have gradually become apparent. The focal nature of the resurgence requires emphasis. More than 40% of the counties in the United States reported no cases of tuberculosis in 1992, a percentage that increases yearly. In 1992, there were 4472 more cases than in 1985, a 20.1% increase nationwide, but the states of New York and California together accounted for 89.1% of the increase. New York City alone accounted for just under 50% of the increase, and contributed 61.4% of the MDR cases in a 1992 nationwide survey (6). Increases were noted in several other large population areas, but case rates in most U.S. cities and states have continued to decline, some having experienced only transient upswings. However, the magnitude of the increases in New York City and other high-prevalence areas has been sufficient to offset small declines in low-prevalence areas. In those areas where increases have been noted, human immunodeficiency virus (HIV) infection, immigration from high-prevalence countries, homelessness, institutional transmission including in hospitals, shelters, and prisons, substance abuse, and eroded public tuberculosis control programs appear to have been the factors principally responsible. Even in areas again enjoying declining case rates, these factors are often important risk factors for tuberculosis. In New York City, fortunately, a large infusion of federal funds for tuberculosis control, primarily to ensure completion of therapy through treatment supervision, has produced a decline in tuberculosis cases (6b). Assuming that significant funds continue to be made available for tuberculosis control, it is likely that national trends will continue to be downward despite a disproportionate contribution from high-risk areas. The discussion on whether or not to use BCG in the United States must be approached with the understanding that the current resurgence of tuberculosis is highly focal geographically and within the population and may be relatively short-lived. This does not preclude the possibility of future resurgences from as yet unanticipated factors. Furthermore, the current resurgence is leaving behind a legacy of infected persons, some with MDR tuberculosis, which will influence case rates for many years to come.

POSSIBLE MECHANISMS OF BCG VACCINATION TO PREVENT TUBERCULOSIS

For the world's most widely used vaccine, BCG is poorly understood. Not only has its efficacy been the subject of heated debate, but its mechanism of action is incompletely known, in part a reflection of gaps in our understanding of the complex immune responses to tuberculosis (7). In the most general terms, current concepts of how BCG works can be summarized as follows.

Contrary to popular belief, BCG immunization is not believed to prevent tuberculous infection, defined as implantation of one or more tubercle bacilli and their replication to 10^4 bacilli, at which point cell-mediated immunity (CMI) and delayed-type hypersensitivity (DTH) are triggered. The period of bacillary replication prior to the triggering of immunity occurs within ordinary scavenging alveolar macrophages. Continued replication depends on the permissiveness of macrophages, that is, their innate and acquired nonspecific capacity to kill tubercle bacilli (8,9). Presumably, in some persons, inhaled organisms replicate within macrophages, but because growth is arrested before reaching 10^4 bacilli, DTH is not triggered, the tuberculin test remains negative, and "infection" does not occur as further evidenced by an extremely small chance of future reactivation disease. When DTH and CMI are triggered, however, their combined effect is to stabilize microbial growth by about the twenty-first day after implantation (8). T cell-activated macrophages are more bacteriocidal, and once bacillary control is established, focal lesions are isolated through granuloma formation. In persons previously infected with *Mycoplasma tuberculosis*, or immunized with BCG, granuloma formation is accelerated, leading to more efficient localization of infection. Improved localization also reduces subsequent hematogenous dissemination and implantation in the lung apex and other organs. Vaccination with BCG presumably reduces the risk for all forms of active tuberculosis, although the mechanisms by which BCG enhances granuloma formation remain uncertain.

CLINICAL TRIALS: FINDINGS OF META-ANALYSIS SUMMARIZED

Uncertainty about the protective efficacy of BCG against tuberculosis has been engendered by conflicting results of several major controlled trials and case-control studies (10,11). A meta-analysis of the published literature of the efficacy of BCG in preventing tuberculosis cases or deaths recently derived overall average protection rates for vaccination and explored sources of variation in protection rates in different studies (12). More than 1200 articles and abstracts were reviewed. Fourteen prospective trials and 12 case-control studies met the inclusion criteria and were analyzed. Data from the trials and the case-control studies were combined separately. Combining data from the trials gave an overall average protective effect of BCG against tuberculosis cases of 51%. When the seven trials that reported deaths from tuberculosis were analyzed, BCG had a 71% protective effect against tuberculous death. The combined 10 case-control studies with 1414 cases of predominantly pulmonary tuberculosis showed a 50% protective effect for BCG compared with no vaccination. Separate analyses from the case-control studies of BCG vaccination of infants showed a protective effect of 64% against tuberculous meningitis and a protective effect of 78% against disseminated tuberculosis.

A random-effects regression model was used to explore reasons for the wide range of efficacy rates for BCG reported in individual studies. In the 13 prospective trials reporting tuberculosis cases, geographical latitude and study validity score explained 66% of the between-study variance. Latitude alone explained 41% of the variance. The efficacy of BCG increased with increasing distance from the equator and with higher study validity score.

A regression model variable such as latitude may be a surrogate for a known or unknown factor capable of influencing BCG's reported efficacy in different study populations. For example, factors that vary by geographical location and could influence effectiveness of BCG include socioeconomic conditions, genetic composition of the population, climate, exposure to sunlight, diet and nutrition, presence of nontuberculous mycobacteria in the environment, completeness of surveillance in BCG studies, and the storage and viability of BCG among others. The study validity score was determined from a scoring system that assessed the potential for bias in study design and methods used to confirm the diagnosis of tuberculosis.

The meta-analysis found that the protection from BCG persisted across many subgroups and study designs. Higher rates of protection were found against severe forms of tuberculosis, although this result may reflect the ability of the investigators of the original studies to identify better these forms of disease. BCG protected against pulmonary tuberculosis as well as against extrapulmonary disease. Age at the time of vaccination did not predict efficacy.

SIDE EFFECTS

A majority of persons receiving an intradermal vaccination with BCG develop a superficial ulcer at the vaccination site. The ulcer may take 2 to 3 months to heal and often leaves a 4- to 8-mm scar (13). Ipsilateral axillary or supraclavicular adenopathy may occur; it usually resolves without treatment. These side effects are usually not considered complications of vaccination with BCG. Their frequency is affected by the strain and dose of BCG used and the age of recipients. In a prospective report of BCG complications, Lotte and colleagues noted a rate of suppurative adenitis and other local complications of 4% among infants receiving BCG and 0.3% among children vaccinated between the ages of one and 20 years old (14). Treatment for these complications ranges from observation to surgical excision of the affected nodes. Persisting or disseminated BCG infection occurred in three to six infants per 10^6 vaccinations with one to 14 cases per 10^6 vaccinations for the older age group. Although disseminated BCG infection has been most commonly reported among children with immunologic disorders, disseminated disease, including fatal BCG infection, has been reported rarely in apparently healthy children (15,16). Disseminated BCG in otherwise healthy children has been successfully treated with antituberculous therapy even after going unrecognized for 4 months (15).

Disseminated BCG has been reported in both HIV-infected adults (17,18) and children (19,20). Three small studies of HIV-infected and uninfected children vaccinated with BCG at birth found no difference in rates of local side effects (significant ulceration or adenopathy) for the two groups (21–23). No cases of disseminated BCG infection were reported in these studies. Besnard and colleagues, however, reported two cases of disseminated BCG infection and 7 cases of large adenopathy among 68 HIV-infected children vaccinated with BCG at birth (20). These complications occurred between 3 to 35 months after vaccination. Thus disseminated BCG infection among HIV-infected individuals occurs, but its incidence remains unclear. Disseminated BCG also has been reported in a person vaccinated years before developing HIV-infection (17). BCG vaccination continues to be recommended for asymptomatic children regardless of their HIV status born in areas where the risk of tuberculosis is high, although the efficacy of BCG vaccination in preventing tuberculosis in HIV-infected individuals is not yet known (24). Kallenius and colleagues also have speculated that vaccination with BCG may help prevent subsequent development of disseminated nontuberculous mycobacterial infections in HIV-infected persons (25).

BCG AND THE TUBERCULIN SKIN TEST

Most early investigators of BCG considered a postvaccination reaction to a tuberculin test to be an indicator of vaccine-induced immunity (26–29), with the lack of a positive reaction indicative of a poor response to vaccination (30). Because of low rates of tuberculin conversion after oral vaccination, subcutaneous and then intradermal administration was recommended (26,31).

Despite this widespread acceptance of postvaccination tuberculin reactions as a marker for BCG-induced immunity, epidemiologic and laboratory data suggest that BCG-induced DTH is an unreliable surrogate market for immunity. Data from the British Medical Research Council BCG trial showed that the incidence of tuberculosis among participants was independent of the amount of tuberculin sensitivity induced by vaccination (32,33). Comstock reviewed the controlled trials of BCG efficacy in 1988 and concluded that postvaccination skin test conversion rates did not correlate with a strain's protective effect (34). Studies in schoolchildren demonstrated that postvaccination tuberculin reactivity could be maintained by repeated tuberculin testing. In guinea pigs, this phenomenon did not correlate with the preservation of acquired resistance (35,36).

Studies in guinea pigs (37) and mice (38) immunized with BCG found no significant relationship between the degree of postvaccination tuberculin sensitivity and the degree of immunity to a challenge with virulent *M. tuberculosis*. The removal of the Ly^{2+} T cells from a pool of harvested T cells from BCG-immunized mice transferred to T cell-deficient mice prevented the development of immunity to virulent *M. tuberculosis* but not of DTH to purified protein derivative (PPD). This result suggests that different T-cell populations were responsible for immunity and hypersensitivity (39).

Difficulty in interpreting tuberculin skin testing as a marker for *M. tuberculosis* infection in individuals vaccinated with BCG has been an argument against its use in the United States. An oft heard comment is that the tuberculin test is lost as a marker if BCG is given. Review of the extensive literature shows that prior BCG produces skin test reactivity, thereby reducing the utility of the tuberculin skin test. However, analysis of data from past studies for relevance to the current situation is difficult for many reasons. Antigens used for tuberculin testing have varied in their purity, dose, handling, and method of administration. Tuberculin skin testing today is most often carried out using PPD administered by the Mantoux method, which involves intracutaneous injection of a standardized amount of antigen. Other kinds of tuberculin, for example, old tuberculin, and other methods of administration, such as multiple puncture techniques, have been used in some studies.

The timing for reading results and criteria used for considering a tuberculin test negative or positive range widely among studies. Some results were read in millimeters of induration, whereas others were graded (Heaf grade 0 through 4) or simply described as negative or positive. Studies have been done in populations with different background rates of tuberculosis and in geographical areas with different rates of exposure to environmental mycobacteria.

Tuberculin sensitivity 6 months after BCG vaccination in different studies varies widely, from less than 50% (40) to more than 95% (41). Criteria for interpreting tuberculin sensitivity are not uniform across studies. The size of the tuberculin reaction after BCG vaccination varies with the age at vaccination (42), duration and number of skin tests since vaccination (35), and dose and BCG vaccine used (43). The tuberculin skin test is larger at 12 months in persons given an interim skin test at 10 weeks or 6 months (36). Studies using different BCG vaccines in schoolchildren in Copenhagen found that 9 to 11 weeks after BCG the mean tuberculin reactivity varied from 13 to 20 mm depending on the vaccine administered (43).

Tuberculin sensitivity induced by the same BCG vaccine varies with the population tested. After receiving Danish BCG, several thousand schoolchildren in Denmark and Greece had Mantoux tests (10 TU). Although the tuberculin reactions grouped symmetrically around single central values, in Denmark the average size was 16.7 mm, whereas in Greece it was 10.8 mm (29).

Postvaccination reactions tend to be smaller in persons vaccinated as infants and decrease with time (42,44,45). Menzies and Vissandjee tested schoolchildren and young adults 10 to 25 years after BCG and found that only 7.9% of those vaccinated in infancy had significant tuberculin reactions, in contrast to 18% among those vaccinated between ages one and 5 years (42). Horwitz and colleagues found, in children tested 2 months and 5 years after BCG, that small reactions tended to decrease in size and large reactions remained almost unchanged (46). In populations where there are high rates of exposure to tuberculosis and BCG is given at birth, prevalence of positive tuberculin tests declines over 3 to 5 years, then rises, presumably as a result of infection with *M. tuberculosis* (47).

Large tuberculin reactions (> 15 mm) are likely to represent infection with tuberculosis in persons with a history of remote BCG vaccination and residence in an area with high rates of tuberculosis. A study of foreign-born persons in Montreal provides support for considering incidence of tuberculosis in the country of origin in interpretation of tuberculin test results. In immigrants from countries with low rates of tuberculosis, the researchers found higher rates of positive tuberculin reactions in BCG-vaccinated persons than those not vaccinated. BCG-vaccinated persons coming from countries with high incidence of tuberculosis had higher rates of positive tuberculin reactions than did BCG-vaccinated persons from low-incidence areas. In persons from high-incidence areas, skin test reactivity was similar in persons with and without previous BCG. These results suggest that many BCG-vaccinated persons with large tuberculin reactions coming from countries with a high incidence of tuberculosis have been infected with *M. tuberculosis* (48).

Sensitivity to tuberculin can result from infection with *M. tuberculosis*, infection with nontuberculous mycobacteria, and vaccination with BCG. Tuberculin sensitivity as measured by skin testing can be seen as an expression of the weighted sum of mycobacterial experience in that individual, with *M. tuberculosis* infection causing larger reactions on average than those due to nontuberculous mycobacteria or BCG. Although postvaccination tuberculin reactions may overlap in size with those indicative of infection with *M. tuberculosis* and persist for 15 or more years (49), tuberculin reactions caused by previous vaccination with BCG are on average smaller than those attributed to natural infection (41,50). Booster reactions to PPD (increase in size of tuberculin skin test when tests are repeated) may be seen in persons with a history of BCG vaccination, tuberculosis, and infection with nontuberculous mycobacteria.

The tuberculin test is highly imperfect, and many skin test results are neither sensitive nor specific. Significant variation among observers in reading results has been shown in some studies. Host factors unrelated to mycobacterial infections affect the test and can also vary over time. Performing the test can influence the results of subsequent tests. Prior BCG vaccination adds another variable to the interpretation of an already problematic test. Especially in the BCG-vaccinated individual, the tuberculin test should be viewed as one of many pieces of data that can be used in deciding the probability that an individual is infected with *M. tuberculosis*. With a good history including the patient's risk for tuberculosis, history of BCG with age at vaccination, number of doses of BCG, years since BCG vaccination, number and timing of tuberculin skin tests, size of the reaction, and host factors (immunosuppressive drugs or diseases), the tuberculin test still has some value in patients who have previously received BCG (57).

The possible expanded use of BCG highlights the difficulties in our current methods to screen for *M. tuberculosis* infection. The development of an alternative test for tuberculosis infection based on a specific antigen or an effective vaccine that did not induce DTH to tuberculin would be important advances that would eliminate the skin test issue from the risk–benefit analysis in the decision to use BCG or other vaccine to prevent tuberculosis.

One strategy for persons recently vaccinated with BCG would be follow-up tuberculin testing at 6 to 12 months after vaccination to establish the degree of tuberculin sensitivity induced in that individual. This test would establish that individual's baseline of tuberculin sensitivity. Most studies show that absent new infection with mycobacteria, this sensitivity will wane over time in most persons. Depending on factors already noted, a portion of the population may have little or no tuberculin sensitivity a year or more after BCG vaccination. Regular, periodic skin testing after vaccination, despite the risk of preserving tuberculin reactivity, identifies those individuals with small or negative reactions and still may be more sensitive in detecting new infections in most individuals than chest roentgenographs or clinical symptoms.

STRAINS

One explanation for the observed variation in the efficacy of BCG in preventing tuberculosis is that different "strains" of BCG have been used in different trials. Strain is defined in most papers as the BCG vaccine maintained in a particular laboratory (52). Of the lyophilized seed stocks most commonly used today for vaccine production, only the Pasteur strain was derived from a single colony isolate and is a strain in the traditional sense of the word (53). Although investigators have long believed that there are many strains of BCG, recent work using IS986 gene probes in 35 vaccines from 11 strains found only two distinct banding patterns (54). *Mycobacterium bovis* BCG has few copies of the IS986 gene present (54b), making the relationship between strain and banding patterns unclear.

Interpreting data on BCG immunogenicity and protective effect from laboratory studies is difficult because results vary with the in vitro (38) test or animal model (55) used. The dose of BCG used for vaccination and the interval between vaccination and challenge also influence the reported protection provided by different strains (56). In vivo and in vitro differences in the allergenic potency of BCG strains may reflect variations in production methods more than inherent strain differences. Two products prepared from the same strain in separate laboratories may differ more than two products prepared from different strains in the same laboratory (57). The many variables involved in the use of animal models to assess the protective effect of tuberculosis vaccines make confirming results described in one animal model with a different model difficult, if not impossible (58). Furthermore, Crowle has argued that animal or animal cell experiments may not accurately reflect human immunity to *M. tuberculosis* infection (59).

Limited information from studies in human beings and human cell lines suggests that strain is not an important determinant of BCG efficacy. T-cell clones from nine individuals vaccinated with Danish BCG were studied to examine their ability to respond to a variety of mycobacterial antigens. All T-cell clones responded to four different BCG vaccines, regardless of their ability to respond to other mycobacterial antigens (60).

Two prospective trials of BCG efficacy in human beings assessed the impact of strain on the prevention of tuberculosis. In the Madras trial in south India, both the Danish and Paris strains showed no efficacy in preventing pulmonary tuberculosis (52). There was no difference in efficacy between the two vaccines. The British Medical Research Trial, using the Danish and vole bacillus (*Mycobacterium microti*) vaccines, found both strains to be highly effective in preventing tuberculosis (61). Despite the divergent efficacy results in these two studies, Madras researchers concluded that the British and Madras Danish strains were genetically identical (62). The only data from a prospective study to suggest that strain may influence protective efficacy comes from a study in infants from Hong Kong (13). In this study, the Paris strain was more effective in preventing tuberculosis than the Glaxo strain; the absolute difference in efficacy between the vaccines could not be determined because of the absence of a control group.

The meta-analysis of BCG efficacy described above demonstrated that the ability of BCG to induce immunity is retained across a gamut of study conditions, BCG pedigrees, populations, and vaccine preparations as well as a 60-year time span (12). Strain did not explain the variation in protection noted among the studies. Other possible explanations for the range of protection noted in the trials include genetic or physiologic differences in the study populations, presence of nontuberculous mycobacteria in the environment, the risk of primary tuberculosis (as opposed to reactivation disease), exogenous reinfection, and the study design used (10,11).

CURRENT USE OF BCG

Rationale for Continued BCG Use in Different Countries

Strategies for BCG use vary by country. Since 1953, BCG has been given in the United Kingdom to adolescent schoolchildren and has been recommended for infants belonging to groups at high risk for tuberculosis such as Asian immigrants. It is estimated that 3600 BCG vaccinations were needed in England and Wales to prevent one reported case of tuberculosis in 1989 in contrast to 460 vaccinations in 1969 (63). Given the United Kingdom's current low rate of tuberculosis, their policy is under review. In a risk–benefit analysis, it has been suggested that when the risk of tuberculosis in a community is less than 0.1% per year, the risk of adverse reactions from BCG may exceed its potential benefit. Sweden has discontinued routine use of BCG. Some countries, such as Japan, give BCG to infants and administer repeat doses to schoolchildren who have negative tuberculin reactions. The value of repeat doses of BCG to maintain protective efficacy is unknown.

For developing countries with high rates of tuberculosis, the World Health Organization (WHO) has supported universal infant BCG immunization along with active case finding and treatment for the control of this disease. Globally, an estimated 71% of infants born in 1989 received BCG as part of the WHO Expanded Programme on Immunization (64). The only listed contraindication to BCG use in these countries has been symptomatic HIV infection or other serious immunodeficiency disease.

In many developing countries, children are often exposed at a young age to tuberculosis, usually within the household. The annual risk of infection with tuberculosis may be 2 to 3% or higher. Diagnosis of tuberculosis is often difficult in young children, who rarely produce bacteriologically positive sputum. Treatment is expensive and inaccessible to many segments of the population. Rates of tuberculosis in many parts of the world are increasing because of the HIV-induced immunosuppression in populations with high background rates of tuberculosis. Vaccination with BCG is often the only tuberculosis prevention method available for these children. WHO/UNICEF continue to recommend BCG, preferably at birth, for all infants born in high-risk countries, including those with asymptomatic HIV infection (65).

BCG Use for Bladder Cancer

Mycobacteria can stimulate the immune response to heterologous antigens. Live BCG induces an inflammatory response that activates macrophages and stimulates T and B lymphocytes and natural killer cells. After BCG was shown to inhibit tumor growth in experimental animals, investigators began to study the possible role of BCG in the prevention and treatment of malignancies in human beings (66). BCG is thought to augment the immune response to tumor-associated antigens. Hundreds of published papers describe studies testing different BCG vaccines (including heat killed) in varying doses against multiple kinds of malignancies, alone and in combination with other therapies. Routes of BCG administration tested in cancer patients have included intralesional, intradermal, subcutaneous, intraperitoneal, intravesical (67), oral, intrapleural (68), and aerosol administration (69). At present, BCG is used regularly for only one kind of malignancy. In 1991, the U.S. Food and Drug Administration approved BCG for treatment of carcinoma of the bladder after a multi-institutional study showed that immunotherapy with intravesical BCG provided better protection than intravesical doxorubicin against recurrence of superficial bladder cancer (70). Not surprisingly, cystitis and local symptoms following large doses of intravesical BCG have been common (> 90%), but serious adverse reactions are infrequently documented (71). In a retrospective review of 1278 patients, fever above 103°F was reported in about 4%, granulomatous prostatitis in 1.3%, and BCG pneumonitis or hepatitis in about 1% (72). Miliary BCG infection also has been reported (73). Local and systemic infection with BCG generally responds to treatment with antituberculous drugs (71,74,75).

The question of whether BCG could stimulate tumor growth has been studied in an animal model (76). Several epidemiologic studies in patients have looked at cancer rates in persons with and without prior BCG (77–80). No protective effect of BCG against cancer has been noted and a slight excess of cases of lymphosarcoma and Hodgkin's disease among the vaccine recipients was reported in some studies.

Considerations for Wider BCG Use in the United States

Recommendations for BCG use in the United States should consider several factors. The rates of tuberculosis in most segments of the population remain low. Exposure to tuberculosis can be inapparent, but many individuals and groups likely to come into contact with tuberculosis can be identified. Populations in the United States with high rates of new infections with tuberculosis include intravenous drug users, the homeless (especially those living in shelters), persons who live and work in prisons and other closed institutions, health care workers in some geographical areas, and household contacts of persons with tuberculosis.

Since 1988, BCG has been recommended only for tuberculin-negative children with ongoing exposure to INH- and rifampin-resistant tuberculosis, or who are unable to take INH and have continued exposure to someone with infectious tuberculosis, or who belong to groups where the rate of new *M. tuberculosis* infections exceeds 1% per year (81). With increasing numbers of tuberculosis cases, especially due to MDR organisms, the role of BCG in tuberculosis control needs to be reevaluated (4).

Rates of resistance to INH among newly acquired tuberculosis infections exceed 30% in some geographical areas. Prophylaxis with INH can be expected to have little or no benefit in these persons. It is assumed that BCG will have the same protective efficacy against tuberculosis caused by MDR forms of tuberculosis, although this has never been proven with a scientific study.

In the past, BCG vaccination of health care workers has been effective in preventing tuberculosis (82,83) and a recent decision analysis suggests that vaccination may prevent more cases among house staff at high risk for tuberculosis than currently used methods (5). Furthermore, many cases of nosocomial-acquired tuberculosis have been due to MDR tuberculosis for which chemoprophylaxis regimens with proven benefit do not exist. Assuming an average efficacy rate of 50% as determined by meta-analysis, BCG would be cost effective for the homeless as well (84).

The tuberculosis case rate in Central Harlem in 1990 was 233/100,000 (85), 20 times the rate for the United States as a whole and higher than in many countries with national BCG vaccination programs. The treatment of active tuberculosis in this locale is fraught with high loss to follow-up and failure rates (86); tuberculin screening and chemoprophylaxis are unlikely to fare any better. BCG vaccination may be a cost-effective addition to case finding and treatment programs for this and similar populations.

The management of persons with high risk of tuberculosis exposure in the United States in the past two to three decades has involved regular screening with the tuberculin test and administration of preventive therapy with INH when skin test conversion is observed. Difficulties with this approach have included poor compliance with regular skin testing and with INH prophylaxis for converters, and problems with interpreting the tuberculin test because of boosting and other factors discussed earlier.

Currently in the United States, BCG should not be given to persons infected with HIV. Therefore, screening for HIV infection would be prudent before giving BCG. The persistence of mycobacteria for months or years after BCG vaccination produces a dilemma about its use in HIV-negative persons who practice behaviors that place them at high risk for HIV infection. BCG is not contraindicated in persons infected with *M. tuberculosis*, but few data suggest that BCG provides benefit for this population (87).

Acceptance of BCG Acceptance of BCG may be a barrier to its use in the United States. In general, in the United States high vaccination rates of targeted groups are achieved only when integrated into infant and childhood immunization programs or are mandated (for school or university entry, by hospital or other institution, or by law). For example, acceptance of the hepatitis B vaccine by high-risk health care workers was low when receipt of vaccine was voluntary despite its high reported efficacy and low complication rate. There will likely be reluctance to use BCG for several reasons: general skepticism about its efficacy, lack of familiarity with its use, and concern about using a live vaccine that will be contraindicated in some individuals. Also, it may be difficult to identify and reach some high-risk groups. If screening for HIV infection is recommended prior to vaccination with BCG, concern about confidentiality may also discourage the vaccine's use.

FUTURE PROSPECTS

New developments include the use of BCG as an adjuvant with other antigens for immunotherapy and as a carrier of protective antigens in recombinant vaccines. The use of other mycobacterial species for immunoprophylaxis and immunotherapy and the development of subunit vaccines are also under study.

The vaccine has a long record of safety, has been given to more than 3 billion persons, and is the most effective adjuvant known for the induction of cell-mediated immunity in humans (88). These properties make BCG an attractive candidate for a multi-antigen vaccine. Plasmids can be transferred between *Escherichia coli* and mycobacterial species, and the insertion of additional protective antigens to *M. tuberculosis* or other pathogens into BCG vaccines is theoretically possible. An enhanced vaccine against tuberculosis, however, might require the insertion of multiple protective genes and deletion of suppressor genes (89).

Some investigators believe that the "protective antigens" are common to all mycobacterial species, while tissue damaging ones are specific to *M. tuberculosis* species, including BCG (90,91). Hence, a nonpathogenic mycobacterial species may be able to elicit protective immunity in humans. *Mycobacterium vaccae*, a nonpathogenic species found in the soil, has been used for both immunoprophylaxis and immunotherapy. Children exposed to patients with leprosy and who had been vaccinated with killed *M. vaccae* were more likely to react to leprosin A than their unvaccinated counterparts. If leprosin A reactivity is a marker for immunity, as the investigators believe, then this vaccine may induce protective immunity (92). When given as immunotherapy in conjunction with chemotherapy for active tuberculosis, *M. vaccae* recipients gained more weight than did patients treated with chemotherapy alone (93). Limited information also suggests that *M. vaccae* immunotherapy may reduce mortality in tuberculous patients (92).

Living bacilli may not be necessary to induce immunity. Cell wall antigens may possess the protective epitopes necessary to create a subunit vaccine, thereby eliminating the risk of disseminated disease posed by a live mycobacterial vaccine (88). However, subunit vaccines need to be able to stimulate a cell-mediated response; the lack of adjuvant properties has been felt to be responsible for the poor performance of nonliving vaccines in the past (59). Killed *Mycobacterium leprae* given with live BCG has been used for immunotherapy in patients with lepromatous leprosy. In vitro evidence suggests that the immunosuppression of this disease can be reversed in some patients with this therapy (88). In studies of guinea pigs, a vaccine derived from secreted proteins of *M. tuberculosis* protected animals from challenge with aerosolized virulent *M. tuberculosis* (94). The ability of these and other new vaccines to prevent and treat tuberculosis in human beings remains to be determined.

CONCLUSIONS

In reviewing the efficacy of BCG vaccination to prevent tuberculosis, we elected not to focus on selected individual clinical trials but have concluded from the results of a recent meta-analysis of many trials over several decades that BCG is likely to be at least 50% effective in preventing pulmonary and extrapulmonary tuberculosis (12). These data together with the substantial published experience in the areas of BCG safety, the effects of vaccination on tuberculin skin testing, and tuberculosis immunology comprise the scientific basis for considering wider use of BCG in the United States. However, the longstanding BCG controversy goes well beyond the scientific, involving strong emotional viewpoints rooted in historical precedence in this and other countries, a long-standing public health strategy based on chemoprophylaxis, speculation on future epidemiologic trends in tuberculosis, and perceptions—both of the risks of potentially drug-resistant tuberculosis and the possible protective effects of vaccination. Physicians trained in North America have been taught that the effectiveness of BCG is unproven and its use is inappropriate in countries like the United States where the prevalence of tuberculosis has been relatively low. This widely held perception is unlikely to change without clear recommendations from authoritative governmental and academic sources followed by a major educational initiative. Whether the results of the recent meta-analysis will change any viewpoints remains to be seen. In the view of the authors, however, BCG should be used more often in the United States than is now the case, administered under clear guidelines to specific HIV-negative high-risk populations or individuals.

Homeless persons and residents of institutions at high risk for tuberculosis, especially in areas where MDR tuberculosis is common, should be offered BCG as an alternative to periodic skin testing and chemoprophylaxis. Among the homeless, skin testing is difficult and chemoprophylaxis is often not possible without extraordinary resources that might better be reserved for disease treatment. Workers in hospitals, shelters, correctional facilities, and others potentially exposed to unsuspected MDR tuberculosis, where the efficacy of chemoprophylaxis is uncertain, should also be offered BCG with the understanding that vaccination is not 100% protective and should not replace efforts to minimize exposure to tuberculosis. The use of BCG does not preclude regular tuberculin testing or future chemoprophylaxis under appropriate circumstances. BCG-vaccinated persons exposed to tuberculosis who have documented large increases in skin test reactivity (10 to 15 mm increases, for example, with or without prior waning of skin test reactivity) should be offered chemoprophylaxis.

Although additional large clinical trials of BCG are not warranted, epidemiologic data on vaccinated persons at high risk for both HIV and tuberculous infections, such as injecting drug users, should be collected to determine the efficacy of vaccination and the risk of BCG dissemination among vaccinated persons who subsequently become HIV-infected. Studies in other high-risk populations, such as health care workers and employees in correctional facilities in high prevalence areas for tuberculosis, could help answer other unresolved questions including the impact of BCG on the tuberculin skin test in U.S. adults. Even if BCG is used more widely, effective, uninterrupted treatment and case finding will remain the foundation of tuberculosis control in the United States.

REFERENCES

1 **Centers for Disease Control.** Management of persons exposed to multidrug-resistant tuberculosis. MMWR 1992;41:61–69.

2 **American Thoracic Society.** Control of tuberculosis in the United States. Am Rev Respir Dis 1992;146:1623–1633.

3 **Centers for Disease Control.** Draft guidelines for preventing the transmission of tuberculosis in health-care facilities, 2nd ed. Fed Regist 1993;58:52810–52854.

4 **Koch-Weser D.** BCG vaccination. Can it

contribute to tuberculosis control? Chest 1993;103:1641–1642.

5 **Greenberg PD, Lax KG, Schechter CB.** Tuberculosis in house staff. A decision analysis comparing the tuberculin screening strategy with BCG vaccination. Am Rev Respir Dis 1991;143:490–495.

6 **Bloch A, Cauthen GM, Onorato M, et al.** Nationwide survey of drug-resistant tuberculosis in the United States. JAMA 1994; 271:665–671.

6b Hamburg MA, Frieden TR. Tuberculosis transmission in the 1990s. N Engl J Med 1994;330:1750–1751.

7 Piessens WF. Introduction to the immunology of tuberculosis. Rev Infect Dis 1989;11: 3436–3442.

8 Dannenberg AM. Delayed-type hypersensitivity and cell-mediated immunity in the pathogenesis of pulmonary tuberculosis. Immunol Today 1991;12:228–233.

9 Nardell EA. Pathogenesis of tuberculosis. In: Reichman LB, Herschfield ES, eds. Tuberculosis: a comprehensive international approach. New York: Marcel Dekker, 1993: 103–122.

10 Fine PEM, Rodrigues LC. Modern vaccines: mycobacterial diseases. Lancet 1990; 335:1016–1020.

11 Clemens JD, Chuong JJH, Feinstein AR. The BCG controversy: a methodological and statistical reappraisal. JAMA 1983;249: 2362–2369.

12 Colditz GA, Brewer TF, Berkey CS, et al. Efficacy of BCG vaccine in the prevention of tuberculosis: meta-analysis of the published literature. JAMA 1994;271:698–702.

13 ten Dam HG. BCG vaccination. In: Reichman LB, Hershfield ES, eds. Tuberculosis: a comprehensive international approach. New York: Marcel Dekker, 1993: 251–274.

14 Lotte A, Wasz-Hockert O, Poisson N. Second IUATLD study on complications induced by intradermal BCG-vaccination. Bull Int Union Against TB Lung Dis 1988; 63:47–59.

15 Tardieu M, Truffot-Pernot C, Carriere JP, Dupic V, Landrieu P. Tuberculous meningitis due to BCG in two previously healthy children. Lancet 1988;1:440–441.

16 Pedersen FK, Engbaek HC, Hertz H, Vergmann B. Fatal BCG infection in an immunocompetent girl. Acta Paediatr Scand 1978;68:519–523.

17 Armbruster C, Junker W, Vetter N, Jaksch G. Disseminated Bacille Calmette-Guerin infection in AIDS patient 30 years after BCG vaccination. J Infect Dis 1990;162: 1216.

18 Boudes P, Sobel A, Deforges L, Leblic E. Disseminated *Mycobacterium bovis* infection from BCG vaccination and HIV infection. JAMA 1989;262:2386.

19 Ninane J, Grymonprez A, Burtonboy G, Francois A, Cornu G. Disseminated BCG in HIV infection. Arch Dis Child 1988;63: 1268–1269.

20 Besnard M, Sauvion S, Offredo C, et al. Bacillus Calmette-Guerin infection after vaccination of human immunodeficiency virus-infected children. Pediatr Infect Dis J 1993;12:993–997.

21 Centers for Disease Control and Prevention. BCG vaccination and pediatric HIV infection-Rwanda, 1988–1990. MMWR 1991;40:833–836.

22 Lallemant-Le Coeur S, Lallemant M, Cheynier D, Nzingoula S, Drucker J, Larouze B. Bacillus Calmette-Guerin immunization in infants born to HIV-1-seropositive mothers. AIDS 1991;5:195–199.

23 Ryder RW, Oxtoby MJ, Mvula M, et al. Safety and immunogenicity of Bacille Calmette-Guerin, diphtheria-tetanus-pertussis, and oral polio vaccines in newborn children in Zaire infected with human immunodeficiency virus type 1. J Pediatr 1993;122:697–702.

24 ten Dam HG. BCG vaccination and HIV infection. Bull Int Union Against TB Lung Dis 1990;65:38–39.

25 Kallenius G, Hoffner SE, Svenson SB. Does vaccination with Bacille Calmette-Guerin protect against AIDS? Rev Infect Dis 1989;11:349–351.

26 Rosenthal SR. Vaccination against tuberculosis by BCG (bacillus of Calmette and Guerin). Am Pract 1948;2:462–466.

27 Park WH, Kereszturi C, Mishulow L. Effect of vaccination with BCG on children from tuberculous families. JAMA 1933;101: 1619–1626.

28 Frappier A, Guy R. The use of BCG. Can Med Assoc J 1992;146:529–535.

29 Palmer CE. BCG vaccination and tuberculin allergy. Lancet 1952;1:935–940.

30 Rosenthal SR, Blahd M, Leslie EI. Ten years' experience with BCG. J Pediatr 1945; 26:470–480.

31 Aronson JD. Protective vaccination against tuberculosis with special reference to BCG vaccination. Am Rev Tuberculosis Pulm Dis 1948;58:255–281.

32 BCG vaccination and tuberculin testing. Tubercle 1969;50:203–204. (Editorial).

33 BCG and the tuberculin test. Lancet 1969; 1:192–193. (Editorial).

34 Comstock GW. Identification of an effective vaccine against tuberculosis. Am Rev Respir Dis 1988;138:479–480.

35 **Guld J, Waaler H, Sundaresan TK, Kaufmann PC, ten Dam HG.** The duration of BCG-induced tuberculin sensitivity in children and its irrelevance for revaccination. Bull Wld Hlth Org 1968;39:829–836.

36 **Olakowski T, Mardon K.** The restorative influence of repeated tuberculin testing on tuberculin sensitivity in BCG-vaccinated schoolchildren. Bull World Health Organ 1971;45:649–655.

37 **Sarber RW, Hemans MJ.** The significance of the tuberculin skin reaction in antituberculous vaccine assay. Am Rev Tuberculosis Pulm Dis 1952;66:351–356.

38 **Gheorghiu M, Lagrange PH.** Viability, heat stability and immunogenicity of four BCG vaccines prepared from four different BCG strains. Ann Immunol (Inst Pasteur) 1983;134C:125–147.

39 **Orme IM, Collins FM.** Adoptive protection of the Mycobacterium tuberculosis-infected lung. Cell Immunol 1984;84:113–120.

40 **Shaw LW.** Field studies on immunization against tuberculosis. I. Tuberculin allergy following BCG vaccination of school children in Muscogee County, Georgia. Public Health Rep 1951;66:1415–1426.

41 **Hewell B, McClellan M.** Tuberculin allergy after BCG vaccination. Am Rev Tuberc 1954;70:1064–1082.

42 **Menzies R, Vissandjee B.** Effect of Bacille Calmette-Guerin vaccination on tuberculin reactivity. Am Rev Respir Dis 1992;145:621–625.

43 **Vallishayee RS, Shashidhara AN, Bunch-Christensen K, Guld J.** Tuberculin sensitivity and skin lesions in children after vaccination with 11 different BCG strains. Bull World Health Organ 1974;51:489–494.

44 **Kroger L, Katila ML, Korppi M, Brabder E, Pietikainen M.** Rapid decrease in tuberculin skin test reactivity at preschool age after newborn vaccination. Acta Paediatr 1992;81:678–681.

45 **Joncas JH, Robitaille R, Gauthier T.** Interpretation of the PPD skin test in BCG-vaccinated children. Can Med Assoc J 1975;113:127–128.

46 **Horwitz O, Bunch-Christensen K.** Correlation between tuberculin sensitivity after 2 months and 5 years among BCG vaccinated subjects. Bull World Health Organ 1972;47:49–58.

47 **Young TK, Merdad S.** Determinants of tuberculin sensitivity in a child population covered by mass BCG vaccination. Tubercle Lung Dis 1992;73:94–100.

48 **Menzies R, Vissandjee B, Amyot D.** Factors associated with tuberculin reactivity among the foreign-born in Montreal. Am Rev Respir Dis 1992;146:752–756.

49 **Comstock GW, Edwards LB, Nabangxang H.** Tuberculin sensitivity eight to fifteen years after BCG vaccination. Am Rev Respir Dis 1971;103:572–575.

50 **Aronson JD, Parr EI, Saylor RM.** The specificity and sensitivity of the tuberculin reaction following vaccination with BCG. Am J Hyg 1941;33:42–49.

51 **Snider DE.** Bacille Calmette-Guerin vaccination and tuberculin skin tests. JAMA 1985;253:3438–3439.

52 **Tuberculosis Prevention Trial, Madras.** Trial of BCG vaccines in south India for tuberculosis prevention. Indian J Med Res 1980;72(suppl):1–74.

53 **Osborn TW.** Changes in BCG strains. Tubercle 1983;64:1–13.

54 **Formukong NG, Dale JW, Osborn TW, Grange JM.** Use of gene probes based on the insertion sequence IS986 to differentiate between BCG vaccines strains. J Appl Bacteriol 1992;72:126–133.

54b **Hermans PWM, van Soolinger D, Dale JW, et al.** Insertion element IS986 from *Mycobacterium tuberculosis*: a useful tool for diagnosis and epidemiology of Tuberculosis. J Clin Microbiol 1990;28:2051–2058.

55 **Wiegeshaug EH, Harding G, McMurray D, et al.** A co-operative evaluation of test systems used to assay tuberculosis vaccines. Bull World Health Organ 1971;45:543–550.

56 **Dubos R, Pierce CH.** Differential characteristics in vitro and in vivo of several substrains of BCG. I–IV. Am Rev Tuberculosis Pulm Dis 1956;74:655–717.

57 **Bunch-Christensen K.** Evaluation of BCG vaccines in children: the effect of strain and dose. J Biol Stand 1977;5:159–164.

58 **Wiegeshaus E, Balsubramanian V, Smith DW.** Immunity to tuberculosis from the perspective of pathogenesis. Infect Immun 1989;57:3671–3676.

59 **Crowle AJ.** Immunization against tuberculosis: what kind of vaccine? Infect Immun 1988;56:2769–2773.

60 **Mustafa AS, Kvalheim G, Degre M, Godal T.** *Mycobacterium bovis* BCG-induced human T cell clones from BCG-vaccinated healthy subjects: antigen specificity and

lymphokine production. Infect Immun 1986;53:491–497.

61 Hart PD, Sutherland I. BCG and vole bacillus vaccines in the prevention of tuberculosis in adolescence and early adult life. Br Med J 1977;2:293–295.

62 **Tuberculosis Prevention Trial.** Trial of BCG vaccines in south India for tuberculosis prevention: first report. Bull World Health Organ 1979;57:819–827.

63 **Citron KM.** BCG vaccination against tuberculosis: international perspectives. Br Med J 1993;306:222–223.

64 World Health Organization. Expanded Programme on Immunization Update. Global situation: immunization coverage. WHO, Geneva, Switzerland. November 1993.

65 Global Programme on AIDS and Expanded Programme on Immunization. Joint WHO/UNICEF statement on early immunization for HIV-infected children. Wkly Epidemiol Rec 1989;64:48–49.

66 **Bast RC Jr, Zbar B, Borsos T, Rapp HJ.** BCG and cancer. N Engl J Med 1974; 290:1413–1418;1458–1468.

67 **Morales A, Eidinger D, Bruice AW.** Intracavitary bacillus Calmette-Guerin in the treatment of superficial bladder tumors. J Urol 1976;116:180–183.

68 **Lowe J, Iles PB, Shore DF, Langman MJS, Baldwin RW.** Intrapleural BCG in operable lung cancer. Lancet 1980;1:11–13.

69 **Garner FB, et al.** Aerosol BCG treatment of metastatic carcinoma in the lung. Cancer 1975;35:1088–1094.

70 **Lamm DL, Blumenstain BA, Crawford ED, et al.** A randomized trial of intravesical doxorubicin and immunotherapy with bacille Calmette-Guerin for transitional cell carcinoma of the bladder. N Engl J Med 1991;325:1205–1209.

71 **Marans HY, Bekirov HM.** Granulomatous hepatitis following intravesical bacillus Calmette-Guerin therapy for bladder carcinoma. J Urol 1987;137:111–112.

72 **Lamm DL, Stogdill VD, Stogdill BJ, Crispen JG.** Complications of bacillus Calmette-Guerin immunotherapy in 1,278 patients with bladder cancer. J Urol 1986; 135:272–274.

73 **McParland C, Cotton DJ, Gowda KS, Hoeppner VH, Martin WT, Weckworth PF.** Miliary *Mycobacterium bovis* induced by intravesical bacille Calmette-Guerin immunotherapy. Am Rev Respir Dis 1992;146: 1330–1333.

74 **Sparks FC, Silverstein MJ, Hunt JS, Haskell CM, Pilch YH, Morton DL.** Complications of BCG immunotherapy in patients with cancer. N Engl J Med 1973;289: 827–830.

75 **Aungst CW, Sakal JE, Jager BV.** Complications of BCG vaccination in neoplastic disease. Ann Intern Med 1975;82:666–669.

76 **Bansal SC, Sjogren HO.** Effects of BCG on various facets of the immune response against polyoma tumors in rats. Int J Cancer 1973;11:162–171.

77 **Comstock GW.** BCG vaccination and cancer. Tubercle 1991;72:304–305.

78 **Snider DE, Comstock GW, Martinez I, Caras GJ.** Efficacy of BCG vaccination in prevention of cancer: an update. J Natl Cancer Inst 1978;60:785–788.

79 **Skegg DEG.** BCG vaccination and the incidence of lymphomas and leukaemia. Int J Cancer 1978;21:18–21.

80 **Kendrick MA, Comstock GW.** BCG vaccination and the subsequent development of cancer in humans. J Natl Cancer Inst 1981; 66:431–437.

81 Centers for Disease Control. Use of BCG vaccines in the control of tuberculosis: a joint statement by the ACIP and the Advisory Committee for the Elimination of Tuberculosis. MMWR 1988;37:663–664;669–675.

82 **Ferguson RG.** BCG vaccination in hospitals and sanatoria of Saskatchewan. Am Rev Tuberc 1946;54:325–339.

83 **Rosenthal SR, Afremow ML, Nikurs L, et al.** BCG vaccination and tuberculosis in students of nursing. Am J Nurs 1963;63:88–93.

84 **Nettleman MD.** Use of BCG vaccine in shelters for the homeless. A decision analysis. Chest 1993;103:1087–1090.

85 **Hamburg MA.** The challenge of controlling tuberculosis in New York City. NY State J Med 1992;92:291–293.

86 **Brudney K, Dobkin J.** Resurgent tuberculosis in New York City. Human immunodeficiency virus, homelessness, and the decline of tuberculosis control programs. Am Rev Respir Dis 1991;144:745–749.

87 **Coetzee AM, Berjak J.** BCG in the prevention of tuberculosis in an adult population. Proc Mine Med Officers' Assoc 1968;48:41–53.

88 **Bloom BR, Jacobs WR.** New strategies for leprosy and tuberculosis and the development of bacillus Calmette-Guerin into a

multivaccine vehicle. Ann NY Acad Sci 1989;596:155–173.

89 **Collins FM.** Antituberculous immunity: new solutions to an old problem. Rev Infect Dis 1991;13:940–950.

90 **Grange JM.** Immunotherapy of tuberculosis. Tubercle 1990;71:237–239.

91 **Stanford JL, Rook GA, Bahr GM, et al.** *Mycobacterium vaccae* in immunoprophylaxis and immunotherapy of leprosy and tuberculosis. Vaccine 1990;8:525–530.

92 **Stanford JL, Grange JM.** New concepts for the control of tuberculosis in the twenty-first century. J R Coll Physicians Lond 1993;27:218–223.

93 **Stanford JL, Bahr GM, Rook GAW, et al.** Immunotherapy with *Mycobacterium vaccae* as an adjunct to chemotherapy in the treatment of pulmonary tuberculosis. Tubercle 1990;71:87–93.

94 **Pal PG, Horwitz MA.** Immunization with extracellular proteins of *Mycobacterium tuberculosis* induces cell-mediated immune responses and substantial protective immunity in a guinea pig model of pulmonary tuberculosis. Infect Immun 1992;60:4781–4792.

Immunization in Adults in the 1990s

PIERCE GARDNER
THEODORE EICKHOFF

The rapidly changing health care system in the United States promises a greater focus on preventive health measures, including immunizations. The Childhood Immunization Initiative will approximately double the funding to support immunization of children and will consolidate and secure the gains that have brought most diseases targeted by childhood immunizations to record lows in 1993 and 1994. Unfortunately, adult immunization has not been part of the new national priorities, even though the overwhelming predominance of deaths from vaccine-preventable disease is among adults (1). About 50,000 to 70,000 adults die each year from pneumococcal infection, influenza, and hepatitis B (Table 12.1) (2–4), whereas there are currently fewer than 500 deaths per year from diseases targeted by childhood immunizations. Even allowing for the fact that the protective efficacy of the pneumococcal and influenza vaccines is suboptimal, there is the potential to save over 30,000 lives annually through full implementation of the current immunization recommendations (1). The total annual number of deaths preventable by adult immunizations is similar to annual deaths from automobile accidents or acquired immunodeficiency syndrome (AIDS).

Factors contributing to our poor record of adult immunizations include weak traditions regarding immunization practices, lingering doubts of both health care providers and the public regarding the efficacy and safety of adult vaccines, complex recommendations often based on underlying conditions rather than age, liability concerns, complex record keeping, inadequate reimbursement, and poorly developed systems for immunizing adults both in the private and public sector.

The schedule and general indications for the vaccines used in adults in the United States are presented in Table 12.2. Our discussion will emphasize the vaccines in most common use, new vaccines and areas of controversy or changing recommendations.

Table 12.1.   Estimated Effect of Full Use of Vaccines Currently Recommended for Adults

Disease	Estimated Annual Deaths (no.)	Estimated Vaccine Efficacy* (%)	Current Vaccine Utilization† (%)	Additional Preventable Deaths/Yr‡ (no.)
Influenza	20,000§	70	41	8,260
Pneumococcal infection	40,000	60	20	19,200
Hepatitis B	5,000	90	10‖	4,050
Tetanus-diphtheria	<25	99	40¶	<15
Measles, mumps, and rubella	<30	95	Variable	<30
Travelers' diseases (cholera, typhoid, Japanese encephalitis, yellow fever, poliomyelitis, and rabies)	<10	—	—	<10

* Indicates efficacy in immunocompetent adults. Among elderly and immunocompromised patients, estimated efficacy may be lower.
† The percentage of targeted groups who have been immunized according to current recommendations. Rates vary among different targeted groups. Data for influenza and pneumococcal vaccines were obtained from the 1991 National Health Interview Survey and apply to persons ≥65 years of age.
‡ Calculated as follows: (potential additional vaccine utilization) × (estimated vaccine efficacy) × (estimated annual deaths).
§ Variable (range, 0 to 40,000).
‖ Highly variable (range, 1% to 60%) among different targeted groups.
¶ This estimate is based on seroprevalence data.
SOURCE: Adapted from Gardner P, Schaffner W. Immunization of adults. N Engl J Med 1993; 328:1252–1258.

UNIVERSAL VACCINES FOR ADULTS

Pneumococcal Vaccine

Pneumococcal vaccine was introduced in the United States in 1977. Originally a 14-valent product containing 50 µg each of capsular polysaccharide from the 14 most common capsular types of pneumococci causing bacteremia in the United States, the formulation was changed in 1983 to 25 µg each of 23 capsular polysaccharides, again representing the most common bacteremia types in the country. The vaccine is pure polysaccharide; hence, it is a pure B-cell immunogen. That feature of pneumococcal vaccine is important in understanding immunization policy in this country. Repeated doses do not result in an anamnestic response, but antibody levels usually approximate the same level as that developed after the initial dose (5).

The history of pneumococcal vaccine in the last 25 years is a case study in vaccine evaluation and experimental methodology. Initial field trials conducted in South African gold miners were randomized and placebo controlled; a high level of efficacy was found (6). Two randomized placebo-controlled trials were carried out in the United States to study the effect of the vaccine in elderly or institutionalized populations (7,8). Neither trial showed efficacy, owing in large part to a very low incidence of pneumococcal disease in the control population. Thus, the vaccine was licensed based solely on the South Africa gold miner data. Initial reaction in the United States was, perhaps understandably, apathetic. Recommendations from policy-making bodies such as the Advisory Committee in Immunization Practices were unenthusiastic as well. It was not surprising that the vaccine was very poorly used.

Austrian pointed out the unique problems in evaluating this vaccine (9), which is actually 23 vaccines in one product. If each of the 23 vaccines were 99% effective individually, and if the 1% failure rate of each component were considered to represent a failure of the entire 23-valent product, then the maximum theoretical efficacy of the product would be 0.99^{23}, or 79%. Similarly, if each component were 95% effective, then the efficacy of the entire 23-valent product would be only 31%! Although the assumptions used in this model do not fit the known epidemiology of pneumococcal infection, it cannot be entirely dismissed as a statistical game; rather, it underscores the complexities in evaluating this vaccine. Furthermore, it is known that the host response to individual capsular polysaccharides is variable, and each type has its own failure rate. Several of the capsular types are rather poor immunogens (10).

During the past decade, several additional studies using different methodologies have resulted in substantial documentation of efficacy. There have been a number of case-control studies (11–14), the most comprehensive of which (11) involved over 1000 patients with serious pneumococcal infection, and an equal number of controls. The Centers for Disease Control and Prevention (CDC) have done several studies of pneumococcal vaccine efficacy using an innovative technique referred to as the indirect cohort method, in which the proportion of infections caused by serotypes included in the vaccine among vaccinated persons is compared to that in unvaccinated persons (15–17). These studies all demonstrate that the vaccine is 60 to 70% effective in healthy elderly, about 50% effective in those with underlying disease not associated with marked immunosuppression, but only about 20% effective in those with significant immunosuppression as a result of underlying disease. Thus, the boundaries of efficacy of this vaccine have been much more clearly delineated.

It is important to appreciate the scope of the pneumococcal disease burden in this country. An estimated 500,000 cases of pneumonia, 50,000 cases of sepsis, 3000 cases of meningitis, and 40,000 deaths each year are attributed to *Streptococcus pneumoniae* (4). Age and race are important determinants of risk (18): rates of pneumococcal disease in adults begin to increase significantly in the fifth decade of life (beginning at age 40); African Americans and Native Americans are at higher risk for pneumococcal disease than whites; and about 70% of adults with pneumococcal bacteremia have some identifiable risk factor.

Table 12.2. Vaccines Used in Adults*

Vaccine	Type	Schedule[†]	Indications[‡]	Precautions and Contraindications[§]	Side Effects[§]
Toxoids					
Tetanus-diphtheria	Adsorbed toxoids	Primary: 2 doses (0.5 mL) IM, 1–2 mo apart; third dose 6–12 mo later Booster: q10y	For all adults	First trimester of pregnancy; hypersensitivity or neurologic reaction to previous doses; severe local reaction	Local reactions; occasional fever; systemic symptoms; Arthus-like reaction in persons with multiple previous boosters; rare systemic allergy
Inactivated bacteria vaccines					
Cholera	Phenol-killed *Vibrio cholerae* (4 × 10⁹/mL)	Primary: 0.5 mL IM or SQ, or 0.2 mL intradermally, 2 doses 1 wk to 1 mo apart at least 6 d before travel Booster: 0.5 mL IM or SQ or 0.2 mL intradermally q6mo	No longer required under international health regulations	Safety in pregnancy unknown; previous severe local or systemic reaction	Local reaction of pain, erythema, and induration lasting 1–2 d; occasional fever, malaise
Haemophilus influenzae type B	Polysaccharide conjugated to diphtheria toxoid	Primary: 1 dose (0.5 mL) IM Booster: not recommended	For patients with splenic dysfunction, other at-risk conditions	Safety in pregnancy unknown	Mild local reactions in approximately 10% of patients
Pneumococcal polysaccharide	23 serotypes	Primary: 1 dose (0.5 mL) or SQ or IM Booster: not recommended for most patients	For persons at increased risk of pneumococcal disease and its complications, healthy adults 65 or older	Safety in pregnancy unknown	Erythema and pain at injection site in approximately 50% of patients; systemic reaction in less than 1% of patients; Arthus-like reaction with booster doses

Meningococcal polysaccharide	Tetravalent (A, C, Y, W 135)	Primary: 1 dose (0.5 mL) SQ Booster: unknown	Travel to areas with epidemic meningococcal disease	Safety in pregnancy unknown	Infrequent, mild local reactions
Typhoid	Phenol- and heat-killed *Salmonella typhi*	Primary: 2 doses (0.5 mL) SQ, given 4 or more wk apart Booster: 0.5 mL SQ or 0.1 mL intradermally, q3y	Risk of exposure to typhoid fever	Previous severe local or systemic reaction	Local reaction of pain, swelling and induration lasting 1–2 d; systemic reactions may occur
	Vi capsular polysaccharide (Vi CPS)	Primary: 1 dose (0.5 mL) IM Booster: 0.5 mL IM q2y	Same	Safety in pregnancy unknown	Mild local reactions
Attenuated, live bacteria vaccines					
Typhoid	—	Primary: 4 oral doses Reimmunize q5y	Risk of exposure to typhoid fever	Immunocompromised host ¶; enteric illness; concurrent antimicrobial treatment	Infrequent mild nausea
Bacille Calmette-Guérin	—	Primary: 1 dose intradermally or SQ Booster: none	Debatable benefits for selected adult groups	Immunocompromised host¶	Local progression; disseminated infection
Attenuated live virus vaccines					
Measles	—	Primary: 2 doses SQ Booster: none	For adults born after 1956 without measles (diagnosed by a physician or immunologic test) or live-virus immunization; for revaccination of persons given killed measles vaccine (1963–1967)	Pregnancy; immunocompromised host¶: history of anaphylaxis to eggs or neomycin	Temperature of ≥39.4°C, 5–21 d after vaccination in 5 to 15%; transient rash in 5%; local reaction in 4 to 55% of persons previously immunized with killed vaccine (1963–1967)

Table 12.2. *Continued*

Vaccine	Type	Schedule†	Indications‡	Precautions and Contraindications§	Side Effects§
Mumps	—	Primary: 1 dose SQ Booster: none	For susceptible adults	Pregnancy; immunocompromised host¶; history of anaphylaxis in response to eggs or neomycin	Mild allergic reactions uncommon; rare parotitis
Attenuated live virus vaccines					
Oral polio	Trivalent	1 Oral dose	One-time booster for previously immunized persons; complete the series in partially immunized adults; alternative to inactivated polio vaccine when there is <1 mo before travel exposure; not used for primary immunization in persons 18y or older	Immunocompromised host¶ or immunocompromised contacts of recipients	Rare paralysis
Rubella	—	Primary: 1 dose subcutaneously Booster: none	For adults, particularly women of childbearing age, without documented illness or live vaccine on or after first birthday	Pregnancy; immunocompromised host¶; history of anaphylaxis in response to neomycin	Joint pains, transient arthralgias in up to 40%, beginning 3–25 d after vaccination, persisting 1–11 d; frank arthritis in <2%
Yellow fever	—	Primary: 1 dose (0.5 mL) SQ, 10d to 10y before travel Booster: q10y	As required by individual countries	Avoid in pregnant women, unless engaged in high-risk travel; immunocompromised host¶; hypersensitivity to eggs	Mild headache, myalgia, fever, 5–10 d after vaccination in 2–5%; rare immediate hypersensitivity

Inactivated virus vaccines

Hepatitis B	Recombinant hepatitis B surface antigen	Primary: 2 doses IM in deltoid, 1 mo apart; third dose 5 mo after second. Alternate schedule for Engerix-B: 4 dose series at 0, 1, 2 and 12 mo Booster: not routinely recommended	For health care workers in contact with blood; persons residing for > 6 mo in areas of high endemicity of hepatitis B surface antigen; others at risk	Safety to fetus unknown; pregnancy not a contraindication in high-risk persons	Mild local reaction in 10–20%; occasional systemic symptoms of fever, headache, fatigue, and nausea
Inactivated polio	Enhanced potency trivalent killed polio virus	Primary: 2 doses (0.5 mL) SQ, 4–8 wk apart; third dose 6–12 mo after second	Preferred for persons 18 y or older for primary immunization; one-time booster dose for travelers	Safety in pregnancy unknown; anaphylactic reactions to streptomycin or neomycin	No serious side effects
Influenza	Inactivated whole and split virus	Annual vaccination with current vaccine	For adults with high-risk conditions; healthy persons more than 65 y old; medical care personnel	First trimester of pregnancy a relative contraindication; anaphylaxis in response to eggs	Mild local reaction in less than one third; occasional systemic reaction of malaise, myalgia, beginning 6–12 h after vaccination and lasting 1–2 d; rare allergic reaction
Japanese B encephalitis	—	Primary: 3 doses (1.0 mL) SQ on days 0, 7, and 30 or at weekly intervals Booster: consider 1.0 mL q1–3y	Travel to areas of risk with rural exposure or prolonged residence	Pregnancy; allergy to mice or rodents; immunocompromised host¶	Local mild reaction lasting 1–3 d

Table 12.2. *Continued*

Vaccine	Type	Schedule[†]	Indications[‡]	Precautions and Contraindications[§]	Side Effects[§]
Rabies (human diploid cell vaccine)	—	Preexposure: 1 mL IM in deltoid, on days 0, 7, and 28 or 0.1 mL intradermally, on days 0, 7, and 21 to 28 Booster: q2h or when antibody titer falls below acceptable level	Travel for > 1 mo to areas where rabies is a constant threat	Allergy to previous doses; may be given in pregnancy if indicated; intradermal route should be completed 30 d or more before travel; intradermal route should not be used with concurrent chloroquine administration	Local reaction in approximately 25%; mild systemic reactions of headache, nausea, aches, dizziness in approximately 20%; rare neurologic illness; occasional immune reactions with booster doses occurring 2–21 d after vaccination

*Data are from the Centers for Disease Control and Prevention and the American College of Physicians Task Force on Adult Immunization.

†Manufacturers' full prescribing information should be consulted. Doses given are for adults; doses for children may vary.

‡See the text for details.

§Only major precautions, contraindications, and side effects are listed.

¶Persons who are immunocompromised because of immunodeficiency diseases, leukemia, lymphoma, generalized cancer, or AIDS, or who are receiving immunosuppressive therapy with corticosteroids, alkylating agents, antimetabolites, or radiation.

SOURCES: Update on adult immunization: recommendations of the Immunization Practices Advisory Committee (ACIP). MMWR 1991;40(RR-12). American College of Physicians Task Force on Adult Immunization, Infectious Diseases Society of America. Guide for adult immunization, 3rd ed. Philadelphia: American College of Physicians, 1994.

Common risk factors include chronic cardiac and pulmonary disease, hepatic and renal failure, alcoholism, anatomic and functional asplenia, multiple myeloma, and Hodgkin's disease. The case–fatality rate of bacteremic pneumococcal pneumonia is 15 to 25%; among patients with underlying conditions it is 30% or more, and in the elderly mortality may be 60% or more.

Any discussion of pneumococcal vaccine has been made more urgent in recent years by the steady increase in penicillin resistance among pneumococci throughout the world. In the United States, although the overall rate of relative resistance to penicillin is only about 12%, there are geographical areas in which such resistance is 30 to 40% (19). Resistance to many drug classes is often present, so that multiple drug resistant (MDR) pneumococci are a real, rather than a theoretical, threat. Thus, it is even more important to ensure that persons at high risk of pneumococcal infection are adequately immunized. Recent estimates, however, continue to indicate that only about 20% of those for whom the vaccine is recommended actually receive it (20).

The optimal age at which to administer pneumococcal vaccine is debatable. For healthy persons, it has been recommended at age 65. This recommendation was based on the traditional age of entering the definition of "elderly" rather than on any substantive data. It is clearly established that antibody levels decay gradually after immunization, and it is also clear that the height of the antibody response declines with advancing age (5,14). Thus, it seems reasonable to immunize healthy adults at an earlier age, perhaps 50 to 60 years, at a time when the antibody response would be expected to be more vigorous than at age 65. Unfortunately, no data directly support that suggestion; it is not known whether most persons would be better protected at age 75 if immunization occurred 20 years earlier as compared to 10 years earlier.

The third edition of the *Guide for Adult Immunization* (4), sponsored by the American College of Physicians and the Infectious Diseases Society of America, has strongly recommended that age 50 be used as a convenient marker to review all preventive health measures, including immunization. If risk factors are found that suggest the need for pneumococcal vaccine, it should be given without further delay. Between 30 and 40% of the population aged 50 to 65 years have high-risk conditions for which pneumococcal vaccine is recommended. The duration of protective efficacy of pneumococcal vaccine is not clearly established although in one study 80% of immunocompetent individuals were protected for 9 or more year (17). Therefore, revaccination is not routinely recommended. However, for certain subgroups reimmunization is recommended. These include: 1) individuals who receive the 14-valent vaccine if they are at highest risk of serious or fatal pneumococcal infection (e.g., patients with surgical or functional asplenia); 2) patients with conditions resulting in rapid decreases in antibody levels (e.g., nephrotic syndrome or renal failure) provided six years have elapsed since receiving the first dose of pneumococcal vaccine; and 3) individuals with risk factors requiring pneumococcal immunization before age 65 with reimmunization strongly recommended at age 65 if more than 6 years have elapsed since the first dose of pneumococcal vaccine (4).

The long-term solution to these uncertainties is a "second-generation" pneumococcal vaccine. Conversion of *Haemophilus influenzae*, type B polysaccharide vaccine from a pure B-cell vaccine to a T-cell vaccine by linking the polysaccharide to a protein carrier resulted in a dramatic increase in immunogenicity (21). Evidence indicates that this can be done with pneumococcal polysaccharides as well (22). Numerous technical challenges must be overcome, and the first such product will likely be for pediatric use, with polysaccharides from the most common otitis media capsular types. Within a decade, however, it is reasonable to anticipate a substantially more immunogenic conjugated vaccine for use in adults.

Influenza Vaccine

Influenza vaccines were first used in the United States in 1943 and 1944, during World War II; the initial evaluations were conducted in the U.S. Armed Forces (23). Further research and development of influenza vaccines was carried out in very large part in military populations, with support from the Department of Defense, under the sponsorship of the Commission on Influenza of the Armed Forces Epidemiological Board (24). It was not until after the Asian influenza pandemic of 1957–1958 and the beginnings of the Advisory Committee on Immunization Practices at CDC in the 1960s that recommendations were made to use influenza vaccine in high-risk civilian populations on a regular basis.

Since the reappearance of H1N1 influenza virus in 1976 ("Russian flu"), influenza vaccines have been trivalent preparations, containing 15 μg each of hemagglutinin antigen from an H3N2 strain, an H1N1 strain, and an influenza B strain. Because of the continuing antigenic drifting of influenza viruses, particularly influenza A viruses, the vaccine strains are updated annually, based on the antigenic nature and epidemiologic behavior of influenza strains circulating throughout the world during the preceding year. Not all vaccine strains are changed each year, but it is a rare circumstance in which not even one strain is changed annually to a more current isolate. For the last decade, the degree of antigenic match between the circulating wild strain and the vaccine strain has been remarkably close.

Influenza A (H3N2) strains have generally caused the most severe outbreaks, typically resulting in high levels of school and workplace absenteeism, and excess mortality; the latter is, of course, concentrated in the elderly and chronically ill. Since its reappearance in 1976, influenza A (H1N1) has been typically somewhat less severe, with relative sparing of elderly populations because that age group was exposed to H1N1 strains when they were children. Thus, there is typically little or no excess mortality associated with H1N1 outbreaks. Influenza B outbreaks may be prolonged and sometimes severe, but possibly because there is less antigenic drift in influenza B viruses, disease tends to be milder, and with less dramatic excess mortality.

The best predictor of efficacy of influenza vaccine is the postvaccination level of serum hemagglutination inhibition (HI) antibody (25). A serum HI antibody titter of 1:32 or 1:40 or greater correlates very well with protection against clinical disease, as determined in field trials. In healthy young adult military populations, influenza vaccines have proven 75 to 85% effective in preventing infection when there is a good match between the vaccine strain and the circulating strain (26). Efficacy rates decline when variant strains appear and cause unexpected epidemics (27). Protective efficacy rates decline in the elderly, but among vaccine recipients who contract influenza, the disease may be less severe. In nursing home residents, for example, efficacy in preventing infection may be only 25 to 40%, but the vaccine is more effective, 50 to 80%, in preventing pneumonia, hospitalization, and death (28–30).

It is a sad commentary on our collective failings in adult immunization to note that despite the availability of influenza vaccine, seven epidemics in the United States between 1977 and 1988 resulted in more than 10,000 excess deaths, and over 40,000 excess deaths occurred in two of these outbreaks (31)! Current estimates are that each year approximately 30 to 40% of noninstitutionalized elderly and approximately 10% of younger high-risk persons receive influenza vaccine each year (32). Utilization rates in institutionalized elderly are better than those not institutionalized, probably a result of institution-wide immunization policies or campaigns. Although there is evidence that influenza vaccination rates in the United States have been gradually improving in recent years, we are still failing to immunize the majority of the targeted individuals, and thus missing a major preventive health opportunity.

The populations recommended to receive influenza vaccine each year are well known and widely available each year (31) and need not be reproduced in detail here. Very simply, the elderly and those of any age with significant underlying disease, *and the health care personnel* who provide care to them are the recommended "targets" for influenza vaccine each year.

The safety of influenza vaccines has not been an issue in recent years. One of the reasons influenza vaccines were not widely accepted during the 1960s was that the vaccines in those years were quite reactive. Great strides were made in purifying the product during the 1960s and 1970s, and vaccines for the last 20 years have been relatively free of reactions. Transient local soreness at the injection site is common, of course, and may be seen in up to one-third of vaccinees. Systemic reactions may be seen in vaccinees who have had little or no exposure to the antigens contained in the vaccine; such reactions usually consist of fever, myalgia, and malaise that last for one to two days after administration of vaccine. Because the vaccine virus is grown in eggs, and there are trace residual amounts of egg protein in the vaccine, it is contraindicated in those rare individuals who have true anaphylactic hypersensitivity to eggs.

The swine influenza immunization campaign in 1976 was terminated, perhaps fortuitously, by recognition of an association between use of that vaccine, containing swine influenza antigen, and the subsequent development of Guillain-Barré syndrome (33), which occurred at a rate of approximately

1/100,000 vaccinees. Since 1976, despite careful surveillance, there has been no clear association of influenza vaccination with subsequent Guillain-Barré syndrome (GBS) (31, 34). The specific properties of the swine influenza antigen that may have resulted in this association have never been identified.

Two major challenges must be met before we can consider that the threat of influenza has been neutralized: first, we must develop better strategies to ensure that the vaccine reaches its target population each year; and second, there is a clear need for improved vaccines.

The recent decision by Congress that influenza vaccine should be reimbursable under Medicare is a major step in the direction of improved utilization, particularly if other insurers follow suit. Even this blessing, however, is mixed; reimbursement covers little more than the cost of the vaccine itself; balance billing for administration cost is prohibited.

In recent years a number of simple devices to solve simple logistic problems have been evaluated and found to be useful (35–38). These include telephone reminders to patients, postcard reminders, putting a nurse or nurse-practitioner in charge of giving influenza vaccine to all eligible patients in a practice, chart reminders, vaccinating all eligible patients in a given clinic each fall, and the like. Some practices have developed an annual goal, such as the immunization of at least 80% of eligible patients in the practice each year (37). Financial incentives to achieve that goal may be incorporated as well. Each of these devices may be helpful and has enabled some practices to achieve high levels, 80% or more, of immunization of eligible patients.

Prospects for improved vaccines are promising, as well. Much work has been done on attenuated cold-adapted influenza vaccines that may be given by nasal instillation (39). It would be advantageous, of course, if the vaccine could be given topically rather than parenterally. Although a number of field trials have shown high levels of efficacy with monovalent vaccines, it has not yet proven possible to develop a trivalent product that might need to be changed in composition periodically. Furthermore, the live attenuated vaccine proved no better than inactivated vaccine in an immunogenicity study in an elderly population (40). Interestingly, both vaccines together proved to be more immunogenic in that population than either vaccine alone. This approach to preventing influenza in the elderly should be evaluated more fully.

There have been many efforts in the past to incorporate adjuvants into the vaccine to increase the immune response and to increase the duration of protection (39). Most of these studies were carried out in military populations during the 1950s and 1960s, but they were eventually abandoned because of concerns about possible long-term adverse effects and the fact that aqueous vaccines were steadily improving. The suboptimal efficacy of influenza vaccine in the elderly and improved understanding of immune modulators has stimulated a renewed interest in vaccine adjuvants. Liposome-based adjuvants are currently under study, and there is further interest in evaluating mediators such as interleukin-2 as an influenza vaccine adjuvant. It is entirely reasonable to expect improved influenza vaccines before the end of this decade.

Hepatitis B Vaccine

Hepatitis B is a disease of major global importance. It is estimated that there are over 300 million chronic carriers of hepatitis B surface antigen (HBsAg) in the world, and about one million of them live in the United States. The CDC have estimated that the lifetime risk of hepatitis B in this country is about 5%, but in certain high-risk populations it is close to 100%. Approximately 300,000 cases occur each year, most of them in young adults; from 6 to 10% of these new cases result in chronic carriage of HBsAg (41).

The first hepatitis B vaccine was introduced by Merck, Sharpe and Dohme in 1982, using HBsAg derived from the plasma of antigen-positive donors and then subjected to an extensive purification and inactivation process. The first recombinant DNA vaccine, also produced by Merck, was introduced in 1986, derived from yeast cells into which a plasmid coding for the production of HBsAg had been inserted. A second yeast-derived product was introduced by SmithKline Beecham in 1989. The original plasma-derived vaccine is no longer produced in the United States.

The three-dose intramuscular immunization series results in protective levels of antibody (anti-HBs) in over 90% of healthy young adults (42). Serum anti-HBs levels of 10 mIU/mL or greater are generally considered protective. The initial efficacy trials were carried out with the plasma-derived product in homosexual young men; the vaccine was shown to be close to 100% effective in vaccinees who developed antibody, about 95% of the study group (43). In more recent years, however, it has become apparent that seroconversion rates are lowered by advancing age, male sex as compared to female, obesity, smoking, and by a number of underlying diseases including renal failure, chronic liver disease, and diabetes mellitus (44). Interestingly, administration of vaccine in the buttocks results in a lower seroconversion rate than injection into the deltoid muscle presumably due to less reliable intramuscular delivery of the vaccine. Intradermal administration of hepatitis B vaccine appears to be less reliable in eliciting protective levels of antibody and is not recommended (4). If used, postvaccination tests for anti-HBs response should be performed.

The vaccine has proven to be exceptionally safe (45). Earlier concerns about the possible transmission of human immunodeficiency (HIV) by the plasma-derived vaccine proved to be wholly theoretical and not applicable at all to the recombinant yeast-derived vaccine. Transient soreness at the injection site is seen in 15 to 20% of vaccine recipients, but usually lasts no more than one to two days. Concerns have been expressed about a possible association with GBS, but its rate of occurrence of 0.5/100,000 following the first dose of vaccine is of only borderline significance (41).

Hepatitis B vaccination policy in the United States has changed dramatically since it was introduced. Initial recommendations for use were based on targeting high-risk groups, such as homosexual males, injecting drug abusers, and health care personnel. Not only did this policy of targeting risk groups fail to decrease the hepatitis B burden in the United States, but the number of new cases actually increased (46). During the 1980s, the number of target groups for hepatitis B vaccines gradually expanded, based on the prevalence of serologic markers of hepatitis B virus (HBV) infection in those groups. Thus, in addition to sexually active homosexual men, parenteral drug abusers, and health care personnel with frequent blood contact, the following population groups were also shown to be at increased risk, and therefore recommended to receive hepatitis B vaccine: household or sexual contacts of HBV carriers, patients in hemodialysis units, patients with hemophilia, heterosexuals with multiple partners, prisoners, clients in institutions for the developmentally disabled, and immigrants or refugees from areas of the world with high HBV endemicity, especially southeast Asia.

In the late 1980s, with recognition that perinatal transmission of HBV could be prevented by prompt treatment of infants born to HBsAg-positive mothers with hepatitis B immune globulin and hepatitis B vaccine, attention shifted to screening pregnant women believed to be at increased risk of HBsAg carriage. That policy, too, failed because screening guidelines failed to identify as many as half of carrier mothers (47). Thus, the current policy of universal immunization of infants arose from the gradual recognition that any lesser HBV immunization policy was, in fact, likely to fail.

Nevertheless, it will be 15 years or more before universally immunized infants reach the age at which hepatitis B transmission is likely to occur as a result of sexual activity or other risk behaviors. Thus, the hepatitis B burden in this country is not likely to decrease significantly for a decade or more, unless there is a major effort to reach populations already at risk, outlined previously, and adolescents before they become sexually active.

This vaccine is expensive, and this has been one of the important impediments to its widespread use. It is possible that a universal use policy might have been adopted much earlier if this product were less expensive. Nonetheless, it is one of the more cost effective of a number of common and well-accepted medical interventions (48).

In part owing to the expense of the vaccine, prevaccination screening has been an important issue. The cost savings to be achieved, if any, by prevaccination screening are directly related to the prevalence of HBV markers in the target population. Assuming a vaccine cost of $100 and a screening cost of $20 per person, it would be cost effective to screen only in populations with an expected prevalence of HBV markers of greater than 20%. Conversely, populations with a prevalence of HBV markers less than 20% should be immunized without screening. There is no adverse effect from immunizing a person already immune; the vaccine will likely cause a strong booster response, but nothing more.

In the original field trials, the seroconversion rate among the healthy young male subjects was about 95%. In clinical practice, the seroconversion rate has been somewhat lower, and in some instances, much lower (44). Some of the factors associated with a diminished response rate, such as increasing age, obesity, smoking, injection into the buttocks, and underlying disease have already been mentioned. In individuals over 60 years of age, for example, only 50% of vaccinees develop protective levels of antibody (44).

Recognition of nonresponders has led to recommendations for postvaccination antibody measurement, particularly among health care personnel exposed to blood or blood products, and to repeated courses of vaccination to try to stimulate development of protective levels of antibody. It is not necessary to carry out routine postvaccination testing in all vaccine recipients, but it is prudent to do so for persons whose subsequent clinical management depends on knowing their immune status (e.g., health care personnel who may have accidental needlestick injuries) or in persons above age 30 years or with other conditions associated with an impaired response to the vaccine.

Among nonresponders to the initial three-dose series, 20% will achieve protective levels of antibody after one additional dose; 30 to 50% will respond after a second three-dose series (44). Individuals who have failed to develop protective levels of anti-HBs after six doses of vaccine will probably benefit little if at all from further doses. Whether they remain susceptible to hepatitis B or not is not clear, but they should be considered nonimmune, and if exposed, given passive prophylaxis with hepatitis B immune globulin.

Antibody titers do decline with time and reach low levels in from 30 to 50% of vaccinees after seven years. The persistence of antibody is directly correlated with the level of peak antibody response following the last vaccine dose. Nonetheless, the duration of protection against clinical or viremic disease appears to be at least ten years thus far and may prove to be longer as additional time passes. For immunologically normal persons, therefore, there is currently no recommendation for booster doses, although such a recommendation might emerge in the future. In some health care institutions, however, personnel regularly exposed to blood or blood products have been given a booster dose of vaccine six to seven years after initial immunization. Whether this is prudent practice or simply immunologic overkill is not known.

Because HBsAg is a nonreplicating antigen, there is no contraindication to using this vaccine in pregnancy or in immunocompromised persons. Immunocompromised persons are less likely than immunologically normal persons to develop protective antibody titers following the recommended three-dose series. Additional doses may be given, as previously outlined. Similarly, antibody titers in immunocompromised patients may decline to less than protective levels more rapidly; periodic antibody tests at one- or two-year intervals should prove helpful in determining the need for booster doses.

Tetanus and Diphtheria Toxoids

The combined Td (5 Lf units tetanus toxoid, 2 Lf units diphtheria toxoid) is the preparation of choice in all adults. Although never subjected to formal efficacy trials, these toxoids are considered completely effective in preventing disease and all individuals should be actively immunized. However, because antibodies are induced against the exotoxins and not the bacteria themselves, Td does not prevent colonization with *Clostridium tetani* or *Corynebacterium diphtheriae*.

School immunization requirements have ensured that virtually all children in the United States have received at least three (and as many as five) doses of diphtheria-pertussis-tetanus (DPT) before entering first grade. This is probably the main reason for the dramatic decrease in tetanus incidence (now 45 to 65 cases annually) and diphtheria (five or fewer cases annually since 1980). Tetanus and diphtheria now occur primarily in adults who have never received a complete primary series of DPT or Td (49,50). For persons who have completed a primary series of DPT or Td, subsequent doses of tetanus or diphtheria toxoid reliably boost antibody levels even after intervals of 35 years or longer (51–53). However, seroprevalence studies in the United States indicate that among persons aged 60 years or greater at least 40% lack protective levels of tetanus antitoxin and an even larger percentage lack what are considered protective levels of diphtheria antitoxin (54,55). This is compelling evidence that approximately half of older adults are not in compliance with the current recommendations for primary immunizations or decennial Td boosters. Despite this serologic evidence of adult susceptibility, cases of tetanus or diphtheria are rare among adults who have at any previous time received a complete primary series, and in these rare cases the clinical illness is less severe (49,50).

These epidemiologic observations support an immunization strategy that emphasizes the importance of primary immunization and Td immunization (primary or booster) as part of wound management, but downgrades the importance of the current recommendation for routine Td boosters every ten years. The Task Force for Adult Immunization of the American College of Physicians and Infectious Diseases Society of America have recommended as an alternative strategy that a single Td booster be given at age 50 years to individuals who have completed the full pediatric schedule (including the Td booster at age 16) (4). The Task Force believes that a specific age recommendation may result in better compliance by physicians and patients and would improve immunization rates among older individuals. A cost–benefit analysis strongly supports the single midlife dose booster over the traditional decennial booster policy (56).

The single midlife booster policy would not affect the need to give additional Td boosters (or primary immunization) as part of wound management. It is not known how many Td shots are given as routine decennial boosters versus wound management. However, with almost 100 million emergency room visits in the United States annually, it is likely that most of the approximately 12 million doses of Td and 4 million doses of T (without d) that are used annually in the United States are for wound management. If this is the case, then a change from the poorly observed decennial booster policy to an age-based single midlife booster may actually improve the amount of Td administered routinely to adults.

The reemergence of diphtheria in eastern Europe has raised concerns regarding importations of diphtheria in the United States and the potential for subsequent spread among our poorly immunized adult population. Although 42 cases of diphtheria were reported during the 13-year period from 1980 to 1992, none was associated with secondary spread. Thus, it seems unlikely under foreseeable circumstances that there is a realistic possibility for a major diphtheria outbreak.

Measles, Mumps, and Rubella Vaccines

These three vaccines are usually given as a single combined product (MMR), and hence they will be treated as a group. Prototypes of these three live attenuated vaccines were introduced in the 1960s, and immunization policies have evolved gradually over the last three decades to a point at which all three are very similar, albeit certainly not identical. Each induces long-lasting (probably lifelong) immunity in 90 to 95% of susceptible recipients.

In the 1970s, the incidence of measles, mumps, and rubella decreased sharply in the United States as a result of highly effective immunization programs. In the 1980s, however, these childhood immunization efforts faltered, and as a result all three diseases experienced a resurgence during the 1980s. This was particularly dramatic in the case of measles, with an almost 20-fold increase in cases reported during the peak years of 1989 to 1991 (58). Rubella and mumps cases increased also but to a lesser extent. With intensive efforts to achieve universal immunization of children and young adults, measles, mumps, and rubella have all fallen again to record low levels in 1993 and 1994.

In the immunization era, adults have played a more significant role in the epidemiology of measles, mumps, and rubella (59,60). Over 20% of the measles cases reported in the United States in 1990 occurred in adults 20 years of age or older; 28% of deaths due to measles that year were in that age group. Surveillance data have demonstrated that the cases in adults have occurred primarily among students at college and among travelers to countries in which measles was occurring. Imported cases, both in U.S. citizens and foreign nationals coming from measles-endemic countries, have been an important source of outbreaks (61).

Epidemiologic studies indicate that cases of measles, mumps, or rubella that occur among MMR (or component) recipients usually represent individuals who did not respond to initial immunization (primary vaccine failures) and that waning immunity (secondary vaccine failure) is uncommon. Among the approximate 5% of individuals who do not seroconvert following a first MMR dose, the majority will respond to a second dose. This is the rationale for the current two-dose regimen for children, and for the recommendation that previously immunized young adults attending college or other institutions where crowding may occur and travelers to endemic areas for these diseases receive a second dose of MMR (61). Not all adults born before 1956 are immune and a small number of cases have occurred in such older adults particularly in hospital settings (62). Hence, in the event of a hospital outbreak, consideration should be given to vaccinating staff born before 1956, unless there is a clear history of physician-documented measles or receipt of two doses of vaccine.

Because the epidemiology of these three diseases is so similar, and because of the convenience of giving all three vaccines as the single MMR product, it has proven to be cost effective to use MMR as the preferred product even though there may be clear indication only for a single antigen, such as measles. The measles and mumps viruses are grown in chick embryo cell culture; rubella virus is grown in human diploid cells. The final product may contain minute amounts of egg protein and trace amounts of neomycin used in the virus production process; hence, the vaccine should not be given to those rare individuals who have anaphylactic hypersensitivity to either of those antigens. Alternatively, if benefit–risk considerations weigh heavily in favor of vaccine, desensitization protocols may be used (63).

Reactions to MMR are seen only in persons susceptible to one or more of the antigens in the vaccine and are usually part of the attenuated or subclinical infection that is the immunizing event. No adverse effects are associated with giving a second dose of MMR to persons who may already be immune to one, two, or all three viruses in the vaccine. However, for the rubella vaccine up to 40% of susceptible adult female vaccinees may experience arthralgia in small peripheral joints, usually about the wrist and hands (64). It is rarely severe, always less so than the natural disease, and usually lasts no more than one to two weeks. In a small number of susceptible adult women, however, such postrubella vaccine arthralgias have been reported to persist for 18 months or more (65).

In general, these live virus vaccines should not be given to individuals who are immunocompromised as a result of immunodeficiency disease or malignancy, or who are taking immunosuppressive drugs. There are, however, some important exceptions to that generalization. Susceptible persons with leukemia who are in remission, and who have not been given chemotherapy for three months, and asymptomatic HIV-infected persons may safely be given MMR. Measles may be particularly severe in immunocompromised patients, and each circumstance may need to be judged individually. This is the setting in which it may be advisable to consider using an individual antigen preparation rather than trivalent MMR.

Pregnancy is considered a contraindication of all three live viral antigens in MMR but is a particular concern for rubella. It should be noted, however, that the RA 27/3 strain used in the vaccine is quite attenuated, and the risk of rubella vaccine-associated congenital malformations is vanishingly small. Among 321 susceptible pregnant women who had inadvertently received rubella vaccine within the three months before or after conception, no infant had congenital malformations compatible with the congenital rubella syndrome (66).

TRAVEL AND SPECIAL USE VACCINES

Polio Vaccine

In the United States, there have been no indigenous cases of poliomyelitis caused by the wild-type polio virus for more than 15 years (67). The outstanding successes of the World Health Organization, UNICEF, and national programs in achieving childhood immunization rates of 80% or better throughout the world have made the global eradication of polio a realistic goal by the year 2000 (68,69). In the Western Hemisphere, the last documented case of polio caused by the wild-type virus was in August 1991, in Peru.

These happy observations have rekindled discussion of the relative merits of: 1) the inactivated polio vaccine (IPV), which is free of serious side effects and has recently undergone manufacturing changes that enhanced its immunogenic potency, versus (70) 2) the live attenuated oral polio vaccine (OPV), which provides better intestinal immunity and better "herd" immunity but has the rare side effect of causing a paralytic illness in approximately one per 1.2 million first-dose recipients and one per million contacts of first-dose recipients (71). The risk is even smaller for subsequent OPV doses. Nevertheless, all of the polio cases occurring in the United States in recent years have been vaccine associated (72).

Because the risk of polio is vanishingly small, adults in the United States are not targeted for polio immunization unless they travel to areas of polio risk or work in laboratories where polio virus is used. Intestinal immunity is not an important issue in the absence of circulating wild-type virus; thus, IPV becomes the clear choice for all adults who have not been previously immunized or who are immunocompromised. OPV is inexpensive, is easy to administer, and remains the most used polio vaccine in the United States (although many Canadian provinces have switched to IPV as the standard pediatric vaccine). School immunization requirements ensure a very high level of polio immunization in youngsters and reimmunization of adults is not routinely recommended. For previously immunized individuals anticipating foreign travel to an endemic area, a one-time booster with either IPV or OPV is recommended (73). The immune response to either IPV or OPV is not compromised by the levels of antibody present in commercially available immune globulin (3,4).

Rabies Vaccines

Although the human diploid cell rabies vaccine (HDCV) used in the United States since 1982 has never been subjected to an efficacy trial, no rabies-exposed individual who has received the recommended intramuscular schedule of HDCV and human rabies immune globulin (HRIG) has contracted rabies. A second rabies vaccine, adsorbed (RVA), grown in a diploid cell line of fetal lung tissue was licensed in 1988 but has not been widely used (74). For postexposure prophylaxis, rabies vaccine must be administered intramuscularly in 1.0-mL doses (75). For preexposure prophylaxis both HDCV and RVA can be used intramuscularly; however, HDCV (but not RVA) has the option of being given intradermally at a 0.1-mL dose, which is less costly (74,76). Following intradermal HDCV, seroconversion rates are slightly lower and the duration of immunity may be shorter than after intramuscular immunization with the higher dose. Chloroquine for malaria prophylaxis may interfere with the response to intradermal (but not intramuscular) HDCV immunization. It is advisable to determine the serologic response to preexposure intradermal HDCV two to four weeks after the third dose of vaccine. Nonresponders should receive additional 1.0-mL doses intramuscularly. Individuals with ongoing risks of rabies exposure should have a booster vaccination every two years (or serologic testing and boosters as needed). Wound management and vaccine use are described in detail elsewhere (4,74).

Typhoid Vaccines

Three inactivated typhoid vaccines and an oral live attenuated vaccine are currently produced (77,78). Each of the vaccines provides protective efficacy in the range of 50 to 80%. Choices among the vaccine options are based mainly on considerations of side effects, ease of administration, and cost (78). The three parenteral vaccines are a heat-phenol inactivated vaccine (the older commercially available vaccine) (79); an acetone-treated vaccine (available only for the armed forces) (80); and the newly produced Vi capsular polysaccharide vaccine (ViCPS) (81), which is composed of purified Vi ("virulence") antigen, the capsular polysaccharide elaborated by bloodstream isolates of *Salmonella typhi*. Antibodies to Vi are protective against typhoid fever. ViCPS vaccine has minimal side effects compared to the severe local and systemic reactions attributed to endotoxin in the other parenteral typhoid vaccines. In addition, ViCPS has a single-dose primary immunization schedule compared to the four-dose oral Ty21a vaccine and the two-dose phenol-inactivated vaccine.

The oral Ty21a vaccine is safe and well tolerated but requires that the vaccine-containing capsules be kept at refrigerator temperature and that each capsule be taken with cool liquid on an empty stomach (82,83). Because antibiotics and the antimalarial mefloquine can inhibit the growth of the Ty21a strain in vitro, immunization with Ty21a should be delayed for 24 hours after ingestion of these drugs (73).

Antibody responses to ViCPS are at least as good as to the other typhoid vaccines and the protective efficacy seems comparable (84,85). The ease of administration and the paucity of side effects of ViCPS will likely establish it as the preferred typhoid vaccine for international travelers.

Yellow Fever Vaccine

Yellow fever has not been documented among U.S. travelers in more than 50 years, although European travelers have contracted the disease during visits to

Africa in the 1980s (86,87). Because yellow fever is a severe hemorrhagic illness for which there is no specific treatment and because the vaccine is highly effective and safe, yellow fever vaccine is recommended for travelers to endemic areas and for persons working in laboratories working with the live virus (73). A valid International Certificate of Vaccination is required by certain endemic countries for entry and by other countries for travelers who come from an area where exposure may have occurred. Reimmunization is recommended at ten-year intervals for individuals at continued risk. However, neutralizing antibodies persist for many years following primary immunization (88).

Levels of antibody in commercially available immune globulin do not interfere with the response to yellow fever vaccine (84).

Because the vaccine is a live attenuated virus, the usual contraindications apply regarding immunocompromised individuals and pregnant women. However, disseminated infection with the vaccine strain has not been reported in such individuals and it is believed that the risk must be very small. Serious systemic adverse reactions are extremely rare. Vaccine-associated encephalitis has been reported in approximately one per ten million vaccine recipients and occurs primarily in children younger than four months of age. Because the vaccine is grown in eggs, immediate hypersensitivity reactions may occur in individuals with severe egg allergy.

Cholera Vaccine

Cholera occurs primarily in conditions of severe socioeconomic deprivation and is rare among travelers. Because the current cholera vaccine is only partially effective (about 50%) and confers only short-term protection, immunization is not routinely recommended for travelers (73,90). The World Health Organization no longer recommends cholera vaccination for travelers to or from areas endemic for cholera and no country lists a cholera vaccine requirement, although some travelers report that on occasion local authorities still require documentation of cholera immunization. For such persons, a single 0.2-mL intradermal dose is sufficient to satisfy requirements. Although conditions that compromise the bacterial defense mechanisms of the stomach (e.g., achlorhydia, antacids, and ulcer surgery) might be considered predisposing factors for increasing the risk of acquiring cholera, most authorities still feel the risk to be so small that cholera vaccine is not advised (4).

Japanese Encephalitis Vaccine

Although the inactivated Japanese encephalitis (JE) vaccine has been licensed in Japan for 40 years and was available on an investigational basis in the United States from 1983 to 1987, the JE vaccine manufactured by Biken has only recently been licensed in the United States in response to the needs of the increased number of travelers to Asia and the military (91). JE virus is mosquito borne and transmission occurs primarily during the rainy season (usually the summer and early fall). Seroprevalence studies in endemic areas indicate nearly universal exposure to JE virus by adulthood and cases occur primarily in children. Infection leads to overt encephalitis in only one of 20 to 1000 cases, but the encephalitis is usually severe with fatal outcomes in 25% and neuropsychiatric sequelae in 50% of the cases (92).

Because the risk of acquiring JE is a function of the season, the duration and type of mosquito exposure, and other variables, most of the estimated 2 to 3 million Americans who travel to Asia in a given year are at very little risk. Only ten cases have been reported in Americans since 1991 and, of these, seven were in military personnel or dependents. Although the risk to the average short-term tourist is less than one in a million, the risks increase for long-term visitors, especially those in rural rice-growing areas.

The Biken JE vaccine is derived from infected mouse brain and purified by centrifugation, ultrafiltration, and protamine sulfate treatment. After formalin inactivation, it is further purified by continuous zonal ultracentrifugation and thimersol is added as a preservative. The myelin basic protein content of the vaccine is below 2 ng/mL. In trials evaluating two doses in children, the vaccine efficacy was 80 to 91%. However, immunogenicity studies in the United States have established three doses as necessary to produce protective levels of neutralizing antibody in more than 90% of vaccine recipients (93,94). The duration of protective immunity is not well established. Until better data are available, a booster dose should be considered at intervals of one to three years for individuals who are at recurrent high risk of JE virus exposure.

Adverse reactions reported with extensive use of JE vaccines in Asia over many years are primarily local irritation (20%) and mild systemic symptoms (10%). Because the vaccine is prepared in neural tissue, there have been concerns about neurologic side effects, but a causal relationship between vaccination and rare, temporarily related neurologic events has not been established. Since 1989, however, an apparently new pattern of hypersensitivity reactions characterized by urticaria, angioedema, or both (sometimes after as much as nine days) has been reported to affect up to 1% of immunized travelers (95,96). The pathogenesis of these delayed accelerated reactions baffles conventional explanations of hypersensitivity. These adverse reactions, as well as the three-dose immunization schedule requiring at least 30 days to complete, will tend to appropriately restrict the use of this vaccine to a subset of travelers whose duration of exposure (more than 30 days) or types of activity place them at greater risk for JE.

Meningococcal Vaccine

Routine immunization with the quadrivalent A, C, Y, W-135 meningococcal polysaccharide vaccine is not recommended because the incidence of meningococcal infection is low and because the vaccine does not protect against serogroup B, which causes almost one half of cases in the United States (97,98). Therefore, vaccination is used mainly for travelers to areas of increased risk for meningococcal infection (e.g., Nepal, Brazil, and Saudi Arabia), control of outbreaks caused by the vaccine serogroups in closed or semiclosed populations (e.g., college students, military base personnel), persons with high risk conditions, such as anatomic or functional asplenia or terminal complement deficiency. Many studies have demonstrated the immunogenicity, safety, and clinical efficacy of the group A and C polysaccharides, but the group Y and W-135 polysaccharides, although safe and immunogenic, have not been evaluated for clinical efficacy in population-based trials. The immunologic response (and presumably clinical protection) persists for up to 10 years (99) and currently reimmunization is not recommended. As with other polysaccharide vaccines, it should be possible to improve the immunologic response and duration of protection of future meningococcal vaccines by developing protein conjugates.

Haemophilus influenzae Type b Conjugate Vaccines

Universal immunization of preschool children has led to the rapid conquest of invasive infection by *Haemophilus influenzae* type b in the United States (100). In the past, almost all adults developed immunity to invasive disease by natural exposure to *H. influenzae* type b or cross-reacting antigens in other bacteria. The immunization of children with the currently available *H. influenzae* type b conjugate (Hib) vaccines diminishes colonization rates and, as a consequence, natural immunization of older children and adults may be less uniform in the future.

There are no vaccine efficacy studies in individuals above age five years. Because invasive infection with *H. influenzae* type b is uncommon in the general adult population, the vaccine is not recommended for this group. However, an argument can be made for immunizing adults with underlying conditions that might predispose to invasive *H. influenzae* type b infection including splenectomy, sickle cell disease, Hodgkin's disease, and other hematologic neoplasms and immunosupression (101). Although persons with AIDS appear to have a higher than normal risk of developing invasive *H. influenzae* type b infection (102), the risk is still modest and most AIDS centers have not made the Hib vaccine a routine immunization.

It would seem reasonable to consider giving Hib conjugate vaccine to adults working in pediatric services, day care centers, and other settings where *H. influenzae* type b transmission is common to diminish colonization rates. It should be emphasized that Hib conjugate vaccine provides no protection against unencapsulated *H. influenzae*, which commonly cause recurrent sinusitis and bronchitis in adults.

Bacillus Calmette-Guérin Vaccine

In the United States, efforts to control tuberculosis are directed toward early identification and treatment of infected persons, preventive therapy with isoniazid, and prevention of transmission to others (103,104). Bacillus Calmette-Guérin (BCG) immunization has been discouraged because it interferes with skin test surveillance and also because the efficacy studies in adults have yielded widely varying results and controversy regarding its benefit. Interest in BCG has been rekindled due to the emergence of MDR *Mycobacterium tuberculosis* infection in several urban centers, as well as by the increase in tuberculosis over the past decade after almost a century of steady decline (105). Since 1989, eight nosocomial outbreaks of MDR tuberculosis have occurred in hospital wards serving HIV-infected individuals (106). Each has been characterized by high mortality rates (70 to 90%) in HIV-infected individuals, rapid spread of infection, delays in case recognition and infection control efforts due to atypical presentation, and high tuberculosis skin test conversion rates (30 to 50%) among staff. These alarming outbreaks have been brought under control by intensifying standard hospital infection-control measures but have raised interest in expanding the role of BCG.

An extensive meta-analysis commissioned by the CDC has concluded that BCG provides protective efficacy of at least 50% in adults (107). Therefore, in areas of high tuberculosis incidence, particularly with MDR tuberculosis, BCG immunization of health care workers is being actively considered. Over three million doses of BCG had been given since its introduction over 70 years ago. The bacillus attenuated by Calmette and Guérin has been propagated in laboratories around the world and BCG vaccines now in use are not identical, although there are no clear-cut differences in their protective efficacy or adverse reaction rates. The safety profile is good, although local reactions including regional lymphadenitis are common. BCG should not be given to immunocompromised individuals (including AIDS patients) due to the risk of developing disseminated BCG infection. However, in asymptomatic HIV-infected children, BCG appears to be well tolerated (108,109).

VACCINES SOON TO BE LICENSED

Varicella Vaccine

A live attenuated varicella vaccine (Oka strain) has been licensed for high-risk children in several European countries since 1984 and has been given to healthy children in Japan and Korea since 1989. Administration of more than two million doses in other countries, as well as administration to 11,000 healthy individuals in the United States, has established a good safety record (110,111). In adults, two doses (the second 4 to 8 weeks after the first) are required to achieve 99% seroconversion (112). Among vaccinees of all ages followed up to nine years, less than 1 to 3% have developed chickenpox after exposure to varicella-zoster virus, and the breakthrough cases were mild with fewer vesicles compared to controls.

The attenuated varicella vaccine will be recommended as a universal (one dose) immunogen for children between 12 and 18 months of age. A two-dose schedule will be recommended for adolescents and adults with no prior history of chickenpox (prevaccination serologic testing to determine immunity may be cost effective depending on the relative cost of the test and vaccine). Target groups for immunization will likely include susceptible individuals who are health care workers, day care workers, school teachers, and others in occupations in which varicella-zoster virus transmission is common; international travelers; nonpregnant women of childbearing age; and persons who work or live in closed institutions such as colleges, the military, or correctional institutions.

Hepatitis A Vaccine

Two killed-virus hepatitis A vaccines are nearing licensure (113). Each has been shown to have protective efficacy exceeding 90% and low levels of adverse reactions in trials in children (114,115). The vaccine is likely to be universally recommended for pediatric use. Adults who will be targeted for the hepatitis A vaccine include international travelers, staff members of day care centers and custodial institutions, military personnel, food handlers, members of population groups with high levels of endemic infection (such as Native Americans, Alaskan natives), and persons whose sexual practices (male homosexuality or multiple sex partners) place them at increased risk. It is anticipated that for preexposure prophylaxis, hepatitis A should replace immune globulin for most indications provided the vaccine is not too costly. It has not been established whether immunization will be of value in the postexposure care of persons who have had contact with patients with hepatitis A.

VACCINE DEVELOPMENT AND DELIVERY

The field of vaccine development is burgeoning with the ability to identify molecular mechanisms of pathogenesis for a variety of organisms and use of genetic engineering methods to create new immunogens. The ability to combine multiple antigens on a carrier, the development of new adjuvants that control the type of T-cell response, and the use of novel vaccine delivery systems such as microspheres are but some of the techniques that point to the rapid expansion of this field.

However, the current bottleneck in adult immunization is not the development or the availability of vaccines but the poor record of implementation of current vaccine recommendations. Among the estimated 65,000 annual deaths from invasive pneumococcal disease, influenza, and hepatitis B, more than 34,000 could be prevented by full implementation of the existing vaccine recommendations for adults (1). This level of preventable mortality exceeds both automobile accident deaths and AIDS deaths for 1992. Inexpensive, low-technology vaccine programs can provide an immediate high-impact benefit, and building systems that will effectively immunize the adults of the United States deserves a high priority by health care providers in both the private and public sectors.

REFERENCES

1 Gardner P, Schaffner W. Immunization of adults. N Engl J Med 1993;328:1252–1258.

2 Williams WW, Hickson MA, Kane MA, Kendal AP, Spika JS, Hinman AR. Immunization policies and vaccine coverage among adults: the risk for missed opportunities. Ann Intern Med 1988;108:616–625.

3 Update on adult immunization: recommendations of the Immunization Practices Advisory Committee (ACIP). MMWR 1991;40(RR-12).

4 American College of Physicians Task Force on Adult Immunization, Infectious Diseases Society of America. Guide for adult immunization, 3rd ed. Philadelphia: American College of Physicians, 1994.

5 Musher DM, Groover JE, Rowland JM, et al. Antibody to capsular polysaccharides of Streptococcus pneumoniae: prevalence, persistence, and response to revaccination. Clin Infect Dis 1993;17:66–73.

6 Austrian R, Douglas RM, Schiffman G, et al. Prevention of pneumococcal pneumonia by vaccination. Trans Assoc Am Physicians 1976;89:184–194.

7 Austrian R. Surveillance of pneumococcal infection for field trials of polyvalent pneumococcal vaccines. Bethesda, Maryland: National Institutes of Health 1980:1–84. (Report DAB-VDP-12-84).

8 Austrian R. Some observations on the pneumococcus and on the current status of pneumococcal disease and its prevention. Rev Infect Dis 1981;3(suppl):S1–S17.

9 Austrian R. A reassessment of pneumococcal vaccine. N Engl J Med 1984;310: 651–653. (Editorial).

10 Simberkoff MS, Cross AP, Al-Ibrahim M, et al. Efficacy of pneumococcal vaccine in high-risk patients: results of a Veterans Administration Cooperative Study. N Engl J Med 1986;315:1318–1327.

11 Shapiro ED, Clemens JD. A controlled evaluation of the protective efficacy of pneumococcal vaccine for patients at high risk of serious pneumococcal infection. Ann Intern Med 1984;101:325–330.

12 Sims RV, Steinmann WC, McConville JH, et al. The clinical effectiveness of pneumococcal vaccine in the elderly. Ann Intern Med 1988:108:653–657.

13 Forrester HL, Jahnigen DW, LaForce FM. Inefficacy of pneumococcal vaccine in a high-risk population. Am J Med 1987;83: 425–430.

14 Shapiro ED, Berg AT, Austrian R, et al. The protective efficacy of polyvalent pneumococcal polysaccharide vaccine. N Engl J Med 1991;325:1453–1460.

15 Broome CV, Facklam RR, Fraser DW. Pneumococcal disease after pneumococcal vaccination: an alternative method to estimate the efficacy of pneumococcal vaccine. N Engl J Med 1980;303:549–552.

16 Bolan G, Broome CV, Facklam RR, et al. Pneumococcal vaccine efficacy in selected populations in the United States. Ann Intern Med 1986;104:1–6.

17 Butler JC, Breiman RF, Campbell JF, et al. Pneumococcal polysaccharide vaccine efficacy. JAMA 1993;270:1826–1831.

18 Bennett NM, Buffington J, LaForce FM. Pneumococcal bacteremia in Monroe County, New York. Am J Public Health 1992;82:1513–1516.

19 Applebaum PC. Antimicrobial resistance in Streptococcus pneumoniae: an overview. Clin Infect Dis 1992;15:77–83.

20 Broome CV, Breiman RF. Pneumococcal vaccine—past, present, and future. N Engl J Med 1991;325:1506–1508. (Editorial).

21 Eskola J, Peltola H, Takala AK, et al. Efficacy of Hemohilus influenzae type b polysaccharide-diphtheria toxoid conjugate vaccine in infancy. N Engl J Med 1987;317:717–722.

22 Schneerson R, Robbins JR, Parke JC Jr, et al. Quantitative and qualitative analyses of serum antibodies elicited in adults by Haemophilus influenzae type b and pneumococcus type 6A capsular polysaccharide-tetanus toxoid conjugates. Infect Immun 1986;52:519–528.

23 Davenport FM. The search for the ideal influenza vaccine. Postgrad Med J 1979; 55:78–86.

24 **Davenport FM, Lennette EH, Meiklejohn GM.** Origins and development of the Commission on Influenza. Arch Environ Health 1970;21:267–272.

25 **Dowdle WR.** Influenza immunoprophylaxis after 30 years experience. In: Nayak DP, ed. Genetic variation among influenza viruses. ICN-UCLA Symposia on Molecular and Cellular Biology, vol XXI. New York: Academic Press, 1981: 525–534.

26 **Meiklejohn G.** Viral respiratory disease at Lowry Air Force Base in Denver, 1952–82. J Infect Dis 1983;148:775–784.

27 **Stiver HG, Graves P, Eickhoff TC, et al.** Efficacy of "Hong Kong" vaccine in preventing "England" variant influenza A in 1972. N Engl J Med 1973;289:1267–1271.

28 **Patriarca PA, Weber JA, Parker RA, et al.** Efficacy of influenza vaccine in nursing homes. Reduction in illness and complications during an influenza A (H3N2) epidemic. JAMA 1985;253:1136–1139.

29 **Gross PA, Quinnan GV, Rodstein M, et al.** Association of influenza immunization with reduction in mortality in an elderly population. A prospective study. Arch Intern Med 1988;148:562–565.

30 **Foster DA, Talsma AN, Furomoto-Dawson A, et al.** Influenza vaccine effectiveness in preventing hospitalization for pneumonia in the elderly. Am J Epidemiol 1992;136:296–307.

31 **Centers for Disease Control and Prevention.** Prevention and control of influenza. Part 1. Vaccines. Recommendations of the Immunization Practices Advisory Committee (ACIP). MMWR 1993;42(RR-6):1–14.

32 **Fedson DS.** Clinical practice and public policy for influenza and pneumococcal vaccination of the elderly. Clin Geriatr Med 1992;8:183–199.

33 **Schonberger LB, Bregman LB, Sullivan-Bolyai JZ, et al.** Guillain-Barre Syndrome following vaccination in the National Influenza Immunization Program, United States, 1976–1977. Am J Epidemiol 1979; 110:105–123.

34 **Kaplan JE, Katona P, Hurwitz ES, et al.** Guillain-Barre syndrome in the United States, 1979–1980 and 1980–1981: lack of an association with influenza vaccination. JAMA 1982;248:698–700.

35 **Williams WW, Hickson MA, Kane MA, et al.** Immunization policies and vaccine coverage among adults: the risk for missed opportunities. Ann Intern Med 1988;108:616–625.

36 **Margolis KL, Lofgren RP, Korn JE.** Organizational strategies to improve influenza vaccine delivery. A standing order in a general medical clinic. Arch Intern Med 1988;148:2205–2207.

37 **Buffington J, Bell KM, LaForce FM, Genesee Hospital Medical Staff.** A target-based model for increasing influenza immunizations in private practice. J Gen Intern Med 1991;6:204–209.

38 **Nichol KL.** Improving influenza vaccination rates for high-risk inpatients. Am J Med 1991;91:584–588.

39 **Kilbourne EM.** Influenza. New York: Plenum Publishing, 1987.

40 **Treanor JJ, Mattison HR, Dumyati G, et al.** Protective efficacy of combined live intranasal and inactivated influenza A virus vaccines in the elderly. Ann Intern Med 1992;117:625–633.

41 **Centers for Disease Control. Update on adult immunization.** Recommendations of the Immunization Practices Advisory Committee (ACIP). MMWR 1991;40:(RR-12):1–94.

42 **Gibas A, Watkins E, Dienstag J.** Long-term persistence of protective antibody after hepatitis B vaccination of healthy adults. In: Zuckerman AJ, ed. Viral Hepatitis and Liver Disease. New York: Alan Liss, 1988:998–1001.

43 **Szmuness W, Stevens CE, Zang EA, et al.** A controlled clinical trial of the efficacy of the hepatitis B vaccine (heptavax B): a final report. Hepatology 1981;1:377–385.

44 **Hadler SC, Margolis HS.** Hepatitis B immunization: vaccine types, efficacy, and indications for immunization. In: Remington JS, Swartz MN, eds. Current Clinical Topics in Infectious Diseases. Boston: Blackwell Scientific Publications; 1992: 282–308.

45 **McMahon BJ, Helminiak C, Wainright RB, et al.** Frequency of adverse reactions to hepatitis B vaccine in 43,618 persons. Am J Med 1992;92:254–256.

46 **Alter MJ, Hadler SC, Margolis HS, et al.** The changing epidemiology of hepatitis B in the United States. Need for alternative vaccination strategies. JAMA 1990;263: 1218–1222.

47 **Centers for Disease Control. Hepatitis B virus: a comprehensive strategy for eliminating transmission in the United States through universal childhood vaccination:**

recommendations of the Immunization Practices Advisory Committee (ACIP). MMWR 1991;40(RR-13):1–25.

48 **Krahn MD, Detsky AS.** Universal hepatitis B vaccination: the economics of prevention. Can Med Assoc. J 1992;146:19–21.

49 **Prevots R, Sutter RW, Strebel PM, Cochi SL, Hadler S.** Tetanus surveillance—United States, 1989–1990. MMWR 1992; 41:ss1–ss9.

50 **Advisory Committee for Immunization Practices.** Diphtheria, tetanus and pertussis: recommendations for vaccine use and other preventive measures. MMWR 1991;40(RR-10).

51 **Ruben FL, Nagel J, Fireman P.** Antitoxin responses in the elderly to tetanus-diphtheria immunization. Am J Epidemiol 1978;108:145–149.

52 **Simonsen O, Badsberg JH, et al.** The fall-off in serum concentration of tetanus antitoxin after primary and booster vaccination. Acta Pathol Microbiol Scand 1986;94:77–82.

53 **Christenson B, Bottiger M.** Epidemiology and immunity to tetanus in Sweden. Scand J Infect Dis 1987;19:429–435.

54 **Weiss BP, Strassburg MA, Feeley JC.** Tetanus and diphtheria immunity in an elderly population in Los Angeles. Am J Public Health 1983;73:802–804.

55 **Crossley K, Irvine P, Warren JB, Lee BK, Mead K.** Tetanus and diphtheria immunity in urban Minnesota adults. JAMA 1979;242:2298–3000.

56 **Ballestra DJ, Littenberg B.** Should adult tetanus immunization be given as a single vaccination at age 65? A cost-effectiveness analysis. J Gen Intern Med 1993;8:405–412.

57 **Centers for Disease Control.** Diphtheria outbreak—Russian Federation, 1990–1993. MMWR 1993;42:840–847.

58 **Arkinson WL, Orenstein WA, Krugman S.** The resurgence of measles in the United States, 1989–91. Annu Rev Med 1992;43:451–463.

59 **Sosin DM, Cochi SL, Gunn RA, et al.** The changing epidemiology of mumps and its impact on university campuses. Pediatrics 1989;84:779–784.

60 **Robertson SE, Cochi SL, Bunn GA, et al.** Preventing rubella: assessing missed opportunities for immunization. Am J Public Health 1987;77:1347–1349.

61 **Markowitz LE, Tomassi A, Hawkins CE, et al.** International measles importations,

United States, 1980–85. Int J Epidemiol 1988;17:187–192.

62 **Arkinson WL, Markowitz LE, Adams NC, et al.** Transmission of measles in medical settings—United States, 1985–1989. Am J Med 1991;91(suppl 3B):320S–324S.

63 **Lavi S, Zimmerman B, Koren G, et al.** Administration of measles, mumps, and rubella virus vaccine (live) to egg-allergic children. JAMA 1990;263:269–271.

64 **Preblud SR.** Some current issues relating to rubella vaccine. JAMA 1985;254:253–256.

65 **Tingle AJ, Yang T, Petty RE, et al.** Comparative study of joint manifestations associated with natural rubella infection and RA 27/3 rubella immunization. Ann Rheum Dis 1986;45:110–114.

66 **Centers for Disease Control.** Rubella prevention. Recommendations of the Immunization Practices Advisory Committee (ACIP). MMWR 1990;39(RR-15):1–18.

67 **Kim-Farley RJ, Bart KJ, Schonberger LB, et al.** Poliomyelitis in the USA: virtual elimination of the disease caused by wild virus. Lancet 1984;2:1315–1317.

68 **Hinman AR, Foege WH, de Quadros CA, Patriarca PA, Orenstein WA, Brink EW.** The case for global eradication of poliomyelitis. Bull World Health Organ 1987; 65:835–840.

69 **Wright PF, Kim-Farley RJ, de Quadros CA, et al.** Strategies for the global eradication of poliomyelitis by the year 2000. N Engl J Med 1991;325:1774–1779.

70 **Roberston SE, Traverso HP, Drucker JA, et al.** Clinical efficacy of a new, enhanced-potency, inactivated poliovirus vaccine. Lancet 1988;1:897–899.

71 **Hinman AR, Koplan JP, Orenstein WA, Brink EW, Nkowane BM.** Live or inactivated poliomyelitis vaccine: an analysis of benefits and risks. Am J Public Health 1988;78:291–295.

72 **Nkowane BM, Wassilak SGF, Orenstein WA, et al.** Vaccine-associated paralytic poliomyelitis. United States: 1973 through 1984. JAMA 1987;257:1335–1340.

73 **Health Information for international travel 1993.** Altanta: Centers for Disease Control, 1993; HHS publication no. (CDC) 93.

74 **Centers for Disease Control.** Rabies prevention—**United States, 1991: recommendations of the Immunization Practices Advisory Committee (ACIP).** MMWR 1991;40(RR-3):1–19.

75 **Baer GM, Fishbein DB.** Rabies post-exposure prophylaxis. N Engl J Med 1987; 316:1270–1272.

76 **Bernard KW, Mallonee J, Wright JC, et al.** Pre-exposure immunization with intradermal human diploid cell rabies vaccine: risks and benefits of primary and booster vaccination. JAMA 1987;257:1059–1063.

77 **Levine MM, Ferreccio C, Black RE, et al.** Progress in vaccines against typhoid fever. Rev Infect Dis 1989;11:S552–S567.

78 **Woodruff BA, Pavia AT, Blake PA.** A new look at typhoid vaccination: information for the practicing physician. JAMA 1991;265:756–759.

79 **Ashcroft MT, Nicholson CC, Balwent S, Ritchie JM, Soryan S, William F.** A seven year field trial of two typhoid vaccines in Guyana. Lancet 1967;ii:1056–1060.

80 **Edwards EA, Johnson JP, Pierce WE, Peckinpaugh RO.** Reactions and serologic response to monovalent acetone-inactivated typhoid vaccine and heat-killed TAB vaccine when given by jet-injection. Bull World Health Organ 1974;51:501–505.

81 **Cumberland NS, Roberts JS, Arnold WSG, Patel RK, Bowker CH.** Typhoid Vi: a less reactogenic vaccine. J Int Med Res 1992;20:247–253.

82 **Ferreccio C, Levine MM, Rodriguez H, et al.** Comparative efficacy of two, three, or four doses of Ty21a live oral typhoid vaccine in enteric-coated capsules: a field trial in an endemic area. J Infect Dis 1989;159: 766–769.

83 **Levine MM, Black RE, Ferreccio C, et al.** Large scale field trial of Ty21a live oral typhoid vaccine in enteric-coated capsule formulation. Lancet 1987;i:1049–1052.

84 **Acharya IL, Lowe CU, Thapa R, et al.** Prevention of typhoid fever in Nepal with the Vi capsular polysaccharide of *Salmonella typhi*. N Engl J Med 1987;317:1101–1104.

85 **Keitel WA, Bond NL, Zahradnik JM, Cramton TA, Robbins JB.** Clinical and serological responses following primary and booster immunization with *Salmonella typhi* Vi capsular polysaccharide vaccines. Vaccine 1994;12:195–199.

86 **Centers for Disease Control.** Yellow fever. MMWR 1990;39(RR-10):1–5.

87 **Woodall JP.** Summary of a symposium on yellow fever. J Infect Dis 1981;144:87–91.

88 **Poland JD, Calisher CH, Monath TP, Downs WG, Murphy K.** Persistence of neutralizing antibody 30–35 years after immunization with 17D yellow fever vaccine. Bull World Health Organ 1981;59: 895–900.

89 **Kaplan JE, Nelson DB, Schonberger LB, et al.** The effect of immune globulin on the response to trivalent oral poliovirus and yellow fever vaccinations. Bull World Health Organ 1984;62:585–590.

90 **Gardner P, ed.** Health issues of international travelers. Infect Dis Clin North Am 1992;6:275–502.

91 **Centers for Disease Control.** Japanese encephalitis. MMWR 1993;42(RR-1):1–15.

92 **Rosen L.** The natural history of Japanese encephalitis virus. Ann Rev Microbiol 1986;40:395–414.

93 **Hoke CH, Nisalak A, Sangawhipa N, et al.** Protection against Japanese encephalitis by inactivated vaccines. N Engl J Med 1988;319:609–614.

94 **Poland JD, Cropp CB, Craven RB, Monath TP.** Evaluation of the potency and safety of inactivated Japanese encephalitis vaccine in US inhabitants. J Infect Dis 1990;161:878–882.

95 **Andersen MM, Rønne T.** Side-effects with Japanese encephalitis vaccine. Lancet 1991;337:1044.

96 **Ruff TA, Eisen D, Fuller A, Kass R.** Adverse reactions to Japanese encephalitis vaccine. Lancet 1991;338:881–882.

97 **Pinner RW, Gellin BG, et al.** Meningococcal disease in the United States—1986. J Infect Dis 1991;164:368–374.

98 **Jackson LA, Wenger JD.** Laboratory-based surveillance for meningococcal disease in selected areas, United States 1989–1991. MMWR 1993;42(SS-2):21–30.

99 **Zangwill KM, Stout RW, Carlone GM, et al.** Duration of antibody response after meningococcal polysaccharide vaccination in U.S. Air Force personnel. J Infect Dis 1994;169:847–852.

100 **Adams WG, Deaver KA, Cochi SL, Plikaytis BD, Zell ER, Broome CV, Wenger JD.** Decline of childhood *Haemophilus influenzae* type b (Hib) disease in the Hib vaccine era. JAMA 1993;269:221–226.

101 **Centers for Disease Control.** Recommendations of the Advisory Committee on Immunization Practices (ACIP): use of vaccines and immune globulins in persons with altered immunocompetence. MMWR 1993;42(RR-5):1–18.

102 Steinhoff MC, Auerbach BS, Nelson K, et al. Antibody responses to *Haemophilus influenzae* type b vaccines in men with human immunodeficiency virus infection. N Engl J Med 1991;325:1837–1842.

103 Centers for Disease Control and Prevention. Prevention and control of tuberculosis in U.S. communities with at-risk minority populations. MMWR 1992; 41(RR-5):1–11.

104 American Thoracic Society/Centers for Disease Control. Control of tuberculosis in the United States. Am Rev Respir Dis 1992;146:1623–1633.

105 Bloch AB, Cauthen GM, Onorato IM, et al. Nationwide survey of drug-resistant tuberculosis in the United States. JAMA 1994;271:665–671.

106 Kent JH. The epidemiology of multi-drug-resistant tuberculosis in the United States. Med Clin North Am 1993;77:1391–1409.

107 Colditz GA, Brewer TF, Berkey CS, et al. Efficacy of BCG vaccine in the prevention of tuberculosis. JAMA 1994;271:698–702.

108 Lallemont-Le Coeur S, Lallemont M, Cheynier D, et al. Bacillus Calmette-Guerin immunization in infants born to HIV-1-seropositive mothers. AIDS 1991;5: 195–199.

109 Msellati P, Dabis F, Lepage P, et al. BCG vaccination and pediatric HIV infection-Rawanda, 1988–1990. MMWR 1991;40: 833–836.

110 Kuter BJ, Weibel RE, Guess HA, et al. Oka-Merck varicella vaccine in healthy children: final report of a 2-year efficacy study and 7-year follow-up studies. Vaccine 1991;9:643–647.

111 White CJ, Kuter BJ, Hildebrand CS, et al. Varicella vaccine (VARIVAX) in healthy children and adolescents: results from clinical trials, 1987–1989. Pediatrics 1991; 87:604–610.

112 Gershon AA, Steinberg SP, LaRussa P, Ferrara A, Hammerslag M, Gelb L, NIAID Varicella Vaccine Collaborative Study Group. Immunization of healthy adults with live attenuated varicella vaccine. J Infect Dis 1988;158:132–137.

113 Siegl G, Lemon SM. Recent advances in hepatitis A vaccine development. Virus Res 1990;17:75–92.

114 Innis BL, Snitbhan R, Kunasol P, et al. Protection against hepatitis A by an inactivated vaccine. JAMA 1994;271:1328–1334.

115 Werzberger A, Mensch B, Kuter B, et al. A controlled trial of a formalin-inactivated hepatitis A vaccine in healthy children. N Engl J Med 1992;327:453–457.

Outpatient Management of HIV Infection in the Adult: An Update

STEPHEN L. BOSWELL

EPIDEMIOLOGY

Overview

From 1981 through December 1993, 361,509 cases of acquired immunodeficiency syndrome (AIDS) were reported to the Centers for Disease Control and Prevention (CDC) in the United States. Of these, 140,636 are living. The United States epidemic has grown rapidly. The first 100,000 cases of AIDS were reported in the first eight years of the epidemic, whereas the second 100,000 cases were reported over the subsequent two years. This rapid growth in the epidemic has been characterized by important demographic changes.

As the epidemic has matured, the average age at the onset of human immunodeficiency virus (HIV) infection has declined substantially (1). AIDS is now the sixth leading cause of death among youth ages 15 to 24. Heterosexuals constitute an ever-increasing portion of those reported with AIDS (2). In 1985, 1.9% of AIDS cases reported to the CDC were in persons whose most likely mode of acquiring the disease was heterosexual contact. In 1993, 9.0% of all cases were acquired in this manner. The greatest growth of the epidemic has moved from large metropolitan areas of the east and west coasts to small metropolitan and rural areas throughout the United States (3,4). Ninety-eight percent of all reported cases have involved adults or adolescents and of these 12% have occurred in women.

These observations of the AIDS epidemic are limited by the 7- to 10-year period that characterizes the delay between transmission and development of AIDS in adults. Thus, while 361,509 cases of AIDS were reported through the end of 1993, 800,000 to 1,200,000 persons are infected with HIV. Currently, more people are living with AIDS than were diagnosed in the first 8 years of the epidemic. Further, the longevity of individuals who are HIV infected has increased significantly. Chief among the factors that have contributed to the improved survival of those who are HIV infected are the introduction

301

of prophylaxis of *Pneumocystis carinii* pneumonia (PCP) and antiretroviral therapy (5).

These phenomena—the large number of individuals infected with HIV, the increasing number of these individuals with advanced HIV infection (AIDS), and the increasing longevity of those who are HIV infected—imply that providers will continue to see increasing numbers of HIV-infected patients for the foreseeable future.

Recent Developments

The past year has seen several epidemiologic developments of particular clinical importance. Those noted below by no means include the full list of such developments.

Zidovudine Reduces Risk of Maternal Transmission of HIV   In the United States, approximately 7000 infants are born to HIV-infected mothers each year. One thousand to 2000 of these infants are HIV infected (6). In February 1994, the National Institute of Allergy and Infectious Diseases announced the preliminary results of a phase III double-blind, placebo-controlled randomized clinical trial designed to evaluate the efficacy, safety, and tolerance of zidovudine for the prevention of maternal–fetal HIV transmission (AIDS Clinical Trials Group [ACTG] 076). Zidovudine or placebo was given to HIV-infected pregnant women between 14 and 34 weeks of gestation, continued intrapartum, and then given to their infants during the first six weeks of life. The eligibility criteria and zidovudine regimen involved in this study are given in Tables 13.1 and 13.2.

At the time of this preliminary analysis, 477 women were enrolled and 421 babies had been born. Data were sufficient to analyze 364 infants, 180 in the zidovudine group and 184 in the placebo group. At the time of the announcement, 13 (8.3% ± 4.5%) babies in the zidovudine group and 40 (25.5% ± 7.2%) in the placebo group were HIV infected. All babies who were infected were identified as being infected within the first 24 weeks of life. This represents a 67.5% reduction in transmission risk and was highly statistically significant ($P = .00006$). Mothers and infants experienced minimal short-term side effects attributable to zidovudine. Some infants taking zidovudine experienced a reversible mild anemia. Data on long-term effects of zidovudine therapy on infants in this study are not available (7).

The Food and Drug Administration (FDA) has not approved zidovudine to prevent transmission of HIV during pregnancy and delivery. However, the Public Health Service has made interim recommendations regarding the use of zidovudine for this purpose (Table 13.3) (6). The Public Health Service is developing additional recommendations for the use of zidovudine for HIV-infected pregnant women whose clinical indications differ from the ACTG 076 eligibility criteria, and for counseling and HIV-antibody testing of women of childbearing age. Decisions regarding the use of zidovudine for this purpose should be taken

Table 13.1. Eligibility Criteria for ACTG 076

Mother has not received antiretroviral treatment during current pregnancy
Mother has no clinical indications for maternal antepartum antiretroviral therapy in
the judgment of her health care provider
Mother has a CD4 lymphocyte count >200 cells/mm³ (≥14%) at initial assessment

Table 13.2. Zidovudine Regimen Used in ACTG 076

Oral administration of 100 mg zidovudine five times daily, initiated at 14–34 weeks'
gestation and continued for the remainder of the pregnancy
During labor, IV administration of zidovudine in a loading dose of 2 mg/kg body
weight given over 1 h, followed by continuous infusion
Oral administration of zidovudine to the newborn (zidovudine syrup at 2 mg/kg
body weight per dose q6h) for the first 6 weeks of life beginning 8–12 h after birth

Table 13.3. Interim Recommendations of the Public Health Service Regarding the
Use of Zidovudine to Prevent Maternal Transmission of HIV

All health care workers providing care to pregnant women and women of
childbearing age should be informed of the results of ACTG protocol 076.
HIV-infected pregnant women meeting the protocol eligibility criteria should be
informed of the potential benefits and unknown long-term risks of zidovudine
therapy as administered in ACTG protocol 076.
Providers should inform their patients that this zidovudine regimen substantially
reduced, but did not eliminate, the risk of HIV infection among the infants.
Until the potential risk for teratogenicity and other complications from zidovudine
therapy given in the first trimester can be assessed, zidovudine therapy only for the
purpose of reducing the risk for perinatal transmission should not be instituted
earlier than the 14th week of gestation.

on a case by case basis. The mother should be carefully apprised of the possible
benefits and the unknown risks.

Primary Infection with Zidovudine-Resistant HIV Type 1 Zidovudine resistance has been recognized for many years among patients treated with the drug
for extended periods of time. Recently, the first reports appeared of the horizontal transmission of a zidovudine-resistant strain of HIV type 1 (HIV-1) (8–11).
This may have an important bearing on the clinical approach to newly infected
persons who might have acquired a resistant strain of HIV. It may also bear on
the decision to use zidovudine for prophylaxis of significant occupational exposures (12,13). When the exposure involves an individual with late stage disease,
a stage when zidovudine-resistant virus is more easily found, the theoretical
benefit of zidovudine prophylaxis is significantly lessened.

Revised Adult and Adolescent HIV Classification System and the Expanded Surveillance Case Definition for Severe HIV Disease (AIDS) With the implementation of the new AIDS surveillance definition in January 1993, the number of cases of AIDS increased by more than 50% (14). The most significant change was in the inclusion of CD4 lymphocyte counts in the definition—those HIV-infected individuals with CD4 counts less than 200 cells/mm³ (or alternatively, <14% of total lymphocytes) are now considered to have AIDS. Of the estimated one million persons infected with HIV in the United States, it is estimated that 160,000 individuals without an AIDS-defining condition have CD4 lymphocyte counts less than 200 cells/mm³. The addition of CD4 criteria to this definition should simplify the AIDS case-reporting process and may lessen the confounding effects of treatment on the surveillance of the epidemic.

The expanded definition retains the 23 clinical conditions in the AIDS surveillance case definition published in 1987. In addition, pulmonary tuberculosis, recurrent bacterial pneumonia, and invasive cervical cancer have been added to this list (Table 13.4). Although these conditions occur in persons without HIV infection, data suggest that they occur more frequently and with greater severity in immunosuppressed persons.

Table 13.4. AIDS-Indicator Conditions of the 1993 Expanded Surveillance Case Definition for Severe HIV Disease (AIDS)

Candidiasis of bronchi, trachea, or lungs	Lymphoma, immunoblastic
Candidiasis, esophageal	Lymphoma, primary in brain
Coccidioidomycosis, disseminated or extrapulmonary	*Mycobacterium avium* complex or *Mycobacterium kansasii*, disseminated or extrapulmonary
Cryptococcosis, extrapulmonary	*Mycobacterium tuberculosis*, disseminated or extrapulmonary
Cryptosporidiosis, chronic intestinal (>1 mo duration)	*Mycobacterium*, other species or unidentified species, disseminated or extrapulmonary
Cytomegalovirus disease (other than liver, spleen, or nodes)	*P. carinii* pneumonia
Cytomegalovirus retinitis (with loss of vision)	Progressive multifocal leukoencephalopathy
HIV encephalopathy	Salmonella septicemia, recurrent
Herpes simplex: chronic ulcer(s) (>1 mo duration) or bronchitis, pneumonitis, or esophagitis	Toxoplasmosis of brain
Histoplasmosis, disseminated or extrapulmonary	Wasting syndrome due to HIV
Isosporiasis, chronic intestinal (>1 mo duration)	Recurrent bacterial pneumonia
Kaposi's sarcoma	Pulmonary tuberculosis
Lymphoma, Burkitt's	Invasive cervical cancer

Table 13.5. CDC Classification System for HIV Infection for HIV-Seropositive Adolescents and Adults

CD4 Lymphocyte Count Categories	Clinical Categories		
	A Asymptomatic or PGL	B Symptomatic not (A) or (C) Conditions	C AIDS-Indicator Conditions
1. ≥ 500 cells/mm³	A1	B1	C1
2. 200–499 cells/mm³	A2	B2	C2
3. < 200 cells/mm³	A3	B3	C3

Darkly bordered cells represent AIDS-defining categories; PGL, persistent generalized lymphadenopathy.

Table 13.6. Correlation of Absolute CD4 Lymphocyte Count with Percent CD4 Lymphocytes

CD4 Lymphocyte Count Category	Absolute CD4 Lymphocyte Count (cells/mm³)	Percent CD4 Cells (% of Total Lymphocytes)
1	≥ 500	≥ 29
2	200–499	14–28
3	< 200	< 14

The revised CDC HIV classification system for adolescents and adults categorizes persons on the basis of clinical conditions associated with HIV infection and CD4 lymphocyte counts. The system is based on three ranges of CD4 lymphocyte counts and three clinical categories (Table 13.5). T-lymphocyte immunotyping should be conducted by an experienced laboratory with quality assurance procedures. The lowest accurate, but not necessarily the most recent, CD4 lymphocyte count should be used for classification purposes.

Compared with the absolute CD4 lymphocyte count, the percent CD4 cells is less subject to variation on repeated measurements. Consequently, some clinicians prefer to use this measure for classification purposes (Table 13.6) (15).

Idiopathic CD4 Lymphocytopenia/Severe Unexplained HIV-Seronegative Immune Suppression During the VIIIth International Conference on AIDS held in Amsterdam during the summer of 1992, five cases of individuals with persistently low CD4 lymphocyte counts with no evidence of HIV infection were reported. No evidence of HIV-1, HIV-2, or human T-cell lymphotropic virus 1 or 2 (HTLV-1, HTLV-2) infection was found. A meeting held at the CDC on August 4, 1992, resulted in the identification of 26 cases from Australia, Denmark, England, France, Germany, Spain, and the United States. At this

Table 13.7. CDC Case Definition for Idiopathic CD4 T Lymphocytopenia

CD4 lymphocyte count < 300 cells/mm^3 (or $< 20\%$ of total CD4 lymphocytes) on more than one determination

No laboratory evidence of HIV type 1 or type 2 infection

No defined immunodeficiency or therapy associated with depressed CD4 lymphocyte levels

meeting a new case definition for idiopathic CD4 lymphocytopenia was developed (Table 13.7) (16–23).

Epidemiologic studies suggest that the causes of this syndrome are heterogeneous. The reported cases are epidemiologically, clinically, and immunologically heterogeneous. Although many of the individuals with the syndrome have clear risk factors for HIV infection, others have none. Kaposi's sarcoma and PCP, two of the most prevalent manifestations of AIDS, have been seen in persons with low CD4 lymphocyte counts and without evidence of HIV-1 or HIV-2 infection (24,25). They have also been seen in individuals with normal CD4 lymphocyte counts (26,27).

It remains uncertain whether the reported cases of idiopathic CD4 lymphocytopenia are the result of HIV infection, a new retrovirus, or other yet unidentified causes. The widespread use of T-lymphocyte immunotyping in the wake of the HIV epidemic may have brought cases of sporadic immunosuppression to clinical attention. The phenomenon appears to be extremely rare.

Clinical Progression in the Adult   More than 90% of HIV-infected individuals show a gradual reduction in immune function as depicted by their diminution in absolute CD4 lymphocyte counts. Spontaneous recovery of immune function does not appear to occur, and thus, the vast majority of those who are HIV seropositive can be expected ultimately to develop progressive and fatal HIV disease. Within the San Francisco Department of Public Health's cohort of HIV-seropositive individuals, one of the most extensively studied of such cohorts, 50% of those studied developed AIDS within 10 to 11 years of initial infection (28). Recent data suggest that this time period has been increased by early intervention with antiretroviral agents and appropriate chemoprophylaxis (5,29–31). The timing of the initiation of antiretroviral therapy and the effect of this timing on overall survival remain controversial (32–37).

SCREENING FOR HIV INFECTION

Overview

When AIDS was first recognized in 1981, its diagnosis depended on the identification of a characteristic set of illnesses indicative of profound immune suppression. With the discovery in 1984 of the causative agent of AIDS, HIV-1, serologic tests for HIV infection appeared. When used appropriately, these tests make it possible to accurately and economically identify those destined to develop AIDS before the onset of symptoms. If these tests are used inappropriately, they needlessly increase health care costs and can wreak emotional and physical harm.

Knowledge of HIV status permits infected persons to seek medical treatment including antiretroviral agents, medications that decrease the risk of developing opportunistic infections, and periodic screening for early detection of medical problems associated with HIV infection (e.g., for tuberculosis skin testing). These measures can delay the onset of AIDS in infected persons and prolong the lives of persons with AIDS. Appropriate counseling, an essential part of screening for HIV infection, may help some individuals prevent HIV transmission by modifying their behavior.

Viral and Immunologic Response to HIV

After transmission of HIV there is usually a two to four week period before the acute retroviral syndrome develops (38,39). This illness, which is clinically similar to influenza, typically lasts one to two weeks and resolves spontaneously. It has been estimated that 40 to 60% of infected individuals experience this syndrome (40).

Coincident with the acute illness, high-grade viremia develops, usually measured by p24 antigenemia. Within two to three weeks from the onset of symptoms, antibodies to envelope glycoproteins and p24 antigen begin to appear. Approximately 50% of infected individuals will develop detectable antibody within two months, with 95% of individuals developing antibody within six months of initial infection (41). In close proximity to the appearance of antibody, p24 antigen rapidly declines, usually to undetectable levels. Serum antigen usually remains undetectable until much later in disease when it reemerges often in association with signs and symptoms of immune dysfunction. In the vast majority of individuals antibody will remain detectable for the remainder of their lives.

Testing Methods

Enzyme-Linked Immunosorbent Assay   Many methods can be used to determine whether an individual is infected with HIV-1. The most important methods in clinical practice measure serum antibodies directed against epitopes of HIV-1. HIV-1 antibody testing entered routine clinical use in early 1985 with the appearance of the first commercial antibody test (42). The test, an HIV-1 enzyme-linked immunosorbent assay (ELISA), uses viral antigens coated onto beads, microwells, or dipsticks. When serum or plasma from the test subject is added, anti–HIV-1 antibody, if present, is bound. After the excess is removed by washing, it can be probed by labeled antihuman antibody, the excess of which is removed by washing. This probe is capable of binding human antibody and is linked to an enzyme that cleaves a colorless substrate into a product with color. After the addition of the probe and removal of the excess, the colorless substrate is added. If anti–HIV-1 antibody is present, color will appear. The amount of color, measured spectrophotometrically, correlates with the amount of HIV-1 antibody present.

Although this testing method is easily automated, rapid, inexpensive, and particularly suited for testing large numbers of samples, it has a significant disadvantage—its potential to produce false positive reactions. Nonspecific binding of antibodies present in samples from subjects exposed to multiple infections or vaccines can lead to significant numbers of false positive reactions. In addition, antibodies to impurities in the antigen preparation can lead to cross-reactions and repeatedly false positive tests. This was a particular problem with HIV antigen derived from H9 cells because of HLA cross-reactivity. This potential to produce false positive reactions is the reason that confirmatory or supplementary tests are essential in HIV testing.

Western Blot   The Western blot has become the principle method of confirming HIV-1 infection in the United States. Relative to ELISA, Western blotting is slow, labor intensive, and significantly more costly but is able to measure multiple HIV-1 antibodies simultaneously. The test is performed by separating HIV-1 antigens electrophoretically on a polyacrylamide gel. This separates the antigens by size in a graded fashion along the gel. The proteins are then transferred onto nitrocellulose filter paper, which is then cut into strips. A strip is then incubated in the test subject's serum allowing anti–HIV-1 antibodies, if present, to bind to the HIV-1 antigens dispersed along the paper. Bound antibodies are then detected using a probe capable of binding human antibody, which contains an enzyme or radioactive element. After processing, bands will appear where antibody is bound to antigen. By comparing these bands with those produced by a positive control, it is possible to identify specific HIV-1 antigens that are present.

A universally accepted definition of a positive Western blot does not exist. Most definitions rely on the demonstration of bands from two or three major antigen groups, *gag* (p55, p24, p18), *pol* (p66, p51, p31), *env* (gp160, gp120, gp41). The CDC and the Association of State, Territorial and Public Health Laboratory Directors have established criteria that require the following (43–45):

Positive:	at least two of the bands p24, gp41, gp160/120
Negative:	no HIV-1 related bands
Indeterminate:	any HIV-1 related band(s) not meeting the criteria for a positive result

Currently, these are the most widely accepted criteria for confirming HIV-1 infection using Western blot.

Other Tests   In addition to ELISA and Western blot several other techniques have been used with variable success to test for HIV infection. These tests can be placed into three groups: 1) antibody assays, 2) tests for virus or viral components, and 3) surrogate marker tests.

Antibody assays such as radioimmunoprecipitation and indirect immunoprecipitation are time consuming, costly, and labor intensive. For these reasons they have not been widely adopted in the United States for HIV testing. Rapid antibody screening tests such as latex and red cell agglutination may have potential when used to test individuals in HIV-1 endemic areas but their accuracy in low-prevalence populations has yet to be established.

Tests for virus or viral components include virus culture, p24 antigen assays, and polymerase chain reaction (PCR) assays. Virus culture is time consuming, costly, difficult to standardize, and relatively insensitive. Assays for p24 antigen are hampered by the low prevalence of p24 antigen during the asymptomatic phase of HIV-1 infection. The major drawback to the use of PCR assays is their inherent propensity to produce false positive results. The slightest contamination of the reagents or test specimen can lead to an erroneous (false positive) result. This has occurred in laboratories with even the most experienced personnel.

Surrogate markers are so named because they do not directly test for virus or antibody to the virus. Commonly available surrogate marker tests include CD4 lymphocyte counts, β2-microglobulin and neopterin levels. These tests can be used effectively to assess prognosis among HIV-infected patients and to make therapeutic decisions regarding infection prophylaxis and the initiation of antiretroviral therapy. They should not be used as an indirect method of determining whether a patient is HIV infected.

Test Interpretation

When testing for the presence of HIV antibodies, it is also necessary to understand the antibody responses to HIV infection and the characteristics of ELISA and Western blot testing in detecting these antibodies. It is also necessary to have a thorough understanding of the concepts of sensitivity, specificity, positive predictive value, negative predictive value, and prevalence. A central theme to the appropriate use of HIV testing is that it be reserved for those individuals who are at increased risk of HIV infection. When applied to populations of low HIV prevalence the positive predictive value of HIV testing drops significantly.

The CDC currently recommend that serologic testing be performed in selected populations (46). Guidelines for selecting those who should be tested are given in Table 13.8. Testing should be offered in a supportive environment with appropriate counseling before and after the test is performed. It should be voluntary and should be accompanied by a formal informed consent (required in most states).

Table 13.8. CDC Recommendations for HIV Serologic Testing

Persons who have sexually transmitted diseases

High-risk individuals: IV drug users, sexually active homosexual and bisexual men, hemophiliacs, regular sexual partners of persons in these categories and persons with known HIV infection; lower incidence groups include prostitutes and persons who received transfusions during 1978–1985

Persons who consider themselves at risk or request the test

Women at risk who are of childbearing age or who are pregnant. Women at increased risk include: IV drug users; prostitutes; women who have had male sexual partners who are IV drug users, bisexual or HIV infected; women living in communities or born in countries with a high prevalence HIV infection in women; and women who received blood transfusions during 1978–1985

Individuals with clinical or laboratory findings suggesting HIV infection. These include generalized lymphadenopathy; unexplained dementia; chronic, unexplained fever or diarrhea; unexplained weight loss; or diseases that commonly complicate HIV infection such as chronic or generalized herpes, thrush, and recurrent or refractory vaginal candidiasis, oral hairy leukoplakia, and "opportunistic" tumors including Kaposi's sarcoma and B-cell lymphoma

Patients with active tuberculosis

Recipient and source of blood and body fluid exposures. Body fluids besides blood considered at risk include: semen, vaginal secretions, cerebrospinal fluid, synovial fluid, pleural fluid, peritoneal fluid, pericardial fluid, amniotic fluid and any bloody body fluid. Body fluids not considered at risk are feces, nasal secretions, sputum, saliva, sweat, tears, urine, and vomitus unless they contain visible blood.

Health care workers who perform exposure-prone invasive procedures

Patients who are 15–55 years of age and who are admitted to the hospital where the seroprevalence rate is $\geq 1\%$ or where AIDS patients account for $\geq 1/1000$ discharges

Donors of blood, semen, and organs

In general, results are reported as *positive, indeterminate,* or *negative.* When a blood sample is tested for HIV it is initially tested using an ELISA. If this test is negative, no further testing is done and the sample is reported as HIV *negative.* If the test is positive, a second ELISA is often performed and if this is positive, a Western blot is performed. There are several different standards by which HIV Western blot results are interpreted. These are discussed earlier in this chapter.

An *indeterminate* result most frequently occurs when a positive ELISA occurs in conjunction with a single band (usually p24) on Western blot. In high-risk individuals this may reflect ongoing seroconversion, but low-risk persons with this result are virtually never infected. Repeat testing should occur within 2 to 6 months of the initial indeterminate result. If the individual is HIV infected, a positive ELISA will usually be accompanied by two or more positive bands on Western blot. Among low-risk individuals the single band will frequently persist. In general, low-risk individuals with indeterminate test results should be reassured that HIV infection is very unlikely (47).

Because of the finite possibility of laboratory error or sample mislabeling, it may be advisable to repeat the test if a positive test result occurs. This is particularly important if the result occurs in an individual with no identifiable risk factor or when the result is obtained from an anonymous testing site.

False negative test results most frequently occur when testing occurs during the window period—usually 2 to 6 months after transmission. Data suggesting high rates of false negative test results have largely been refuted. Alternative methods of identifying HIV infection are available. These include PCR, culture, antigen detection (p24 antigen). These tests should not be used in place of antibody testing. In rare circumstances they may be useful adjuncts to antibody testing.

An essential part of HIV testing is the provision of HIV counseling. Careful instruction should be given to *all* patients in minimizing the risk of HIV transmission. Repeated testing of those who continue to practice high-risk behavior should be conducted periodically, typically at 6- to 12-month intervals.

Counseling

Accurate information regarding the medical, psychological, public health, and social implications of HIV infection should be provided in a sensitive manner. Repetition of this information is an essential component to effective counseling. Assisting the patient in understanding and accepting the changes in his or her sense of self and in life plans and goals is essential to caring for HIV-infected people. It is particularly important to educate the individual as much as possible about the disease and its treatment, so he or she will feel more in control of his or her life. It may be particularly helpful to focus on what the patient can do as opposed to what is out of his or her control. Giving information on long-term survival without implying that AIDS is always fatal is essential. Hope is still one of the strongest weapons we have.

Understanding the patient's existing support network and helping the patient develop additional supports can be very important. It is often helpful if the patient can share experiences with infected peers to minimize isolation, loneliness, fear of HIV infection, and associated issues.

In many communities there now exist special resources to aid HIV-infected patients with legal, social, and financial issues pertaining to the infection. It is important for every physician who cares for these individuals to identify these resources.

Finally, it is essential to discuss death and dying with each patient in an open manner. Often these issues are shunned by others in the patient's support network. The value of being able to get honest and direct answers about death and dying from one's physician cannot be underestimated. During these discussions the physician and patient should strive to come to a common understanding of the patient's wishes regarding this very important issue.

MANAGEMENT OF HIV INFECTION

Overview

The last decade has seen significant advancements in the management of HIV infection. The advances have come as much from a better understanding of the natural history of HIV infection as from new treatments for HIV itself.

Adult HIV infection follows a predictable course. This makes it possible to anticipate many of the complications of HIV infection and has resulted in the successful application of primary prophylaxis of PCP, *Toxoplasma gondii* encephalitis, *Mycobacterium tuberculosis*, and *Mycobacterium avium* complex (MAC) infections. A decade of research has allowed the mapping of laboratory and clinical data onto HIV disease stage. This staging is then used to make treatment decisions aimed at preventing complications and slowing the progression of HIV infection. Our improved understanding of the natural history of this disease has resulted also in case providers more rapidly recognizing HIV-associated complications. These advancements, taken in total, have led to improved survival and quality of life for those who are HIV infected.

As medications to prevent and treat HIV disease proliferate, however, patients are increasingly subjected to drug toxicities and adverse interactions. Managing these medications so as to avoid potential interactions and toxicities requires the careful consideration of laboratory and clinical data.

Laboratory Assessment

Markers of HIV Disease Progression   The staging of HIV infection is essential to its appropriate management. Several clinical and laboratory indicators are useful for this purpose. These indicators are called *surrogate markers* because they are meant to substitute for the end points of disease that have been used extensively in AIDS clinical trials. Surrogate markers have many potential uses, and if interpreted cautiously, may help guide individual treatment, as well as help identify promising new agents for therapy.

The most valuable *laboratory* tests in assessing prognosis in HIV-seropositive individuals are the absolute CD4 lymphocyte count (or percentage of CD4 lymphocytes), serum β_2-microglobulin (a cell surface glycoprotein that is elevated when mononuclear cells are activated and when there is rapid lymphocyte turnover), and serum neopterin (produced during guanosine triphosphate metabolism and increased when mononuclear cells are activated) [48]. Each of these has significant *independent* predictive power. The CD4 lymphocyte count remains the best single indicator of disease progression. Approximately 30% of patients with a cell count less than 200/mm³ develop AIDS within one year of such a finding. It is estimated that 50% of patients with a cell count between 200/mm³ and 400/mm³ develop AIDS within three years. Individuals with cell counts greater than 400/mm³ have about a 15% chance of developing AIDS within three years. However, recent analyses have indicated that the CD4 lymphocyte count is not a complete surrogate marker for death in persons with AIDS or advanced AIDS-related complex (49). Further, data suggest that a significant portion of the beneficial effect of zidovudine in delaying progression to advanced disease cannot be accounted for on the basis of CD4 lymphocyte count alone (50). Finally, CD4 lymphocyte count may be affected by cofactors, including coinfection with other viruses. Among these cofactors is HTLV-1. In a recent study coinfection with human HTLV-1 led to systematically higher CD4 lymphocyte counts at each stage of disease—an observation that may be particularly important for the management of HIV-infected intravenous drug users where coinfection is most common (51,52). Despite these facts, the absolute CD4 lymphocyte count remains the best laboratory marker currently available for advancing disease and death.

Proper interpretation of the CD4 lymphocyte counts requires an understanding of its biologic variation. A CD4 count diurnal increase of approximately 60 cells/mm^3 has been reported between 8 AM and 10 PM blood samples in individuals with Walter Reed stages 1 through 5 infection (15). Although this fluctuation is significantly blunted when compared with the approximately 500 cell/mm^3 change observed for HIV-seronegative individuals, it should be considered when evaluating CD4 measurements. Great variation can often exist within and among laboratories with regard to assessments of CD4 cells (53). This must always be considered when using these laboratory markers in making clinical decisions. In general, significant decisions about clinical care should not be made on the basis of a single CD4 lymphocyte measurement, and evaluation of changes should be made using the same laboratory.

Recent data suggest that the type of immune response that an individual generates to HIV may affect prognosis. TH-1 cells are a subset of CD4 lymphocytes that produce cytokines that assist cellular immune responses. TH-2 cells produce cytokines associated with humoral immune response. Several researchers have demonstrated that a switch from TH-1 response to a TH-2 response is linked to HIV disease progression (54–57). The clinical utility of these observations have yet to be fully delineated.

Viral quantitation can play a role in assessing prognosis. The most prevalent of these markers to date is serum HIV p24 antigen. Several commercial assays can be used to measure HIV p24 antigen. Each is slightly different, and this difference may play a role in assessing the value of this marker as a predictor of disease progression (58). Newer assays involving acid dissociation of p24 antigen appear to improve the sensitivity of this test (59,60). In general, detectable serum HIV p24 antigen can be found in 10 to 20% of HIV-seropositive individuals (61,62). It is often present in the days to weeks prior to seroconversion, then disappears only to reappear late in infection. Among a cohort of homosexual men followed for several years, approximately 5 to 7% developed p24 antigenemia per year (63). Although its presence or absence independently predicts progression to AIDS, the quantitative antigen level does not correlate well with progression. Thus, if it is to enter clinical decision-making, a very high p24 antigen level should be given no more weight than a moderately elevated p24 antigen level. Overall, p24 antigen is a poorer predictor of prognosis than the CD4 lymphocyte count, β_2-microglobulin, or neopterin level. Viral markers, for example, plasma viremia or HIV nucleic acid measurements by PCR technology, are not sufficiently standardized for general use at the current time.

Viral phenotype may also have value as a surrogate marker. One such phenotype marker is the syncytium-inducing capacity of the HIV strain. This refers to an in vitro property of the virus that leads cells in tissue culture to coalesce and is characterized by rapid killing. Several studies have suggested that disease progression occurs more rapidly in patients in whom isolates with the syncytium-inducing phenotype are found (64,65). As with the characterization of immune response, TH-1 versus TH-2, the clinical utility of viral phenotype in staging HIV infection has yet to be determined.

Additional Laboratory Studies   Infection with HIV predisposes individuals to anemia, neutropenia, and thrombocytopenia either as a consequence of the disease itself or the drugs used in treatment. Periodic evaluation of blood counts is essential. The frequency of these evaluations should increase as disease progresses and drug therapy is initiated. Table 13.9 lists many of the commonly performed laboratory tests on initial evaluation of an HIV-seropositive patient. Suggested follow-up laboratory evaluation is described in Table 13.10. If abnormalities in the complete blood cell count arise, it is important to evaluate these, including the assessment of serum iron, folate, and vitamin B_{12} levels when appropriate. A chemistry profile, including lactate dehydrogenase, can be helpful in diagnosing problems attributable to nutritional deficiency, liver disease, muscle disease, PCP, and lymphoma. In patients receiving pentamidine (aerosolized or intravenous), zalcitabine, and didanosine, periodic measurement of serum lipase or amylase is ap-

Table 13.9.   Initial Laboratory Evaluation of an HIV-Seropositive Patient

Complete blood count with differential
T-cell subsets
Electrolytes
Liver function tests, creatinine, blood urea nitrogen
Urinalysis
Syphilis serology
Hepatitis B surface antigen/core and surface antibodies
Human coronary virus antibody
Glucose-6-phosphate dehydrogenase deficiency screen
Papanicolaou (PAP) smear/colposcopy
Posteroanterior and lateral chest x-ray
Purified protein derivative (Mantoux) with anergy controls (two of the following:
    Candida albicans, tetanus toxoid, and mumps)
Serum *T. gondii* IgG antibody titer

Table 13.10. Suggested Laboratory Evaluation of HIV-Seropositive Patients

Test	Use	Typical Frequency
Complete blood count	Diagnosis of anemia, leukopenia, thrombocytopenia associated with HIV or related infections and medications	Asymptomatic individuals: q6–12mo Symptomatic individuals: q3–6mo (may need to be more frequent if the patient is taking zidovudine or other marrow toxic medications)
T-cell subsets	Treatment decisions regarding initiation of antiretroviral therapy and *P. carinii* prophylaxis Assessment of prognosis	q3–6mo
Chemistry	Diagnosis of complications of HIV infection and treatment	q2–6mo among symptomatic patients
	Assessment of nutritional status (e.g., Serum albumin, iron, vitamin B_{12}, etc.)	q12mo
Syphilis serology	Diagnosis of syphilis	As indicated by history
Cytomegalovirus (CMV) serology	Prevention of transfusion-transmitted CMV infections among CMV-seronegative patients	Prior to anticipated transfusions of cellular blood products
Papanicolaou smear/ colposcopy	Early detection of cervical neoplasia	q6–12mo
Purified protein derivative and anergy panel	Diagnosis of latent tuberculosis Guides choice of agent for *Pneumocytis carinii* pneumonia prophylaxis	q12mo until patient is anergic on two consecutive occasions

propriate because clinical and subclinical pancreatitis has been attributed to these drugs.

Serologic testing for syphilis should be conducted because coinfections occur and treatment of syphilis early in HIV infection may be more effective than late treatment. Although evidence is incomplete, the natural history of syphilis may be altered by HIV infection, and therefore, careful attention to past history and treatment for syphilis is necessary for proper management. In an individual who is positive for rapid plasma reagin and treponemal antibody and in whom a prior history of syphilis cannot be documented, further work-up including a lumbar puncture should be considered.

Toxoplasma IgG serology may aid in the diagnosis of brain lesions by identifying those at highest risk of developing cerebral toxoplasmosis. Approximately one third of individuals who have positive *T. gondii* IgG serology will develop symptomatic disease (66). However, *T. gondii* serology may be falsely negative in a significant portion of cases. In one recent review, *T. gondii* serology was negative in 13 of 80 patients with clinical toxoplasmosis (16%). Four of 18 patients with pathologically proved disease (22%) had undetectable antitoxoplasma IgG antibodies by indirect immunofluorescence assay (67). Thus, although the test has clinical utility in some circumstances, it is not foolproof. One interesting use of *T. gondii* serology is its use in identifying those individuals for primary prophylaxis. Data suggest that chemoprophylaxis is possible for those who have been previously exposed to *T. gondii*. Several studies are currently in progress to test various agents for this purpose.

Clinical Assessment

Markers of HIV Disease Progression Clinical markers can be used to identify individuals at high risk of disease progression. The most commonly cited *clinical* predictors of progression to AIDS are thrush, oral hairy leukoplakia, constitutional symptoms (sustained weight loss, fatigue, night sweats, and persistent diarrhea), anergy, and herpes zoster. Persistent generalized lymphadenopathy was once thought to be an important predictor of progression to AIDS in HIV-seropositive homosexual men, but this is no longer the case (68). Herpes zoster, although correlating with disease progression, has little predictive power. The 2-year progression rate to AIDS for men with herpes zoster is approximately 22% (61). This rate is only slightly higher than the rate in asymptomatic HIV-seropositive men (69). Thrush and oral hairy leukoplakia occur later in disease than herpes zoster and tend to be better predictors of progression to AIDS. Among the San Francisco General Hospital cohort of HIV-seropositive men, 39 and 42% of patients with thrush and oral hairy leukoplakia, respectively, progressed to AIDS over a two-year period (61). Within this same cohort, patients who experienced constitutional symptoms virtually all developed AIDS within 2 years. Anergy, another late manifestation of HIV infection, is a significant predictor of progression to AIDS, especially for patients with CD4 lymphocyte counts less than 400 cells/mm^3 (70).

Antiretroviral Therapy Zidovudine prolongs survival in patients with AIDS or advanced AIDS-related complex (ARC) and may delay the progression to AIDS among selected patients who do not yet have AIDS or advanced ARC. Current U.S. FDA recommendations include the use of 500 to 600 mg/d in divided doses at all stages of infection among individuals with fewer than 500

Table 13.11. Recommendations Regarding the Use of Antiretroviral Therapy for HIV-Infected Adults

Clinical Status	CD4 Lymphocyte Count (cells/mm³)	Recommendations
No Previous Antiretroviral Therapy		
Asymptomatic	>500	No therapy
Asymptomatic	200–500	Zidovudine or no therapy
Symptomatic	200–500	Zidovudine
Asymptomatic	<200	Zidovudine
Symptomatic	<200	Zidovudine
Previous Antiretroviral Therapy		
Stable	≥300	Continue zidovudine
Stable	<300	Continue zidovudine or change to didanosine
Progressing	50–500	Change to didanosine or zalcitabine
Progressing	<50	Change to didanosine or zalcitabine
Intolerant to Zidovudine		
Stable or progressing	<50	Change to didanosine or zalcitabine

CD4 cells/mm³. Recent data suggest that the use of zidovudine in patients with 400 to 750 CD4 cells/mm³ may delay progression of HIV infection (37). A large European trial, the Concorde trial, found no difference in survival or progression to advanced disease among asymptomatic individuals after a mean study period of 3 years (35,71). Recently, a retrospective analysis of a large randomized trial of zidovudine versus placebo conducted by the ACTG (protocol 019) found that among asymptomatic adults "the reduction in the quality of life due to severe side effects of therapy approximately equals the increase in the quality of life associated with a delay in the progression of HIV disease" (36). These data have led to great confusion among providers as to the most appropriate use of antiretrovirals in managing HIV-infected patients. To help relieve some of this confusion a consensus view has been developed through the National Institutes of Health. These recommendations are outlined in Table 13.11 (72).

Optimal zidovudine dosing is gradually being clarified. In a study of individuals with advanced HIV infection, a reduced dose of zidovudine (1200 mg/ d for 4 weeks followed by 600 mg/d in divided doses) was not statistically different with respect to delaying time to new opportunistic infections when compared with the much higher dose of 1500 mg/d. Further, the study demonstrated improved survival and less toxicity for those who received the lower dose (73). A second study compared zidovudine at doses of 400 mg, 800 mg, and 1200 mg/d in individuals with advanced HIV disease (74). No significant

Table 13.12. Estimates of the Frequencies of Adverse Reactions Associated with the Use of Antiretroviral Therapies in Adults

Drug (Typical Dosage)	Adverse Reaction	Time Course	Prevalence
zidovudine (AZT) (500 mg/d)	Insomnia	<2 wk	B
	Fever or rash	<2 wk	A
	Nausea	<1 mo	D
	Macrocytosis	>1 mo	E
	Anemia	>1 mo	B–C
	Neutropenia	>1 mo	B–C
	Nail pigmentation*	>1 mo	D
	Myopathy	>6 mo	B
ddI (167–375 mg b.i.d.)	Nausea/vomiting	<2 wk	B
	Hyperuricemia	<1 mo	A
	Pancreatitis	>2 mo	B
	Neuropathy	>3 mo	B–C†
ddC (0.375–0.75 mg t.i.d.)	Fever	<4 wk	B
	Rash	<4 wk	B
	Oral ulcers	<4 wk	B
	Neuropathy	>3 mo	C†
d4T (10–40 mg b.i.d.)	Neuropathy	N/A	C
	Anemia, leukopenia, thrombocytopenia	N/A	A
	Transaminase elevation	N/A	A
	Pancreatitis	N/A	A

A, <1%; B, 1–5%; C, 6–25%; D, 26–50%; E, 51–100%.

*Occurs with increased frequency among African American and Asian individuals.

†Peripheral neuropathy varies as a function of dosage schedule and duration of therapy.

differences were detected in survival or progression rates. Because the intracellular half-life of phosphorylated zidovudine is considerably longer than its serum half-life and because compliance is usually improved by less frequent dosing, it is frequently given in a daily dose of 600 mg (in three divided aliquots).

The principal adverse reactions associated with zidovudine result from bone marrow toxicity (Table 13.12). Anemia and neutropenia occur most frequently. Both the anemia and neutropenia tend to be more severe in more advanced stages of disease and are dose related. In most situations, especially among individuals who are started on zidovudine therapy while asymptomatic, the anemia is mild. It is frequently accompanied by an elevation in the mean corpuscular volume of as much as 30 to 40 Fl. A relatively small percentage of treated individuals, disproportionately represented by those with more advanced disease, may experience a more severe anemia. Evaluation of this anemia typically demonstrates a depressed reticulocyte count, normal serum folate level, and a normal serum vitamin B_{12} level. Bone marrow evaluation shows a low number of red cell precursors. Erythropoietin levels are usually elevated. This anemia may respond to zidovudine dose reduction. However, patients may require blood transfusion or a change in therapy.

Studies evaluating the use of erythropoietin in persons with AIDS have found a reduction in transfusion requirements among those whose endogenous erythropoietin levels at baseline were less than or equal to 500 IU/L (75–77). For individuals with baseline endogenous erythropoietin levels greater than 500 IU/L no reduction in transfusions was observed. Data regarding the use of erythropoietin in earlier stages of HIV infection are not yet available. Therefore, erythropoietin therapy should be reserved for persons with AIDS-associated anemia who have low endogenous erythropoietin levels.

The neutropenia associated with zidovudine use is dose related and becomes more significant in advanced disease. It may be worsened when a patient is placed on additional medications that are also capable of causing neutropenia. This is most frequently seen when patients develop cytomegalovirus (CMV) retinitis requiring ganciclovir therapy. Zidovudine therapy is usually discontinued while induction ganciclovir therapy is begun. Once maintenance ganciclovir therapy is underway it is possible in some patients to slowly reinstitute zidovudine therapy. Granulocyte-macrophage colony-stimulating factor (GM-CSF) or granulocyte colony-stimulating factor (G-CSF) may be useful in managing the neutopenia associated with therapies for HIV and related conditions (78,79). Laboratory data indicate that GM-CSF can promote HIV replication (80,81). Stimulation of HIV replication as a consequence of G-CSF exposure has not been observed. Limited in vitro data suggest that ganciclovir may antagonize the anti–HIV-1 activity of didanosine and zidovudine (82).

At the present time zidovudine, didanosine (ddI), and zalcitabine (ddC) are the only drugs approved by the FDA for the treatment of HIV infection. Zidovudine is the preferred initial monotherapy for antiretroviral naive patients (83,84). In general, didanosine and zalcitabine should be reserved for patients who are unable to tolerate or have "failed" zidovudine monotherapy. Few data are available to address whether didanosine or zalcitabine is superior as an alternative monotherapy in patients failing or intolerant to zidovudine. A recently completed trial suggested comparable effectiveness of didanosine or zalcitabine in terms of disease progression and minimally significant survival benefit in favor of zalcitabine (85). The choice as to the preferred alternative monotherapy is often heavily influenced by drug toxicities.

A fourth nucleoside analogue, d4T, has been made available to patients through a *parallel track program*. This program is intended to make d4T available to patients with advanced HIV infection for whom no satisfactory alternative antiretroviral therapy exists. These patients would include those who: 1) have failed therapy with zidovudine or demonstrated unmanageable intolerance to this therapy or for whom zidovudine is contraindicated *and* 2) have demonstrated failure or intolerance to ddI; *and* 3) are not experiencing drug-related neuropathy due to nucleoside therapy. An advisory committee to the FDA has recommended that it be approved for the treatment of HIV infection but could not give definitive guidelines for its use.

Combinations of antiretroviral agents have been studied and have yielded inconclusive results. The most extensively studied combinations have been pairs of nucleoside analogues (e.g., zidovudine/ddC and zidovudine/ddI), but other combinations involving different classes of drugs are also being studied. Combinations may inhibit the virus at different replicative sites or at the same site. The use of combinations may permit dose reduction of individual agents and reduce the emergence of drug resistance and ultimately prevent virus replication. In vitro data have demonstrated synergistic interactions with many combinations (e.g., zidovudine/didanosine, zidovudine/zalcitabine, zidovudine/didanosine/pyridinone, zidovudine/didanosine/nevirapine), whereas antagonism is seen with others (e.g., zidovudine/ribavirin). The use of some of these combinations may be limited by their overlapping toxicities (e.g., ddC and ddI) (86). Limited in vivo data suggest that some of these combinations can improve surrogate markers (e.g., CD4 lymphocyte count, p24 antigen), but data showing definitive clinical benefit are still lacking (87–91).

A final observation is necessary regarding the combination of acyclovir and zidovudine. Initial interest in this combination arose from a desire to prevent CMV disease in advanced HIV infection and a single report of acyclovir and zidovudine synergy against HIV in vitro (92). Such synergy has never been confirmed. Although there does not appear to be a decrease in the risk of developing CMV disease, several studies have now shown a survival advantage to those who receive acyclovir and zidovudine relative to zidovudine alone (93–95). The reason for this difference remains obscure.

Preventive Treatment

Vaccinations.   Individuals who are HIV seropositive should be properly immunized. Whenever possible, immunization should occur early in HIV infection so as to improve the response rates. Table 13.13 lists immunization recommendations for HIV-seropositive adults. Passive immunotherapy with immune serum globulin has been shown to reduce the frequency of bacterial infection in certain HIV-seropositive children (96). The routine use of immunoglobulin in adults is not currently recommended, however. For HIV-seropositive adults who are traveling to developing countries immune serum globulin should be given to diminish the risk of acquiring hepatitis A infection. Because immune globulin can interfere with the response to live vaccines, it should be given either 2 weeks after or 3 months before live measles or measles-mumps-rubella (MMR) vaccine.

Several contraindications to the use of vaccines should be noted. Because of the theoretical risk to the HIV-seropositive woman and the developing fetus, pregnant women or women likely to become pregnant within 3 months after vaccination should not be given live, attenuated-virus vaccines (MMR) (97). In general, vaccination of pregnant women should occur in the second and third

Table 13.13.   Recommendations for Vaccination of HIV-Seropositive Adults

Vaccine	Recommendations
Diphtheria-tetanus-pertussis	All patients: DT booster q10y
Inactivated polio vaccine	Persons who have never been immunized: three doses of enhanced potency inactivated vaccine Persons previously immunized who are traveling to developing countries; the patient should receive one dose of the inactivated vaccine.
MMR	Persons who were born after 1956: 1. who have not been immunized or 2. were immunized before 1980 and who have neither serologic evidence of infection nor a history of physician-diagnosed measles
Haemophilus influenzae B	Effectiveness uncertain; if given, single dose early in HIV infection
Pneumococcus	All patients: single dose early in HIV infection
Influenza virus	All patients: yearly
Hepatitis B	Patients who do not demonstrate antibody or antigen: series of 3 injections
Typhoid	Patients traveling to developing countries: inactivated parenteral typhoid vaccine; booster doses q3y
Meningococcus	Patients traveling to areas with recognized epidemics or to regions where such disease is endemic especially if prolonged contact with the populace is anticipated
Plague	Patients traveling to areas where there is a high probability of exposure
Japanese encephalitis	Patients traveling to endemic or epidemic areas
Cholera	Rarely indicated for patients traveling to developing countries; may be required by destination country
Rabies	Patients anticipating contact with uncommon wild animals or living for prolonged times in areas where rabies is prevalent
Yellow fever	Contraindicated
Bacille Calmette-Guérin	Contraindicated
Live oral typhoid	Contraindicated
Live oral polio	Contraindicated

SOURCE: Recommendations of the Advisory Committee on Immunization Practices (ACIP): use of vaccines and immune globulins for persons with altered immunocompetence. MMWR 1993.

trimester of pregnancy to minimize the risk of teratogenicity. Because of the risk of exposure to live polio virus by persons recently immunized, oral polio vaccine should not be given to anyone living in the household of an HIV-seropositive individual. There is no substantive evidence of risk to the fetus or HIV-seropositive woman from the use of inactivated virus or bacteria vaccines or toxoids (98).

A growing number of HIV-seropositive patients are sexually active women. Pregnant women should be tested for immunity to rubella. Susceptible women should be immunized immediately after delivery. Newborns of pregnant carriers of hepatitis B virus should receive hepatitis B immune globulin and the hepatitis B vaccine series shortly after delivery.

Chemoprophylaxis

Pneumocystis carinii *pneumonia*. The United States Public Health Service currently recommends prophylaxis for adults with a prior history of PCP, an absolute CD4 lymphocyte count of 200 cells/mm³ or less or when the CD4 lymphocyte count drops to 20% or less of total lymphocytes (99,100). It may also be appropriate to start PCP prophylaxis earlier if certain clinical signs are present. For example, the presence of thrush or fever in an individual with an absolute CD4 lymphocyte count between 200 and 300 cells/mm³ is indicative of an increased risk of developing PCP in the near future (101).

Once it has been determined that PCP prophylaxis is necessary, there are several regimens from which to choose. Many factors should enter into this treatment decision. Systemic therapy may have certain advantages over local therapy. Trimethoprim/sulfamethoxazole (TMP/SMX) may decrease not only the rate of recurrence of PCP but of other infections as well (e.g., isosporiasis and toxoplasmosis) (102). The presence of intrinsic lung disease may adversely affect the distribution of aerosolized pentamidine. Nonuniform distribution of aerosolized pentamidine may contribute to upper lobe pneumonitis with and without pneumothorax (103,104). In addition, rare cases of extrapulmonary *P. carinii* infections may occur more commonly in those receiving local therapy.

Toxicity of individual agents may affect choice of agent and may vary with stage of illness. TMP/SMX may be well tolerated in early HIV disease but may be poorly tolerated as disease advances. Trimethoprim is teratogenic in animals, whereas dapsone appears safe in pregnancy (105,106). Consequently, in a situation where a sexually active HIV-seropositive woman is in need of prophylaxis, dapsone may be a reasonable choice. Little is known about the teratogenicity of aerosolized pentamidine. Dapsone is inexpensive and because of its long half-life can be dosed less frequently (107). Care should be taken when using dapsone in combination with dideoxyinosine (ddI), however. Because dapsone is absorbed better in an acid environment, the current formulation of ddI, which is designed to neutralize gastric acidity, may interfere with absorption of dapsone. A high incidence of PCP has been noted in patients receiving dapsone prophylaxis concomitantly with ddI. It has been recommended that patients who are receiving both ddI and dapsone be advised to take dapsone two hours prior to ddI (108). Dapsone when used in combination with pyrimethamine is effective at preventing PCP and may have the added advantage of preventing first episodes of toxoplasmosis (109). Aerosolized pentamidine requires administration once per month but is frequently costly. Compliance may be improved by matching patient preferences to the medication used. Thus, the process of choosing chemoprophylaxis should be thought of as a dynamic one where several agents may be used for a single patient during the illness. Table 13.14 lists estimates of adverse reactions and relapse rates for dapsone, aerosolized pentamidine (300 mg monthly using a Respirgard II nebulizer or 60 mg q2wk by Fisoneb), and TMP/SMX in adults with HIV infection.

The preferred initial regimen is TMP/SMX (110–115). For those with histories of minor adverse reactions to TMP/SMX, "desensitization" should be considered (Table 13.15). For those who experience significant adverse reactions to TMP/SMX, dapsone is a reasonable alternative because cross-sensitivity is uncommon. Significant glucose-6-phosphate dehydrogenase (G-6-PD) deficiency may discourage the use of dapsone and TMP/SMX in some patients. The highest prevalence of this deficiency in the United States is among African American males (11%), females (3%; 20% are heterozygous), and individuals of Greek, Japanese, Indian, Southeast Asian, and Sephardic Jewish ancestry. In general, aerosolized pentamidine is better tolerated than either TMP/SMX or dapsone but should be considered a second-line alternative to these therapies.

Mycobacterium tuberculosis.   Most individuals who are infected with *M. tuberculosis* are asymptomatic, and disease most frequently represents recrudescence of infection. It is estimated that over 90% of persons reported to have clinical disease are those who have harbored *M. tuberculosis* infection for a year or more (116). The risk of developing active tuberculosis is elevated in HIV-seropositive individuals (117). Screening for *M. tuberculosis* is essential to identify infected persons at high risk of developing disease. These individuals would benefit from preventive therapy. Further, screening can identify persons with clinical disease in need of treatment. Although screening should include all HIV-seropositive individuals, it is particularly important for the homeless and for residents of correctional institutions, mental institutions, nursing homes, and other institutional settings.

Tuberculin skin testing is the most common method of identifying persons infected with *M. tuberculosis*. The administration of 5 units purified protein derivative (PPD) tuberculin intracutaneously (Mantoux test) is the recommended method. The test should be considered positive if the diameter of induration is greater than or equal to 5 mm (116). However, among individuals who show symptoms characteristic of HIV infection, both skin testing and a screening chest radiograph should be performed (116). This combination is recommended because of the higher probability of a false negative skin test result in this population. Table 13.16 lists those individuals who should receive

Table 13.14. Commonly Used Dosages, Adverse Reaction Rates, and Estimates of Relapse Rates for Three Commonly Used Agents for *P. carinii* Pneumonia Prophylaxis

Agent	Dosage	Estimates of Adverse Reaction Rate*	Points to Consider
trimethoprim/ sulfamethoxazole Relapse Rate: 5–10%/y	1DS tab/b.i.d.†	10–20%	Is often difficult to use concomitantly with zidovudine especially among patients with more advanced disease
dapsone Relapse Rate: 50–20%/y	50–100 mg/d	10–17%	May be particularly useful in pregnancy Long half-life may improve compliance Drug reaction to TMP/SMX does not necessarily indicate that a patient cannot take dapsone Concomitant administration with ddC or ddI may increase risk of developing peripheral neuropathy If taken concomitantly with ddI, dapsone should be taken 2 h prior to ddI
dapsone/pyrimethamine Relapse Rate: 5–20%	dapsone: 50 mg/d pyrimethamine: 50 mg/wk	24%	Comparable efficacy to aerosolized pentamidine May have added advantage of preventing *T. gondii* infection in those who have evidence of previous exposure Concomitant administration with ddC or ddI may increase risk of developing peripheral neuropathy If taken concomitantly with ddI, dapsone should be taken 2 h prior to ddI
aerosolized pentamidine Relapse Rate: 15–25%/y	300 mg/mo by Respirgard II Nebulizer or 60 mg q2wk by Fisoneb	5%	Intrinsic lung disease may decrease effectiveness Once monthly treatment may improve compliance Use may alter radiographic appearance of recrudescent disease and may decrease yield of bronchoalveolar lavage Positioning of patient during therapy may affect overall effectiveness

* necessitating discontinuation of medication
† lower doses or less frequent dosing may be equally effective with less toxicity

Table 13.15. Trimethoprim-sulfamethoxazole desensitization schedule

Trimethoprim-sulfamethoxazole pediatric suspension
0.1 cc (0.8 mg trimethoprim/4 mg sulfamethoxazole), P.O.
Double the dose every 2–3 days until full dose reached
Full dose = 20 cc of suspension or 1 DS table

Table 13.16. Persons Who Should Receive Isoniazid Chemoprophylaxis

HIV-infected individuals with a positive Mantoux test
HIV-infected individuals who are anergic and at high risk of tuberculosis (IV drug
  users, the homeless, inmates in correctional institutions, and migrant farm workers)
HIV-infected individual with high risk of tuberculosis regardless of PPD and anergy
  screens (118)
Household members of persons with active tuberculosis

chemoprophylaxis. They should receive this therapy for at least one year. Before therapy is initiated, sputum cultures should be obtained to exclude active pulmonary tuberculosis. The usual preventive therapy is isoniazid (10 mg/kg/d for children, 300 mg/d for most adults) plus pyridoxine. In some settings where the prevalence of isoniazid-resistant organisms is high, alternative chemoprophylaxis regimens should be considered. Patients with no evidence of active disease, a positive Mantoux test, and who have been exposed to multiply-resistant strains of tuberculosis, the CDC recommend that high-dose ethambutol and pyrazinamide, with or without a fluoroquinolone, should be used (119). Those who are unable to tolerate isoniazid may be given rifampin for 6 to 12 months (120).

Mycobacterium avium *complex*. *Mycobacterium avium* complex (MAC) is a common opportunistic infecting organism in advanced HIV infection in the United States. Disseminated MAC infection occurs predominately in patients with a CD4 lymphocyte count less than 100 cells/mm^3 (121). Nearly all patients with disease caused by MAC have positive mycobacterial blood cultures. Necropsy evidence of MAC infection can be found in over 50% of patients who die with AIDS. MAC can be found in the spleen, lymph nodes, liver, lung, adrenals, colon, kidney, and bone marrow. The most common symptoms associated with disseminated MAC infection are listed in Table 13.17. The symptoms fall into two general categories: generalized and gastrointestinal.

Recently, two controlled trials showed rifabutin (300 mg/d) reduces MAC bacteremia by approximately 50% (122). No difference was detected in survival between those given rifabutin prophylaxis and those given placebo. However, several symptoms associated with MAC infection were reduced. On the basis of these studies, the FDA recently approved rifabutin for prophylaxis of disseminated MAC infections among HIV-seropositive patients. The Public Health

Table 13.17. Clinical Syndromes of Disseminated *M. avium* Complex in AIDS

Generalized
Fever, fatigue, weight loss; pancytopenia when bone marrow involvement occurs
Gastrointestinal
Chronic diarrhea and abdominal pain
Chronic malabsorption
Extrabiliary obstructive jaundice secondary to periportal lymphadenopathy

Service recommends that rifabutin prophylaxis be given to patients with a CD4 lymphocyte count less than 100 cells/mm^3 (123). Should rifabutin prophylaxis be considered, one or more blood cultures for MAC should be obtained before prophylaxis is begun in patients with clinical or laboratory features suggestive of disseminated disease. This may decrease the likelihood of inadvertently selecting rifabutin-resistant mutants (124). Further, rifabutin resistance has the potential to lead to mycobacterial resistance to rifampin—one of the most important antituberculosis drugs. Thus, several investigators have recommended that a chest film and tuberculin skin test be performed on all patients being considered for rifabutin prophylaxis so as to exclude active tuberculosis (123). Due to the insensitivity of these tests, a careful examination of several sputa for acid-fast bacilli may be appropriate especially for those at higher risk of tuberculosis (125). Finally, there have been an increasing number of reports of uveitis associated with the use of rifabutin—especially at doses greater than 300 mg/d (126). Particular attention should be paid to the development of eye pain or visual disturbances while taking this drug. Rifabutin induces hepatic microsomal enzymes, which can lead to altered metabolism of many drugs, including oral contraceptives, dilantin, methadone, zidovudine, and warfarin. Careful attention to the possibility of such interactions is essential.

Other agents including the macrolides, clarithromycin and azithromycin, and clofazimine may be effective in preventing MAC infection; clinical trials are currently underway to assess these agents (127,128).

Herpes simplex. Reactivation herpes simplex infections are common, and although these infections are usually self-limiting early in the course of HIV infection, they may produce extensive and persistent ulcerative disease in individuals in whom immune suppression is more advanced. Thus, in individuals who have frequent bouts of overt herpes simplex, suppressive therapy using acyclovir may be warranted (200 mg three times each day or 400 mg twice daily) (129,130). The prolonged use of acyclovir has been associated with acyclovir-resistant herpes simplex from clinical isolates, particularly in immunocompromised hosts (131). It remains unclear whether prolonged continuous herpes simplex virus suppression by acyclovir results in a greater likelihood of developing resistant strains than its intermittent use to treat acute episodes. Among HIV-seropositive individuals who suffer frequent and severe episodes of herpes simplex infections, acyclovir suppression should be considered. If lesions recur or persist despite acyclovir suppression, consideration should be given to the possibility of acyclovir resistance.

Toxoplasma gondii. Toxoplasmosis may also be a preventable opportunistic infection in HIV-seropositive individuals. Data suggest that several agents might be effective in this role. In deciding which agent to use for the prevention of PCP, the *Toxoplasma* serostatus of an individual might be weighed. In addition to its ability to decrease the risk of developing PCP, TMP/SMX has anti-*T. gondii* activity (102). Several studies have now shown it to be effective at decreasing the risk of developing cerebral toxoplasmosis (110,114,115,132). Therefore, among those individuals who are *T. gondii* IgG seropositive and in whom there are no contraindications to the use of TMP/SMX, this drug may be an ideal choice for *P. carinii* prophylaxis. The combination of dapsone (50 mg/d) and pyrimethamine (50 mg/wk) also appears to be effective in preventing PCP and toxoplasmosis (109).

Fungal infections. Fungal disease is a frequent cause of morbidity and mortality among those who are HIV infected. Chief among the diseases caused by fungi are esophageal candidiasis, vaginal yeast infections, cryptococcal meningitis, disseminated histoplasmosis, and coccidioidomycosis.

Oropharyngeal, esophageal, and vaginal candidiasis are particularly common problems among those who are HIV infected (133,134). Topical and systemic agents can treat and suppress these infections but drug-resistant candidiasis caused by *Candida albicans*, *T. glabrata*, and *Candida krusei* is increasingly being reported (135–139). Because these infections usually respond rapidly to topical and systemic treatment, suppression is usually not necessary. However, when recurrent infections occur suppression may be useful (140–142). Topical agents such as nystatin and clotrimazole have been used frequently for this purpose. Evidence supporting their use for prophylaxis of oral and esophageal candidiasis in the HIV-infected adult is anecdotal. Fluconazole at doses of 50 to 100 mg/d or 150 mg weekly has been shown to suppress recurrent oral candidiasis (141–143). Data suggest that fluconazole is useful for the secondary prophylaxis of candidal esophagitis (140). Ketoconazole may be a less expensive alternative to fluconazole but it is absorbed less dependably and is less active against many *Candida* species.

Cryptococcosis is one of the most common opportunistic infections that HIV-infected individuals experience. Cryptococcal meningitis, the most common form of *Cryptococcus neoformans* infection in patients with AIDS, is one of the five most common causes of neurologic disease experienced by HIV-infected individuals (144). Fluconazole, a triazole with good penetration into cerebrospinal fluid (CSF), has been used to treat and suppress cryptococcal meningitis (145–150). Currently, fluconazole (200 mg/d) should be used to prevent relapse of cryptococcal meningitis in patients with AIDS who have completed primary therapy. Alternatives to this regimen include itraconazole (200 mg twice daily) or amphotericin B (1 mg/kg weekly) (151). It should be kept in mind, however, that itraconazole does not penetrate the CSF well and that amphotericin B appears to be clearly inferior to fluconazole as maintenance therapy.

Disseminated histoplasmosis occurs in up to 25% of patients with AIDS living in endemic areas (152). The mortality rate is approximately 50% (153). Maintenance therapy is required. For this purpose itraconazole (200 mg twice daily) has been effective and should be considered first-line maintenance therapy (154). Amphotericin B (1 to 1.5 mg/kg weekly) is a reasonable alternative to itraconazole but has significantly greater toxicity (155). Data supporting the use of fluconazole as an alternative to itraconazole are lacking.

Coccidioidomycosis is an unusual infection among patients with AIDS outside of endemic areas (southwestern United States). In areas endemic for *Coccidioides immitis*, however, the incidence of this infection among these patients may be quite high (156). Fluconazole (400 mg/d) or itraconazole (200 mg twice daily) may be used for maintenance therapy but the data supporting the use of these agents are limited (152,157).

Management of Opportunistic Infections

Pneumocystis carinii *pneumonia*.   *Pneumocystis carinii* pneumonia has been the most frequent AIDS-defining diagnosis reported to the CDC. The development of PCP is a sign of significant immune impairment and is evidence of more advanced disease (AIDS). Much has been learned about the treatment and prevention of PCP in HIV-infected patients. This may account for the fact that the incidence of the disease is decreasing. Therapies for the treatment of PCP are listed in Table 13.18.

Therapy with TMP/SMX (15 to 20 mg/kg/d based on trimethoprim content) remains the preferred treatment regimen for PCP. The drug may be given orally or intravenously. If given intravenously the drug should be diluted in 150 mL of 5% dextrose in water and given over 30 to 60 minutes every 6 hours. The minimum necessary duration of treatment has not been established. Typically 14 to 21 days of therapy are used depending on the clinical course.

Dapsone/trimethoprim is an effective treatment of PCP and is better tolerated than TMP/SMX (158,159). Studies supporting the use of dapsone/trimethoprim are small, and therefore, may not detect significant differences between trial therapies. As a consequence, this regimen should be reserved for people with mild to moderately severe PCP.

Based on small studies and anecdotal experience, primaquine/clindamycin is an effective treatment for PCP (160,161). Clindamycin can be given orally or intravenously. G-6-PD deficiency is a contraindication to the use of this combination. In general, primaquine/clindamycin is reserved for the treatment of mild PCP.

Pentamidine at a dosage of 3 to 4 mg/kg/d has been used successfully to treat PCP. Pentamidine is not absorbed from the gastrointestinal tract and thus must be given parenterally (usually intravenously). Intravenous administration

Table 13.18. Drugs Commonly Used in the Treatment of *P. carinii* Pneumonia in Persons with AIDS

Drug	Typical Dosage	Comments
trimethoprim/ sulfamethoxazole	15–20 mg/kg/d based on trimethoprim content	Should be considered first-line therapy
pentamidine	3–4 mg/kg/d	Reasonable alternative to TMP/SMX; careful monitoring of serum glucose and blood pressure required
dapsone/ trimethoprim	100 mg/d of dapsone; 15–20 mg/kg/d of trimethoprim in 4 divided doses	Used primarily for mild to moderate PCP; usually better tolerated than TMP/SMX and pentamidine
primaquine/ clindamycin	15 mg/d of primaquine base; 450–900 mg of clindamycin given q6h	Methemoglobin levels should be monitored. This is especially true if PCP is more severe as this can contribute significantly to tissue hypoxia.
trimetrexate	30–45 mg/m²/d	Major toxicities include neutropenia, thrombocytopenia, and increased hepatic enzymes. Must be given with leucovorin. May be a reasonable alternative for patients with severe disease who are unable to tolerate TMP/SMX or pentamidine IV.
atovaquone (566C80)	2250 mg/d in 3 divided doses	Should be taken with food because this increases its absorption significantly. May be poorly absorbed in patients with diarrhea and should be avoided in this situation.

should be carefully performed in a setting where proper monitoring of blood pressure and serum glucose can occur. The drug should be dissolved in 250 mL of 5% dextrose in water and administered at a constant infusion rate over at least one hour. The dosing interval should be increased for patients with impaired renal function. The minimum duration of treatment with pentamidine has not been established in a systematic fashion, but in one retrospective analysis 21 days of therapy appeared superior to 14 days (162).

Trimetrexate has recently been approved by the FDA for the treatment of PCP. This drug is a powerful antifolate drug that binds to the dihydrofolate reductase of *P. carinii*. Concurrent therapy with leucovorin attenuates its hematologic toxicity. In a phase III multicenter trial of the ACTG, trimetrexate was compared to TMP/SMX in patients with severe episodes of PCP [(A-a)DO$_2$ > 30 mm Hg]. In this study, there was no statistically significant difference between the two drugs during treatment. However, at 7 weeks into the study, a statistically significant difference in mortality appeared (16 ± 4% for TMP/SMX versus 29 ± 5% for trimetrexate). The mortality attributable to PCP was not different, however. Trimetrexate is a reasonable alternative for patients with severe pneumonia who cannot tolerate TMP/SMX or pentamidine.

Atovaquone, a hydroxynaphthoquinone, was recently approved by the FDA for treatment of PCP. Atovaquone is variably absorbed and requires a fatty meal to enhance absorption. Thus, its use in patients who are anorexic or who have significant diarrhea should be avoided. Therapeutic failure with this agent has been associated with low plasma levels of the drug. Atovaquone is a reasonable alternative to treatment with TMP/SMX in patients who are intolerant of the latter compound. It is tolerated better than TMP/SMX but appears to be less effective (163). Unpublished data reveal a similar effectiveness when atovaquone is compared to pentamidine (164). A new suspension formulation of atovaquone is currently being evaluated and promises to be more consistently and completely absorbed than the current tablet. An intravenous formulation is also being developed.

Several studies have found survival benefit when corticosteroids are used in patients with PCP who have significant a-A gradients. These reports led to National Institutes of Health (NIH) consensus recommendations on the use of corticosteroids in HIV-infected patients with PCP. These recommendations are summarized in Table 13.19.

Toxoplasma gondii *encephalitis.* *Toxoplasma gondii* is a major cause of opportunistic infection of the central nervous system (CNS) among patients with advanced HIV infection. It is the most frequent cause of focal intracerebral lesions in patients with AIDS. The lung, eye, heart, peritoneum, stomach, pancreas, colon, pituitary, adrenal glands, testes, and muscle may also be involved. Eighty percent of patients who develop CNS toxoplasmosis have CD4 counts of less than 100 cells/mm^3 (165,166).

Table 13.19. NIH Consensus Conference Recommendations for the Use of Corticosteroids in the Treatment of *P. carinii* Pneumonia

Corticosteroid therapy should be given to all patients with proven PCP who have an arterial oxygen tension < 70 mm Hg on room air or an a-A gradient > 35 mm Hg.
Steroid therapy should be started within 72 h of initiation of antipneumocystis therapy.
The dosage should be 40 mg oral prednisone or the equivalent of methylprednisolone given IV b.i.d. on days 1 through 5, 40 mg given daily on days 6 through 10, and 20 mg given daily on days 11 through 21.
The diagnosis of PCP should be confirmed rapidly.

Serologic testing for IgG antibody to *T. gondii* can be helpful in determining who may be at risk for disease. Approximately one third of HIV-infected individuals who have IgG antibody to *T. gondii* will develop toxoplasmosis during their lifetime (167). Unfortunately, the lack of IgG antibody does not always rule out this diagnosis. In one recent study, up to 22% of biopsy-proven cerebral toxoplasmosis cases were IgG negative (67). IgM and IgA *Toxoplasma* antibodies are seldom helpful in diagnosis.

Neuroimaging studies can be helpful in differentiating *T. gondii* infection of the CNS from CNS lymphoma, two conditions often difficult to differentiate. In general, CNS toxoplasmosis will appear as numerous ring-enhancing lesions (usually greater than three), whereas CNS lymphoma usually has fewer than three lesions. Magnetic resonance imaging is more sensitive for CNS lesions and therefore is often helpful in identifying the most accessible lesion for brain biopsy should this become necessary.

The standard treatment of *T. gondii* infection is pyrimethamine and sulfadiazine (or other trisulfapyrimidines) (168). This combination, given with folinic acid to decrease the likelihood of bone marrow toxicity associated with pyrimethamine, is frequently poorly tolerated and a change in dosage or therapy is required in 40% of patients (67). The combination of pyrimethamine and clindamycin is the most extensively studied alternative regimen. In two prospective controlled trials of clindamycin and pyrimethamine, no significant difference in clinical outcome was observed when compared to pyrimethamine and sulfadiazine (169,170). Table 13.20 lists currently recommended therapy for *T. gondii* encephalitis in patients with AIDS.

Several investigational agents hold promise in the treatment of *T. gondii* infection. These include several of the new macrolides (including azithromycin, roxithromycin and clarithromycin) and atovaquone. Studies are also underway

Table 13.20. Guidelines for Therapy of Central Nervous System Toxoplasmosis in Patients with AIDS

Primary Therapy	
pyrimethamine	200 mg loading dose, then 50–75 mg
and	PO daily
folinic acid	10–50 mg PO daily
plus	
sulfadiazine *or*	1.0–1.5 g PO q6h
clindamycin	600–900 mg PO or IV q6h
Maintenance Therapy	
pyrimethamine	25–50 mg PO daily
folinic acid	10–20 mg PO daily
plus	
sulfadiazine *or*	500 mg PO q6h
clindamycin	300 mg PO q6h

Table 13.21. Features of Tuberculosis in Advanced HIV Infection

Pulmonary
Common
  Hilar and/or mediastinal adenopathy
  Localized infiltrate in lower and middle lung fields
Unusual
  Cavitation
  Apical infiltrate

Extrapulmonary
  Peripheral lymph nodes and bone marrow are the extrapulmonary sites most likely
    to harbor *M. tuberculosis*
  M. tuberculosis can also be found in blood, bone, urine, joint, liver, spleen, CSF,
    skin, gastrointestinal mucosa, and ascites
  Important syndromes: tuberculoma, *M. tuberculosis* bacteremia

to determine the usefulness of interferon-gamma and interleukin-2 as adjunctive therapy.

Mycobacterium tuberculosis. To date, evidence suggests that most cases of tuberculosis among patients with symptomatic HIV infection are due to reactivation. There are several important differences between tuberculosis as it presents in those who are HIV seronegative and those who have symptomatic HIV infection. In general, the risk of developing active tuberculosis is higher for those who are HIV infected. When it occurs it is more rapidly progressive and more likely to be extrapulmonary. Table 13.21 lists some of the important clinical features of tuberculosis in advanced HIV infection.

Anergy is common among patients with advanced HIV infection (>5 mm of induration to PPD is considered evidence of tuberculous infection). Among those with symptomatic HIV infection 10 to 40% of patients will be anergic at the time of diagnosis of tuberculosis. Although tuberculin skin testing should still be performed, it is essential that appropriate specimens be obtained. These might include sputum, urine, blood, lymph node material, bone marrow, and liver. Acid-fast bacilli found in a sputum smear is the main indicator of a potential for transmitting *M. tuberculosis*. The presence of a pulmonary cavity on chest radiograph further heightens the risk of transmission.

Chest radiographs of patients infected with pulmonary tuberculosis and HIV are remarkable for their infrequent cavitation and increased frequency of lower lobe infiltrates, miliary infiltrates, pleural effusions, and adenopathy. Upper lobe disease, typical of adults with reactivation disease, occurs primarily in HIV-infected patients who are not profoundly immunodeficient.

Mycobacterial culture methods have traditionally depended on seeing mycobacterial growth on solid media. A more rapid radiometric culturing method has been developed (BACTEC) and has significantly decreased the period of time for the detection of mycobacteria.

The response rate of these patients to antituberculous therapy is generally as favorable as in HIV-negative patients, provided multiple drug resistance is not present. Treatment failures with standard regimens of two to four drugs have been uncommon. Although multiple drug resistant strains are unusual, several recent outbreaks have been reported in New York City and Miami.

The CDC recommend initiating antituberculous chemotherapy whenever acid-fast bacilli are found in a specimen from a patient with HIV infection and clinical evidence of mycobacterial disease. Because it is often difficult to distinguish MAC from *M. tuberculosis*, therapy should continue until culture results are final. Recently, nucleic acid hybridization assays using specific probes for *M. tuberculosis* and *M. avium*, and other mycobacterial species, have significantly decreased this waiting period, often to a matter of days.

In areas where drug resistance rates are less than 4%, the currently recommended adult regimen includes oral isoniazid 300 mg/d, rifampin 600 mg orally daily, and pyrazinamide 25 mg/kg/d for the first 2 months. Ethambutol 25 mg/kg/d should be added if extrapulmonary tuberculosis is suspected. In all other areas treatment should include the standard three-drug regimen plus ethambutol or streptomycin (15 mg/kg/d). After the initial treatment period isoniazid and rifampin should be continued for at least 9 months or 6 months after culture conversion, whichever is longer. For those with bone or joint disease, therapy should continue for 18 months. If isoniazid or rifampin resistance is present, therapy should continue for at least 12 months beyond culture conversion and should include pyrazinamide. If there is a reasonable possibility of resistance to isoniazid and rifampin, the initial drug regimen should include isoniazid, rifampin, pyrazinamide, and additional second-line drugs or quinolones so that the patient is receiving at least three drugs to which local multidrug resistant *M. tuberculosis* strains are likely to be susceptible (171). The appropriate duration of therapy is not known currently. The CDC recommend that patients with drug-resistant *M. tuberculosis* infection should receive directly observed therapy and that susceptibility testing be performed on all isolates (171).

Mycobacterium avium *complex*. The treatment of disseminated MAC infection has improved markedly in the last decade. No single class of drugs has contributed more to this improvement than the macrolides, clarithromycin and azithromycin. Recent studies have found significantly decreased quantitative blood cultures of MAC in patients treated with regimens containing clarithromycin (127,128,172). However, in vitro resistance to clarithromycin can occur quickly when clarithromycin is used alone. For this reason clarithromycin-containing combinations of drugs are presently being studied.

Other antimicrobial agents including ciprofloxacin, ofloxacin, sparfloxacin, and liposome-encapsulated aminoglycosides are also being studied in the treatment of disseminated MAC infection. In addition, various cytokines (interleukin-2, interferon-γ, GM-CSF) are also being studied in combination with conventional antimicrobial agents (173–176).

Table 13.22. Dosing of Ganciclovir during Induction and Maintenance Therapy

Induction	5 mg/kg IV q12h × 14–21 days*
Maintenance	5 mg/kg IV qd or 6 mg/kg IV 5 d/wk*

* Administer as a 1-h infusion.

Cytomegalovirus infection. One of the most important opportunistic infections affecting people with advanced HIV infection is CMV. CMV antibody can be found in over 95% of HIV-infected homosexual men and approximately 75% of HIV-infected heterosexuals. Among HIV-infected patients, CMV disease occurs almost exclusively in those with CD4 lymphocyte counts less than 100 cells/mm^3 (with more than 75% of cases occurring in those with CD4 lymphocyte counts less than 50 cells/mm^3). Thus, CMV is a "late" opportunist in this patient population. The organs most frequently affected by CMV are the retina and gastrointestinal tract, and less commonly the nervous system, lungs, adrenals, and biliary system.

Ganciclovir (DHPG) was the first antiviral agent approved by the FDA for the treatment of CMV disease. At the present time ganciclovir is available only for intravenous infusion (Table 13.22). The induction dose is 5 mg/kg administered intravenously every 12 hours but must be adjusted for creatinine clearance. Lifelong maintenance therapy is required to delay reactivation. The drug is given twice daily during initial induction (usually lasting 2 to 3 weeks), whereas maintenance therapy is usually given once daily (5 mg/kg administered intravenously once daily).

The most serious adverse effect of ganciclovir is neutropenia. Approximately 40% of ganciclovir recipients experience neutrophil counts less than 1000 cells/mm^3. Ten to 20% of patients develop neutrophil counts of under 500 cells/mm^3. The dosage should be reduced when the neutrophil count drops below 750 cells/mm^3. Recent data from uncontrolled trials of G-CSF and GM-CSF in patients with dose-limiting neutropenia suggest that coadministration of recombinant myeloid colony-stimulating factors can permit continued ganciclovir treatment. Both drugs can cause profound increases in neutrophil counts. In general, G-CSF is preferred over GM-CSF because of its lesser toxicity including pain at the site of injection, fever, arthralgias, and myalgias. Dosage is adjusted according to response.

Foscarnet was the second antiviral drug to be approved by the FDA for the treatment of CMV disease. Data suggest that in patients with good renal function foscarnet is as effective as ganciclovir in the treatment of CMV retinitis and that there may be improved survival attributable to the use of foscarnet rather than ganciclovir (177,178). The recommended initial therapy with foscarnet is 60 mg/kg administered intravenously every 8 hours (preliminary data suggest that 90 mg/kg given every 12 hours may also be effective). Maintenance therapy with foscarnet is usually 90 to 120 mg intravenously daily or 5 d/wk.

The drug is distributed widely throughout the body and is cleared primarily via the kidneys. The dose must be adjusted for creatinine clearance.

The most common serious adverse effect of foscarnet is nephrotoxicity. This can occur in 10 to 25% of patients and can necessitate dialysis in rare instances. Intravenous sodium loading has been reported to reduce the risk of nephrotoxicity with this drug. Hypocalcemia is also a common serious toxicity of foscarnet therapy. Foscarnet combines with free, unbound calcium, resulting in transient ionized hypocalcemia. This may lead to the occasional arrhythmias, seizures, and mental status changes. A self-limited hyperphosphatemia and mild anemia can occur. Hypokalemia, hypomagnesemia, and nephrogenic diabetes insipidus have been reported. Dermatologic reactions to foscarnet have occurred including a generalized erythematous rash and oral and penile ulcerations (179–182).

Lethal overdose of this drug has occurred and for this reason foscarnet must be administered intravenously via an infusion pump. Serum creatinine, calcium, magnesium, potassium, and hemoglobin should be monitored two to three times per week during induction therapy and weekly during maintenance. Nephrotoxic drugs such as aminoglycosides, amphotericin B, and parenteral pentamidine should be avoided, especially during foscarnet induction therapy.

Due to the eventual emergence of CMV resistant to monotherapy using ganciclovir or foscarnet, interest has developed in combination therapy. In vitro data suggest that ganciclovir and foscarnet behave synergically against CMV (183). Early in vivo data indicate this approach may be effective and well tolerated (184–188). Other experimental compounds are being studied for treatment or prophylaxis of CMV infection. These include oral ganciclovir, BW256U (an acyclovir precursor), and CMV immunoglobulin. Ganciclovir ocular implants are being studied for the treatment of CMV retinitis and may be useful for local control of CMV infection (189).

REFERENCES

1 **Rosenberg RS, Biggar RJ, Goedert JJ.** Declining age at HIV infection in the United States. N Engl J Med 1994;330:789–790.

2 Heterosexually acquired AIDS—United States, 1993. MMWR 1994;43:155–160.

3 Update: acquired immunodeficiency syndrome—United States, 1991. MMWR 1992;41:463–468.

4 HIV immunodeficiency and AIDS—Georgia, 1991. MMWR 1992;41:876–878.

5 **Osmond D, et al.** Changes in AIDS survival time in two San Francisco cohorts of homosexual men, 1983 to 1993. JAMA 1994;271:1083–1087.

6 Zidovudine for the prevention of HIV transmission from mother to infant. MMWR 1994;43:285–287.

7 **National Institute of Allergy and Infectious Diseases.** Clinical alert: important therapeutic information on the benefit of zidovudine for the prevention of the transmission of HIV from mother to infant. 1994.

8 **Fitzgibbon JE, Gaur S, Frenkel LD, et al.** Transmission of human immunodeficiency virus type 1 with a zidovudine-resistance mutation. N Engl J Med 1993; 329:1835–1841.

9 **Hermans P, Sprecher S, Clumeck N.**

Primary infection with zidovudine-resistant HIV. N Engl J Med 1993;329:1123. (Letter).

10 **Masquelier B, Lemoigne E, Pellegrin I, et al.** Primary infection with zidovudine-resistant HIV. N Engl J Med 1993;329: 1123–1124. (Letter).

11 **Sonnerburg A, Johansson B, Ayehanie S, et al.** Transmission of zidovudine-resistant HIV-1. AIDS 1993;7: 1684–1685. (Letter).

12 **Tokars JI, Marcus R, Culver DH, et al.** Surveillance of HIV infection and zidovudine use among health care workers after occupational exposure to HIV-infected blood. The CDC Cooperative Needlestick Surveillance Group. Ann Intern Med 1993; 118:913–919.

13 **Gerberding J.** Is antiretroviral treatment after percutaneous HIV exposure justified? Ann Intern Med 1993;118:979–980. (Editorial).

14 1993 Revised classification system for HIV infection and expanded surveillance case definition for AIDS among adolescents and adults. MMWR 1993;41(RR-17):1–19.

15 **Malone JL, Simms TE, Gray GC, et al.** Sources of variability in repeated T-helper lymphocyte counts from human immunodeficiency virus type 1-infected patients: total lymphocyte count fluctuations and diurnal cycle are important. J Acquir Immune Defic Syndr 1990;3:144–151.

16 **Update:** CD4+ T-lymphocytopenia in persons without evident HIV infection— United States. MMWR 1992;41:578–579.

17 **Fauci AS.** CD4+ T-lymphocytopenia without HIV infection—no lights, no camera, just facts. N Engl J Med 1993; 328:429–431. (Editorial; Comment).

18 **Spira TJ, Jones BM, Nicholson JK, et al.** Idiopathic CD4+ T-lymphocytopenia— an analysis of five patients with unexplained opportunistic infections. N Engl J Med 1993;328:386–392.

19 **Sheppard H, Winkelstein W, Lang W, et al.** CD4+ T-lymphocytopenia without HIV infection. N Engl J Med 1993;328: 1847–1848. (Letter).

20 **Smith DK, Neal JJ, Holmberg SD.** Unexplained opportunistic infection and CD4+ T-lymphocytopenia without HIV infection: an investigation of cases in the United States. N Engl J Med 1993; 328:373–379.

21 **Laurence J.** CD4+ T-lymphocytopenia without HIV infection. N Engl J Med 1993;328:1848–1849. (Letter).

22 **Duncan RA, von Reyn RC, Alliegro GM, et al.** Idiopathic CD4+ T-lymphocytopenia—four patients with opportunistic infections and no evidence of HIV infection. N Engl J Med 1993; 328:393–398.

23 **Ho DD, Cao Y, Zhu T, et al.** Idiopathic CD4+ T-lymphocytopenia—immunodeficiency without evidence of HIV infection. N Engl J Med 1993;328:380–385.

24 **Laurence J, Siegal FP, Schattner E, et al.** Acquired immunodeficiency without evidence of infection with human immunodeficiency virus types 1 and 2. Lancet 1992;340(8814):273–274.

25 **Castro A, Pedreira J, Soriano V, et al.** Kaposi's sarcoma and disseminated tuberculosis in HIV-negative individual. Lancet 1992; 339 (8797):868. (Letter).

26 **Friedman KAE, Saltzman BR, Cao YZ, et al.** Kaposi's sarcoma in HIV-negative homosexual men. Lancet 1990;335(8682): 168–169. (Letter).

27 **Jacobs JL, Libby DM, Winters RA, et al.** A cluster of *Pneumocystis carinii* pneumonia in adults without predisposing illnesses. N Engl J Med 1991;324:246–250.

28 **Lemp GF, Payne SF, Neal D, et al.** Survival trends for patients with AIDS. JAMA 1990;263:402–406.

29 **Hamilton JD, Hartigan PM, Simberkoff MS, et al.** A controlled trial of early versus late treatment with zidovudine in symptomatic human immunodeficiency virus infection. Results of the Veterans Affairs Cooperative Study. N Engl J Med 1992; 326:437–443.

30 **Fischl MA, Richman DD, Hansen N, et al.** The safety and efficacy of zidovudine (AZT) in the treatment of subjects with mildly symptomatic human immunodeficiency virus type 1 (HIV) infection. A double-blind, placebo-controlled trial. The AIDS Clinical Trials Group. Ann Intern Med 1990;112:727–737.

31 **Volberding PA, Lagakos SW, Koch MA, et al.** Zidovudine in asymptomatic human immunodeficiency virus infection. A controlled trial in persons with fewer than 500 CD4-positive cells per cubic millimeter. The AIDS Clinical Trials Group of the National Institute of Allergy and Infectious Diseases. N Engl J Med 1990;322: 941–949.

32 **Corey L, Fleming TR.** Treatment of HIV infection—progress in perspective. N Engl J Med 1992;326:484–486. (Editorial).

33 **Vella S, Giulliano M, Pezzotti P, et al.** Survival of zidovudine-treated patients

with AIDS compared with that of contemporary untreated patients. Italian Zidovudine Evaluation Group. JAMA 1992;267:1232–1236.

34 Vella S, Giuliano M, Dally LG, et al. Long-term follow-up of zidovudine therapy in asymptomatic HIV infection: results of a multicenter cohort study. The Italian Zidovudine Evaluation Group. J Acquir Immune Defic Syndr 1994;7:31–38.

35 Seligmann M, Warrell DA, Aboulker JP, et al. Concorde: MRC/ANRS randomised double-blind controlled trial of immediate and deferred zidovudine in symptom-free HIV infection. Lancet 1994;343:871–881.

36 Lenderking WR, Gelber RD, Cotton DJ, et al. Evaluation of the quality of life associated with zidovudine treatment in asymptomatic human immunodeficiency virus infection. N Engl J Med 1994;330:738–743.

37 Cooper DA, Garell JM, Kroon S, et al. Zidovudine in persons with asymptomatic HIV infection and CD4+ cell counts greater than 400 per cubic millimeter. The European-Australian Collaborative Group. N Engl J Med 1993;329:297–303.

38 Clark SJ, Saag MS, Decker WD, et al. High titers of cytopathic virus in plasma of patients with symptomatic primary HIV-1 infection. N Engl J Med 1991;324:954–960.

39 Fox R, Eldred LJ, Fuchs EJ, et al. Clinical manifestations of acute infection with human immunodeficiency virus in a cohort of gay men. AIDS 1987;1:35–38.

40 Hulsebosch HJ, Claassen FAP, van Ginkel CJW, et al. Human immunodeficiency virus exanthem. J Am Acad Dermatol 1990;23:483–486.

41 Horsburgh CRJ, Ou CY, Jason J, et al. Duration of human immunodeficiency virus infection before detection of antibody. Lancet 1989;2 (8664):637–640.

42 Update: Serologic testing for antibody to human immunodeficiency virus. MMWR 1987;36:833.

43 Interpretation and use of the Western blot assay for serodiagnosis of human immunodeficiency virus type 1 infections. MMWR 1989;38:1–7.

44 The Consortium for Retrovirus Serology Standardization. Serological diagnosis of human immunodeficiency virus infection by Western blot testing. JAMA 1988;260:674–679.

45 O'Gorman MRG, Weber D, Landis SE, et al. Interpretive criteria of the Western blot assay for serodiagnosis of human immunodeficiency virus type 1 infection. Arch Pathol Lab Med 1991;115:26–30.

46 Public Health Service guidelines for counseling and antibody testing to prevent HIV infection and AIDS. MMWR 1987; 36:509–515.

47 Jackson JB, MacDonald KL, Cadwell J, et al. Absence of HIV infection in blood donors with indeterminate Western blot tests for antibody to HIV-1. N Engl J Med 1990;322:217–222.

48 Fahey JL, Taylor JM, Detels R, et al. The prognostic value of cellular and serologic markers in infection with human immunodeficiency virus type 1. N Engl J Med 1990;322:166–172.

49 DeGruttola V, Wulfsohn M, Fischl MA, et al. Modeling the relationship between survival and CD4 lymphocytes in patients with AIDS and AIDS-related complex. J Acquir Immune Defic Syndr 1993;6:359–365.

50 Choi S, Lagakos SW, Schooley RT, et al. CD4+ lymphocytes are an incomplete surrogate marker for clinical progression in persons with asymptomatic HIV infection taking zidovudine. Ann Intern Med 1993;118:674–680.

51 Schechter M, Harrison LH, Halsey NA, et al. Coinfection with human T-cell lymphotropic virus type I and HIV in Brazil. Impact on markers of HIV disease progression. JAMA 1994; 271:353–357.

52 Volberding PA. HIV, HTLV-I, and CD4+ lymphocytes. Troubles in the relationship. JAMA 1994;2:392–393. (Editorial).

53 Sax PE, Boswell SL, White GM, et al. Clinical implications of interlaboratory variability in CD4 cell counts in patients with HIV infection. Int Conf AIDS 1993; 9:557 (Abstract no. PO-B43-2532).

54 Clerici M, Shearer GM. A TH1 → TH2 switch is a critical step in the etiology of HIV infection. Immunol Today 1993;14:107–111.

55 Shearer GM, Clerici M. T helper cell immune dysfunction in asymptomatic, HIV-1-seropositive individuals: the role of TH1-TH2 cross-regulation. Chem Immunol 1992;54:21–43.

56 Shearer G, Clerici M. TH1 and TH2 cytokine production in HIV infection. Int Conf AIDS 1992;8:We53 (Abstract no. WeA 1047).

57 Vyakarnam A, Matear PM, Martin SJ, et al. HIV replication inhibited by TH1 but

not TH2 CD4+ T cell clones specific for HIV-1 gag p24. Int Conf AIDS 1993;9:31 (Abstract no. WS-A15-2).

58 **Bremer JW, Haywood MD, Chu L, et al.** Which HIV antigen EIA do you use? Your therapeutic and clinical evaluations may depend upon the choice. In: Sixth International Conference on AIDS. San Francisco, 1990.

59 **Bollinger RCJ, Kline RL, Francis HL, et al.** Acid dissociation increases the sensitivity of p24 antigen detection for the evaluation of antiviral therapy and disease progression in asymptomatic human immunodeficiency virus-infected persons. J Infect Dis 1992;165:913–916.

60 **Lillo FB, Cao Y, Concedi DR, et al.** Improved detection of serum HIV p24 antigen after acid dissociation of immune complexes. AIDS 1993; 7:1331–1336.

61 **Moss AR, Bacchetti P, Osmond D, et al.** Seropositivity for HIV and the development of AIDS or AIDS related condition: three year follow up of the San Francisco General Hospital cohort. Br Med J 1988;296:745–750.

62 **de Wolf F, Goudsmit J, Paul DA, et al.** Risk of AIDS related complex and AIDS in homosexual men with persistent HIV antigenaemia. Br Med J 1987;295:569–572.

63 **Polk BF, Fox R, Brookmeyer R.** Predictors of AIDS in a cohort of seropositive homosexual men. N Engl J Med 1987;316:61.

64 **Janvier B, Mallet F, Cheynet V, et al.** Zidovudine resistance, syncytium-inducing phenotype, and HIV disease progression in a case-control study. The VA Cooperative Study Group. J Acquir Immune Defic Syndr 1993;6:891–897.

65 **Koot M, Keet IP, Vos AH, et al.** Prognostic value of HIV-1 syncytium-inducing phenotype for rate of CD4+ cell depletion and progression to AIDS. Ann Intern Med 1993;118:681–688.

66 **Grant IH, Gold JMW, Armstrong D.** Risk of CNS toxoplasmosis in patients with AIDS. In 26th Interscience Conference on Antimicrobial Agents and Chemotherapy. New Orleans, 1986.

67 **Porter SB, Sande MA.** Toxoplasmosis of the central nervous system in the acquired immunodeficiency syndrome. N Engl J Med 1992;327:1643.

68 **Osmond D, Chaisson R, Moss A, et al.** Lymphadenopathy in asymptomatic patients seropositive for HIV. N Engl J Med 1987;317:246. (Letter).

69 **Greenspan H, Greenspan JS, Hearst NG, et al.** Relation of oral hairy leukoplakia

to infection with HIV and the risk of developing AIDS. J Infect Dis 1987;155(3): 475.

70 **MacDonell KB, Chmiel JS, Goldsmith J, et al.** Prognostic usefulness of the Walter Reed staging classification for HIV infection. J Acquir Immune Defic Syndr 1988; 1:367–374.

71 **Aboulker JR, Swart AM.** Preliminary analysis of the Concorde trial. Lancet 1993;341:889–890.

72 **Sande MA, Carpenter CC, Cobbs CG, et al.** Antiretroviral therapy for adult HIV-infected patients. Recommendations from a state-of-the-art conference. National Institute of Allergy and Infectious Diseases State-of-the-Art Panel on Anti-Retroviral Therapy for Adult HIV-Infected Patients. JAMA 1993; 270:2583–2589.

73 **Fischl MA, Parker CB, Pettinelli C, et al.** A randomized controlled trial of a reduced daily dose of zidovudine in patients with the acquired immunodeficiency syndrome. The AIDS Clinical Trials Group. N Engl J Med 1990; 323: 1009–1014.

74 Double blind dose-response study of zidovudine in AIDS and advanced HIV infection. Nordic Medical Research Councils' HIV Therapy Group. Br Med J 1992;304:13–17.

75 **Fischl M, Galpin JE, Levine JD, et al.** Recombinant human erythropoietin for patients with AIDS treated with zidovudine. N Engl J Med 1990;322:1488–1493.

76 **Henry DH, Jemsek JG, Levin AS, et al.** Recombinant human erythropoietin and the treatment of anemia in patients with AIDS or advanced ARC not receiving ZDV. J Acquir Immune Defic Syndr 1992;5:847–848. (Letter).

77 **Lancaster DJ, Palte S, Ray D.** Recombinant human erythropoietin in the treatment of anemia in AIDS patients receiving concomitant amphotericin B and zidovudine. J Acquir Immune Defic Syndr 1993;6:533–534. (Letter).

78 **Kaplan LD, Kahn JO, Crowe S, et al.** Chemotherapy with or without GM-CSF in patients with AIDS-associated non-Hodgkin's lymphoma. In: Fifth International Conference on AIDS. Montreal, 1989. Abstract.

79 **Grossberg HS, Bonnem EM, Buhles WC.** GM-CSF with ganciclovir for the treatment of CMV retinitis in AIDS. N Engl J Med 1989;320:1560. (Letter).

80 **Pluda JM, Yarchoan R, Smith PD, et al.** Subcutaneous recombinant granulocyte-

macrophage colony-stimulating factor used as a single agent and in an alternating regimen with azidothymidine in leukopenic patients with severe human immunodeficiency virus infection. Blood 1990;76:463–472.

81 **Hammer SM, Gillis JM, Pinkston P, et al.** Effect of zidovudine and granulocyte-macrophage colony-stimulating factor on human immunodeficiency virus replication in alveolar macrophages. Blood 1990; 75:1215–1219.

82 **Medina DJ, Hsiung GD, Mellors JW.** Ganciclovir antagonizes the anti-human immunodeficiency virus type 1 activity of zidovudine and didanosine in vitro. Antimicrob Agents Chemother 1992;36: 1127–1130.

83 **Kahn JO, Lagakos SW, Richman DD, et al.** A controlled trial comparing continued zidovudine with didanosine in human immunodeficiency virus infection. The NIAID-AIDS Clinical Trials Group [ACTG 116B/117]. N Engl J Med 1992; 327:581–587.

84 **Remick S, Follansbee S, Olson R, et al.** Safety and tolerance of zalcitabine in a double-blind comparative trial. In: Ninth International Conference on AIDS. Berlin, Germany, 1993.

85 **Abrams DI, Goldman AI, Launer C, et al.** A comparative trial of didanosine or zalcitabine after treatment with zidovudine in patients with human immunodeficiency virus infection. The Terry Beirn Community Programs for Clinical Research on AIDS. N Engl J Med 1994;330: 657–662.

86 **LeLacheur SF, Simon GL.** Exacerbation of dideoxycytidine-induced neuropathy with dideoxyinosine. J Acquir Immune Defic Syndr 1991;4:538–589.

87 **Meng TC, Fischl MA, Boota AM, et al.** Combination therapy with zidovudine and dideoxycytidine in patients with advanced human immunodeficiency virus infection. A phase I/II study. Ann Intern Med 1992;116:13–20.

88 **Fauci AS.** Combination therapy for HIV infection: getting closer. Ann Intern Med 1992;116:85–86. (Editorial).

89 **Relter WM, Berger DS, Vorce D.** Combination zidovudine and didanosine therapy for patients remaining persistently HIV p24 antigenpositive despite zidovudine monotherapy. In: VIIIth International Conference on AIDS. Amsterdam, 1992.

90 **Yarchoan R, Lietzau JA, Nguyen BY, et al.** A randomized pilot study of alternating or simultaneous zidovudine and didanosine therapy in patients with symptomatic human immunodeficiency virus infection. J Infect Dis 1994;169:9–17.

91 **Collier AC, Coombs RW, Fischl MA, et al.** Combination therapy with zidovudine and didanosine compared with zidovudine alone in HIV-1 infection. Ann Intern Med 1993;119: 786–793.

92 **Mitsuya H, Broder S.** Strategies for antiviral therapy in AIDS. Nature 1987; 325:773–778.

93 **Cooper DA, Pehrson PO, Pedersen C, et al.** The efficacy and safety of zidovudine alone or as cotherapy with acyclovir for the treatment of patients with AIDS and AIDS-related complex: a double-blind randomized trial. European-Australian Collaborative Group. AIDS 1993;7:197–207.

94 **Youle MS, Gazzard BG, Johnson MA, et al.** Effects of high-dose oral acyclovir on herpesvirus disease and survival in patients with advanced HIV disease: a double-blind, placebo-controlled study. AIDS 1994;8:641–649.

95 **Salvato P, Thompson C, Stroud S, et al.** Zidovudine alone versus zidovudine and acyclovir as treatment for patients with HIV disease. Int Conf AIDS 1992;8: 2441.

96 **Intravenous immune globulin for the prevention of bacterial infections in children with symptomatic human immunodeficiency virus infection.** The National Institute of Child Health and Human Development Intravenous Immunoglobulin Study Group. N Engl J Med 1991; 325:73–80.

97 **Recommendations of the Advisory Committee on Immunization Practices (ACIP): use of vaccines and immune globulins for persons with altered immunocompetence.** MMWR 1993:42(RR-4):1–18.

98 **General recommendations on immunization [published erratum appears in MMWR 1989 May 5;38:311].** MMWR 1989; 38:205–214.

99 **Guidelines for prophylaxis against** *Pneumocystis carinii* **pneumonia for persons infected with human immunodeficiency virus.** MMWR 1989;5:1–9.

100 **Recommendations for prophylaxis against** *Pneumocystis carinii* **pneumonia for persons infected with human immunodeficiency virus.** U.S. Public Health Service Task Force on Antipneumocystis

Prophylaxis in Patients with Human Immunodeficiency Virus Infection. J Acquir Immune Defic Syndr 1993;6:46–55.

101   Phair J, Hoepelman AI, Eeftinck SJK, et al. The risk of *Pneumocystis carinii* pneumonia among men infected with human immunodeficiency virus type 1. Multicenter AIDS Cohort Study Group. N Engl J Med 1990;322:161–165.

102   Carr A, Tindall B, Brew BJ, et al. Low-dose trimethoprim-sulfamethoxazole prophylaxis for toxoplasmic encephalitis in patients with AIDS. Ann Intern Med 1992;117:106–111.

103   Abd AG, Nierman DM, Ilowite JS, et al. Bilateral upper lobe *Pneumocystis carinii* pneumonia in a patient receiving inhaled pentamidine prophylaxis. Chest 1988;94:329–331.

104   Jules-Elysee KM, Stover DE, Zaman MB, et al. Aerosolized pentamidine: effect on diagnosis and presentation of *Pneumocystis carinii* pneumonia. Ann Intern Med 1990;112:750–756.

105   Kahn G. Dapsone is safe during pregnancy. J Am Acad Dermatol 1985;13:838–839. (Letter).

106   Tuffanelli DL. Successful pregnancy in a patient with dermatitis herpetiformis treated with low-dose dapsone. Arch Dermatol 1982;118:876. (Letter).

107   Jorde UP, Horowitz HW, Wormser GP. Utility of dapsone for prophylaxis of *Pneumocystis carinii* pneumonia in trimethoprim-sulfamethoxazole-intolerant, HIV-infected individuals. AIDS 1993;7:361–367.

108   Safety information about dapsone and ddI. 1991, AIDS Clinical Trials Group.

109   Girard PM, Landman R, Gaudebout C, et al. Dapsone-pyrimethamine compared with aerosolized pentamidine as primary prophylaxis against *Pneumocystis carinii* pneumonia and toxoplasmosis in HIV infection. The PRIO Study Group. N Engl J Med 1993;328:1514–1520.

110   Schneider MM, Hoepelman AI, Eeftinck SJK, et al. A controlled trial of aerosolized pentamidine or trimethoprim-sulfamethoxazole as primary prophylaxis against *Pneumocystis carinii* pneumonia in patients with human immunodeficiency virus infection. The Dutch AIDS Treatment Group. N Engl J Med 1992;327:1836–1841.

111   Carr A, Tindall B, Penny R, et al. Trimethoprim-sulphamethoxazole appears more effective than aerosolized pentamidine as secondary prophylaxis against *Pneumocystis carinii* pneumonia in patients with AIDS. AIDS 1992;6:165–171.

112   Ruskin J, LaRiviere M. Low-dose co-trimoxazole for prevention of *Pneumocystis carinii* pneumonia in human immunodeficiency virus disease. Lancet 1991;337:468–471.

113   Martin MA, Cox PH, Beck K, et al. A comparison of the effectiveness of three regimens in the prevention of *Pneumocystis carinii* pneumonia in human immunodeficiency virus-infected patients. Arch Intern Med 1992;152:523–528.

114   Wormser GP, Horowitz HW, Duncanson FP, et al. Low-dose intermittent trimethoprim-sulfamethoxazole for prevention of *Pneumocystis carinii* pneumonia in patients with human immunodeficiency virus infection. Arch Intern Med 1991;151:688–692.

115   Hardy WD, Feinberg J, Finkelstein DM, et al. A controlled trial of trimethoprim-sulfamethoxazole or aerosolized pentamidine for secondary prophylaxis of *Pneumocystis carinii* pneumonia in patients with the acquired immunodeficiency syndrome. AIDS Clinical Trials Group Protocol 021. N Engl J Med 1992;327:1842–1848.

116   Screening for tuberculosis and tuberculous infection in high-risk populations. Recommendations of the Advisory Committee for Elimination of Tuberculosis. MMWR 1990;39:1–7.

117   Selwyn PA, Hartel D, Lewis DA, et al. A prospective study of the risk of tuberculosis among intravenous drug users with HIV infection. N Engl J Med 1989;320:545.

118   Jordan TJ, Lewit EM, Montgomery RL, et al. Isoniazid as preventive therapy in HIV-infected intravenous drug abusers. A decision analysis. JAMA 1991; 265:2987–2991.

119   Management of persons exposed to multidrug-resistant tuberculosis. MMWR 1992;41(RR-11):61–71.

120   A double-blind placebo-controlled clinical trial of three antituberculosis chemoprophylaxis regimens in patients with silicosis in Hong Kong, Hong Kong Chest Service/Tuberculosis Research Centre, Madras/British Medical Research Council. Am Rev Respir Dis 1992; 145:36–41.

121   Ellner JJ, Goldberger MJ, Parenti DM. *Mycobacterium avium* infection and AIDS: a therapeutic dilemma in rapid evolution. J Infect Dis 1991;163:1326–1335.

122 Nightingale SD, Cameron DW, Gordin FM, et al. Two controlled trials of rifabutin prophylaxis against *Mycobacterium avium* complex infection in AIDS. N Engl J Med 1993;329:828–833.

123 Masur H. Special Report: Recommendation on prophylaxis and therapy for disseminated *Mycobacterium avium* complex disease in patients infected with the human immunodeficiency virus. N Engl J Med 1993;329:898–903.

124 Bernard EM, Edwards FF, Kiehn TE, et al. Activities of antimicrobial agents against clinical isolates of *Mycobacterium haemophilum*. Antimicrob Agents Chemother 1993;37:2323–2326.

125 Reichman LB, McDonald RJ, Mangura BT. Rifabutin prophylaxis against *Mycobacterium avium* complex infection. N Engl J Med 1994;330:437–438. (Letter).

126 Shafran SD, Deschene J, Miller M, et al. Uveitis and pseudojaundice during a regimen of clarithromycin, rifabutin, and ethambutol. MAC Study Group of the Canadian HIV Trials Network. N Engl J Med 1994;330:438–439. (Letter).

127 Dautzenberg B, Saint MT, Meyohas MC, et al. Clarithromycin and other antimicrobial agents in the treatment of disseminated *Mycobacterium avium* infections in patients with acquired immunodeficiency syndrome. Arch Intern Med 1993;153:368–372.

128 Dautzenberg B, Truffot C, Legris S, et al. Activity of clarithromycin against *Mycobacterium avium* infection in patients with the acquired immune deficiency syndrome. A controlled clinical trial. Am Rev Respir Dis 1991;144:564–569.

129 Straus SE, Seidlin M, Takiff H, et al. Oral acyclovir to suppress recurring herpes simplex virus infections in immunodeficient patients. Ann Intern Med 1984;100:522–524.

130 Douglas JM, Critchlow C, Benedetti J, et al. A double-blind study of oral acyclovir for suppression of recurrences of genital herpes simplex virus infection. N Engl J Med 1984; 310:1551–1556.

131 Sacks SL, Wanklin RJ, Reece DE, et al. Progressive esophagitis from acyclovir-resistant herpes simplex. Clinical roles for DNA polymerase mutants and viral heterogeneity? Ann Intern Med 1989;111:893–899.

132 Tournerie C, Charreau I. Cotrimoxazole (TMP-SMX) for primary prophylaxis of *Toxoplasma* encephalitis in advanced HIV patients. The MRC/ANRS International Coordinating Committee for the European Australian Alpha Trial. Int Conf AIDS 1993;9:56 (Abstract no. WS-B13-2).

133 Carpenter CC, Mayer KH, Fisher A, et al. Natural history of acquired immunodeficiency syndrome in women in Rhode Island. Am J Med 1989; 771–775.

134 Tavitian A, Raufman JP, Rosenthal LE. Oral candidiasis as a marker for esophageal candidiasis in the acquired immunodeficiency syndrome. Ann Intern Med 1986;104:54–55.

135 Stellbrink HJ, Albrecht H, Fenske S, et al. *Candida krusei* sepsis in HIV infection. AIDS 1992;6:746–748. (Letter).

136 Sanguineti A, Carmichael JK, Campbell K. Fluconazole-resistant *Candida albicans* after long-term suppressive therapy. Arch Intern Med 1993;153:1122–1124.

137 Warnock DW, Burke J, Cope NJ, et al. Fluconazole resistance in *Candida glabrata*. Lancet 1988;2(8623):1310. (Letter).

138 Powderly WG. Mucosal candidiasis caused by non-albicans species of *Candida* in HIV-positive patients. AIDS 1992;6:604–605. (Letter).

139 Redondo-Lopez V, Lynch M, Schmitt C, et al. *Torulopsis glabrata* vaginitis: clinical aspects and susceptibility to antifungal agents. Obstet Gynecol 1990;76:651–655.

140 Lavilla P, Gil A, Valencia ME, et al. Fluconazole preventive therapy for candida esophagitis in AIDS. San Francisco: University of California, 1990:238.

141 Stevens DA, Greene SI, Lang OS. Thrush can be prevented in patients with acquired immunodeficiency syndrome and the acquired immunodeficiency syndrome-related complex. Randomized, double-blind, placebo-controlled study of 100-mg oral fluconazole daily. Arch Intern Med 1991;151:2458–2464.

142 Leen CL, Dunbar EM, Ellis ME, et al. Once-weekly fluconazole to prevent recurrence of oropharyngeal candidiasis in patients with AIDS and AIDS-related complex: a double-blind placebo-controlled study [published erratum appears in J Infect 1990;21:183]. J Infect 1990;21:55–60.

143 Just-Nubling G, Gentschew G, Meissner K, et al. Fluconazole prophylaxis of recurrent oral candidiasis in HIV-positive patients. Eur J Clin Microbiol Infect Dis 1991;10:917–921.

144 Chuck SL, Sande MA. Infections with

Cryptococcus neoformans in the acquired immunodeficiency syndrome. N Engl J Med 1989;321:794–799.

145 Powderly WG, Saag MS, Cloud GA, et al. A controlled trial of fluconazole or amphotericin B to prevent relapse of cryptococcal meningitis in patients with the acquired immunodeficiency syndrome. The NIAID AIDS Clinical Trials Group and Mycoses Study Group. N Engl J Med 1992;326:793–798.

146 Stern JJ, Hartman BJ, Sharkey P, et al. Oral fluconazole therapy for patients with acquired immunodeficiency syndrome and cryptococcosis: experience with 22 patients. Am J Med 1988;85:477–480.

147 Stern JJ, Pietroski NA, Ruckley RM, et al. Parenteral and oral fluconazole for acute cryptococcal meningitis in AIDS: experience with thirteen patients. Ann Pharmacother 1992; 26:876–882.

148 Larsen RA, Leal MA, Chan LS. Fluconazole compared with amphotericin B plus flucytosine for cryptococcal meningitis in AIDS. Ann Intern Med 1990;113:183–187.

149 Saag MS, Powderly WG, Cloud GA, et al. Comparison of amphotericin B with fluconazole in the treatment of acute AIDS-associated cryptococcal meningitis. The NIAID Mycoses Study Group and the AIDS Clinical Trials Group. N Engl J Med 1992; 326:83–89.

150 Sugar AM, Saunders C. Oral fluconazole as suppressive therapy of disseminated cryptococcosis in patients with acquired immunodeficiency syndrome. Am J Med 1988;85:481–489.

151 DeGans J, Eefinek schattenkerk JKM, VanKetel RJ. Itraconazole as maintenance treatment for cryptococcal meningitis in the acquired immune deficiency syndrome. Br Med J 1988;290:559.

152 Gallant JE, Moore RD, Chaisson RE. Prophylaxis for opportunistic infections in patients with HIV infection. Ann Intern Med 1994;120:932–944.

153 Graybill JR. Histoplasmosis and AIDS. J Infect Dis 1988;158:623–628.

154 Wheat J, Hafner R, Wulfsohn M, et al. Prevention of relapse of histoplasmosis with itraconazole in patients with the acquired immunodeficiency syndrome. The National Institute of Allergy and Infectious Diseases Clinical Trials and Mycoses Study Group Collaborators. Ann Intern Med 1993;118:610–616.

155 McKinsey DS, Gupta MR, Riddler SA, et al. Long-term amphotericin B therapy for disseminated histoplasmosis in patients with AIDS. Ann Intern Med 1989;111:655–659.

156 Bronnimann DA, Adam RD, Galgiani JN, et al. Coccidioidomycosis in the acquired immunodeficiency syndrome. Ann Intern Med 1987;106:372–379.

157 Galgiani JN, Catawzaro A, Cloud GA, et al. Fluconazole therapy for coccidioidal meningitis. The NIAID-Mycoses Study Group. Ann Intern Med 1993;119:28–35.

158 Medina I, Mills J, Leoung G, et al. Oral therapy for *Pneumocystis carinii* pneumonia in the acquired immunodeficiency syndrome. N Engl J Med 1990;323: 776–782.

159 Leoung GS, Mills J, Hopewell PC, et al. Dapsone-trimethoprim for *Pneumocystis carinii* pneumonia in the acquired immunodeficiency syndrome. Ann Intern Med 1986; 105:45–48.

160 Black JR, Feinberg J, Murphy RL, et al. Clindamycin and primaquine as primary treatment for mild and moderately severe *Pneumocystis carinii* pneumonia in patients with AIDS. Eur J Clin Microbiol Infect Dis 1991;10:204–207.

161 Noskin GA, Murphy RL, Black JR, et al. Salvage therapy with clindamycin/ primaquine for *Pneumocystis carinii* pneumonia. Clin Infect Dis 1992;14:183–188.

162 Haverkos HW. Assessment of therapy for *Pneumocystis carinii* pneumonia. Am J Med 1984;76:501–508.

163 Hughes W, Leoung G, Kramer F, et al. Comparison of atovaquone (566C80) with trimethoprim-sulfamethoxazole to treat *Pneumocystis carinii* pneumonia in patients with AIDS. N Engl J Med 1993;328:1521–1527. (See Comments).

164 Smith GH. Treatment of infections in the patient with acquired immunodeficiency syndrome. Arch Intern Med 1994;154: 949–973.

165 Eliaszewicz M, Lecomte I, De Sa M. Relation between decreasing serial CD4 lymphocyte counts and outcome of toxoplasmosis in AIDS patients: a basis for primary prophylaxis. Int Conf AIDS 1990;6:242 (Abstract no. Th.B.481).

166 Matheron S, Dournon E, Garakhanian S, et al. Prevalence of toxoplasmosis in 365 AIDS and ARC patients before and during zidovudine treatment. Int Conf AIDS 1990;6:241 (Abstract no. Th.B.476).

167 Grant IH, Gold JWM, Rosenblum M, et al. *Toxoplasma gondii* serology in HIV-infected patients: the development of central nervous system toxoplasmosis in AIDS. AIDS 1990;4:519–521.

168 Luft BJ, Remington JS. Toxoplasmic encephalitis in AIDS. Clin Infect Dis 1992; 15:211–222.

169 Katlama C. Evaluation of the efficacy and safety of clindamycin plus pyrimethamine for induction and maintenance therapy to toxoplasmic encephalitis in AIDS. Eur J Clin Microbiol Infect Dis 1991;10:189–191.

170 Dannemann BR, McCutchan JA, Israelski DM, et al. Treatment of toxoplasmic encephalitis in patients with AIDS: a randomized trial comparing pyrimethamine plus clindamycin to pyrimethamine plus sulfonamides. Ann Intern Med 1992;116:33–43.

171 Initial therapy for tuberculosis in the era of multidrug resistance. Recommendations of the Advisory Council for the Elimination of Tuberculosis [published erratum appears in MMWR 1993;42:536]. MMWR 1993;42(RR-7):1–8.

172 Young LS, Wiriott L, Wu M, et al. Azithromycin for treatment of *Mycobacterium avium-intracellulare* complex infection in patients with AIDS. Lancet 1991;338(8775):1107–1109.

173 Bermudez LE, Martinelli J, Petrofsky M, et al. Recombinant granulocyte-macrophage colony-stimulating factor enhances the effects of antibiotics against *Mycobacterium avium* complex infection in the beige mouse model. J Infect Dis 1994;169:575–580.

174 Bermudez LE, Inderlied C, Young LS. Stimulation with cytokines enhances penetration of azithromycin into human macrophages. Antimicrob Agents Chemother 1991;35:2625–2629.

175 Squires KE, Brown ST, Armstrong D, et al. Interferon-gamma treatment for *Mycobacterium avium-intracellular* complex bacillemia in patients with AIDS. J Infect Dis 1992; 166:686–687. (Letter).

176 Squires KE, Murphy WF, Madoff LC, et al. Interferon-gamma and *Mycobacterium avium-intracellulare* infection. J Infect Dis 1989;159:599–600.

177 Palestine AG, Polis MA, De Smet MD, et al. A randomized, controlled trial of foscarnet in the treatment of cytomegalovirus retinitis in patients with AIDS. Ann Intern Med 1991; 115:665–673.

178 Mortality in patients with the acquired immunodeficiency syndrome treated with either foscarnet or ganciclovir for cytomegalovirus retinitis. Studies of Ocular Complications of AIDS Research Group, in collaboration with the AIDS Clinical Trials Group. N Engl J Med 1992;326:213–220.

179 Van Der Pijl JW, Frissen PHJ, Reiss P, et al. Foscarnet and penile ulceration. Lancet 1990;1:1455–1456.

180 Gilquin J, Weiss L, Kazatchkine MD. Genital and oral erosions induced by foscarnet. Lancet 1990;1:287.

181 Green ST, Nathwani D, Godberg DJ, et al. Generalised cutaneous rash associated with foscarnet usage in AIDS. J Infect 1990;21:227–228.

182 Farese RV, Schambelan M, Hollander H, et al. Nephrogenic diabetes insipidus associated with foscarnet treatment of cytomegalovirus retinitis. Ann Intern Med 1990;112:955–956.

183 Manischewitz JF, Quinnan GVJ, Lane HC, et al. Synergistic effect of ganciclovir and foscarnet on cytomegalovirus replication in vitro. Antimicrob Agents Chemother 1990;34:373–375.

184 Nelson MR, Barter G, Hawkins D, et al. Simultaneous treatment of cytomegalovirus retinitis with ganciclovir and foscarnet. Lancet 1991;338:250. (Letter).

185 Kuppermann BD, Flores-Aguillar M, Quiceno JI, et al. Combination ganciclovir and foscarnet in the treatment of clinically resistant cytomegalovirus retinitis in patients with acquired immunodeficiency syndrome. Arch Ophthalmol 1993;111: 1359–1366.

186 Dieterich DT, Poles MA, Lew EA, et al. Concurrent use of ganciclovir and foscarnet to treat cytomegalovirus infection in AIDS patients. J Infect Dis 1993; 167:1184–1188.

187 Peters M, Schurmann D, Pohle HD, et al. Combined and alternating ganciclovir/foscarnet in HIV-related cytomegalovirus encephalitis. Lancet 1992;340(8825):970. (Letter).

188 Coker RJ, Tomlinson D, Horner P, et al. Treatment of cytomegalovirus retinitis with ganciclovir and foscarnet. Lancet 1991;338(8766):574–575. (Letter).

189 Robinson M, Smith D, Betts R, et al. Ganciclovir implant for CMV retinitis treatment. Berlin, Germany, 1993:423.

Antimicrobial Prophylaxis in Patients Undergoing Solid Organ Transplantation

NESLI BASGOZ
ROBERT H. RUBIN

Despite the considerable advances made in the prevention, diagnosis and treatment of infectious diseases, infection remains the leading cause of morbidity and mortality among solid organ transplant recipients. This is a reflection of the fact that infection and rejection are inextricably intertwined in transplantation, linked by the immunosuppressive therapy required to maintain allograft function. Any intervention that decreases the risk of rejection, permitting the use of less intensive immunosuppressive therapy, will result in a decreased risk of infection; any intervention that decreases the risk of infection, permitting safer use of immunosuppressive therapy, will decrease the risk of rejection. Thus, the therapeutic prescription for the transplant recipient has two components: the immunosuppression that prevents or treats allograft rejection and the antimicrobial strategy that makes this safe (1).

In developing an effective strategy for solid organ transplantation, the infectious disease physician must keep in mind several important tenets:

1. *Prevention must always be stressed over treatment for two reasons.* The inflammatory response to infection is attenuated by the immunosuppressive drugs given to the transplant patient. This may abolish the typical signs and symptoms of infection and render the usual serologic or skin tests much less sensitive. These factors make early diagnosis more difficult, in a patient population in which the effects of established infection may be devastating.

Even if diagnosed promptly, the antimicrobial agents used to treat these infections often have unacceptable toxicities, particularly with the current, cyclosporine-based immunosuppressive regimens (2). Three types of interactions may occur between cyclosporine and a variety of antimicrobial agents. Several drugs, most notably rifampin, upregulate the metabolism of cyclosporine by the hepatic cytochrome p-450 enzyme system, thus decreasing cyclosporine levels and potentially leading to allograft rejection. Other drugs such as erythromycin and presumably the newer macrolides, ketoconazole, itraconazole and, to a lesser extent, fluconazole, downregulate the hepatic

344

metabolism of cyclosporine, leading to higher levels of the drug. This may lead to clinical manifestations of cyclosporine toxicity, particularly renal insufficiency, as well as overimmunosuppression. Finally, there is a non–dose-related, presumably idiosyncratic, synergistic nephrotoxicity between cyclosporine and many other medications. This last interaction is of particular concern because, although the first two interactions can be dealt with by close monitoring of cyclosporine levels in blood and dosage adjustments, this one cannot be. Synergistic nephrotoxocity has been seen with a long list of antimicrobial agents, including amphotericin B, aminoglycosides, vancomycin, high-dose trimethoprim/sulfamethoxazole (TMP/SMX), pentamidine, and itraconazole.

2. *Prevention can be accomplished by giving antimicrobial drugs in two different modes.* The first is the prophylactic mode, in which the antimicrobial is given to everyone. This requires an infection that is common enough and antimicrobials that are safe enough to make prophylaxis worthwhile. The second is the preemptive mode, in which antimicrobials are given not to all but to a subgroup of patients before they develop symptomatic disease. The preemptive mode requires the use of a clinical characteristic or laboratory finding that identifies a subgroup of individuals at high risk, who would be expected to derive maximal benefit from the treatment (3). The third mode, the therapeutic mode, or treatment of established infection, will not be discussed in this review.

3. *The risk of any infection, including opportunistic infection, in the solid organ transplant patient is primarily determined by the interaction of the epidemiologic exposures of the patient and the patient's net state of immunosuppression.* If an exposure is great enough, even a normal host can develop life-threatening infection; on the other hand, if the net state of immunosuppression is high enough, even minor exposures to agents present in the normal environment can cause major infections (1,4).

The exposures of importance for the transplant patient can be divided into two categories—those occurring in the patient's community and those occurring in the hospital.

In the community, there are four major concerns: 1) encounters with the geographically restricted endemic mycoses (e.g., *Histoplasma capsulatum, Coccidioides immitis,* or *Blastomyces dermatitidis;* 2) *Mycobacterium tuberculosis;* 3) agents acquired through food such as *Salmonella* species, *Campylobacter, Listeria,* or *Strongyloides stercoralis;* and 4) respiratory tract pathogens such as influenza and respiratory syncytial virus.

In the hospital, nosocomial epidemics of opportunistic infections due to *Aspergillus* species, *Legionella* species, and gram-negative rods such as *Pseudomonas aeruginosa* are of great concern (1,5). Two epidemiologic patterns have been described: domicilary and nondomiciliary. Domiciliary exposures occur on the ward where the patient is housed, with such epidemics being characterized by clustering of cases in time and space. These exposures can largely be prevented by high-efficiency particulate air (HEPA) being filtered into the patient's room. Nondomiciliary exposures occur when the patients are taken off the ward, for example, to the operating room or radiology department

(6). Infections resulting from these exposures may go undiscovered because of a lack of clustering on a single ward, and thus may go on to exceed in number infections of the classical domiciliary epidemic. These outbreaks are highly associated with construction within the hospital environment. Because HEPA filters are not available at all sites, increasing emphasis must be placed on special masks or special transport vehicles that provide a portable source of filtered air to decrease the risk of infection. The principle here is that the transplant patient is a "sentinel chicken" within the hospital environment, with any excess exposures to infectious agents reflected first in this patient population (5). Constant epidemiologic surveillance is critical to preventing catastrophic outbreaks of life-threatening infection.

The net state of immunosuppression is a complex function that is determined by the interaction of a number of factors. The major factors are the dose, duration, and temporal sequence in which immunosuppressive agents are given. The other factors include leukopenia; injury to the mucocutaneous defenses of the body surface; indwelling lines or foreign bodies; metabolic abnormalities such as malnutrition, hyperglycemia, and uremia; and infection with one of the immunomodulating viruses, cytomegalovirus (CMV), Epstein-Barr virus (EBV), hepatitis B and C viruses (HBV and HCV) as well as the human immunodeficiency virus (HIV). Immunomodulating viruses appear particularly important; approximately 90% of solid organ transplant patients who develop opportunistic infections due to organisms such as *Aspergillus* species or *Legionella* species do so in the presence of concurrent immunomodulating viral infection. Indeed, the occurrence of such opportunistic infections in the absence of such viral infection is often a clue to the presence of an epidemiologic hazard (1,4).

TEMPORAL SEQUENCE OF INFECTION FOLLOWING SOLID ORGAN TRANSPLANTATION

In addition to the tenets described above, there is one additional, overriding principle that guides antimicrobial prophylaxis in solid organ transplant patients. That is that in patients given the current, standard three-drug immunosuppressive regimens (corticosteroids, cyclosporine A, and azathioprine), there is an expected temporal sequence in which infections occur posttransplant (Figure 14.1). Although the clinical course in individual patients may vary from this sequence somewhat, it is consistent enough that knowledge of such a temporal sequence is key not only to designing preventive strategies but also to prescribing empiric therapy for these patients. Major exceptions to this sequence usually indicate the presence of an unusual risk factor, such as an epidemiologic exposure or one of the other, nonmedication-related factors contributing to the net state of immunosuppression, as described previously. For purposes of discussion, it is useful to divide the posttransplant course into three time periods (1).

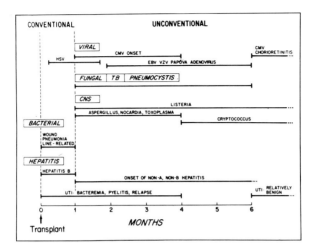

Figure 14.1. Temporal sequence of of Infection following solid organ transplantation[a]
a. From Rubin (1).

First month posttransplant. In this time period, the major causes of infection are the same bacteria and fungi that cause infection in nonimmunosuppressed patients undergoing similar surgeries. They are usually either related to technical complications of the surgery or to the technology necessary to perform the surgery, such as indwelling Foley catheters, the endotracheal tube or intravenous lines. Solid organ transplant patients are the most vulnerable of all surgical patients when it comes to technical problems in their management, and the presence of these problems almost invariably leads to infection.

A less common, but potentially disastrous, form of bacterial infection in all solid organ recipients is infection that was not recognized or not eradicated pretransplant and is conveyed with the allograft. This may result in rupture of the vascular anastomosis in the kidney or liver transplants, in pneumonia or rupture of the tracheal anastomosis in lung transplants, and in bacteremia (or fungemia) in any of the solid organ transplants. Prevention of these infections requires careful attention to the potential donor pretransplant.

Of note, the classical opportunistic infections are not seen in the first month posttransplant, when the daily dose of immunosuppression is the highest, underlining the fact that it is the duration of immunosuppression, or the "area under the curve," rather than simply the daily dose that is the major determinant of the net state of immunosuppression. The rare instances in which opportunistic infections occur during this period suggest unusually intense epidemiologic exposures, often within the hospital. All efforts should be made to identify the exposure before it causes an outbreak. Antimicrobial strategies during this first period are centered on three issues: eradication of infections that preexisted transplantation, surgical wound prophylaxis, and protection from epidemiologic hazards.

One to six months posttransplant.   The etiologies of infection during this time period are very different from those during the first postoperative month. The most important causes of infectious disease syndromes in this time period are the immunomodulating viruses. For example, CMV itself is the cause of more than two-thirds of febrile episodes during this period. In addition to the syndromes directly attributable to viral infection, these viruses have a variety of indirect effects (7). They contribute markedly to the net state of immunosuppression and predispose to the occurrence of opportunistic infection with such organisms as *Pneumocystis carinii*, *Aspergillus fumigatus*, and *Listeria monocytogenes*. In addition, they may be involved in the pathogenesis of allograft injury and rejection. For these reasons, antimicrobial strategies during this period are centered on the prevention of viral infection and *P. carinii*, as well as on epidemiologic protection against *Aspergillus*.

More than six months posttransplant.   Patients who are alive, with a functioning allograft and thus requiring continuous immunosuppression, can be divided into three groups. Taking kidney transplants as an example, about 75% have good allograft function, are on decreased doses of immunosuppression, and are free of chronic viral infections. These patients develop infections that are similar to those observed in the community: influenza, bacterial pneumonia (*Streptococcus pneumoniae*, *Haemophilus influenzae*, and mycoplasma) and urinary tract infection (UTI).

About 10 to 15% of patients who have survived to this time have chronic viral infections with CMV, EBV, HBV, or HCV, or much less commonly, HIV. Because immunosuppressive therapy prevents host defenses from effectively clearing these infections, patients not only develop the complications of these infections but do so with a shortened latent period. These complications include organ failure (hepatic failure and cirrhosis with HBV or HCV), malignancy (hepatocellular carcinoma or EBV-associated lymphoproliferative disease), or the acquired immunodeficiency syndrome (AIDS).

Finally, 5 to 15% of these patients, ones we call the "chronic n'er-do-wells," are characterized by relatively poor allograft function and one or more episodes of acute or chronic rejection, requiring additional immunosuppression. These patients are at highest risk for opportunistic infections such as those due to *P. carinii*, *Cryptococcus neoformans*, *L. monocytogenes*, or *Nocardia asteroides*, and may warrant long-term antimicrobial prophylaxis with low-dose TMP/SMX and fluconazole.

ANTIMICROBIAL STRATEGIES AGAINST SPECIFIC INFECTIONS

Antimicrobial Strategies against Bacterial Infection

The most common bacterial infections in solid organ transplant recipients can be divided into three general categories: 1) infections due to conventional bacteria; 2) infections acquired through the gastrointestinal tract, such as *Salmonella* species, *L. monocytogenes*, and *Campylobacter jejuni*; and 3) infections due to mycobacteria.

The first category is that of infections due to the same bacteria that cause infection in nonimmunosuppressed patients undergoing similar surgeries. Thus, perioperative prophylactic antibacterials targeted to urinary tract organisms and staphylococci are effective in preventing wound infections in renal transplant patients (8–10). For most patients, our standard is cefazolin begun "on call" and continued for less than 24 hours postoperatively. In this population particularly, all efforts to avoid or remove conduits for these infections should be made. Although controlled data in prophylaxis outside of the renal transplant setting are lacking, similar principles appear applicable. Antibiotics chosen should cover staphylococci and the resident flora of the transplanted site, as discussed below for liver transplantation. In the case of lung transplantation, we monitor the sputum of the candidates at least twice monthly before transplantation and then individualize the prophylactic regimen to the colonizing flora of the individual. In addition, given the risk of conveying preexisting bacterial infection with the allograft, the organ donor should be carefully evaluated first by evaluating all of the premortem clinical and culture data available, and then by performing routine cultures of the blood and allograft at the time of harvest.

After the first month, the most common form of bacterial infection in renal transplant recipients is urinary tract infection (UTI). Without prophylaxis, the incidence of UTI in this population has been 35 to 79% (11,12). UTI in the first few months after transplant is frequently associated with signs of pyelonephritis, bacteremia, and a high rate of relapse when treated with a standard course of antibiotics (13,14). UTI has been virtually eradicated from the renal transplant population by the use of prophylaxis with either low-dose TMP/SMX (one single-strength tablet at bedtime) (15) or ciprofloxacin (250 mg at bedtime) (16) for 6 to 12 months posttransplant. TMP/SMX has the added advantage of providing prophylaxis against infection with *P. carinii*, *N. asteroides*, and *L. monocytogenes* (1). In a small percentage of patients, UTIs recur after the period of greatest risk and after routine prophylaxis has been completed. This should prompt a search for anatomic factors predisposing to infection, for example, nephrolithiasis, prostatic hypertrophy, bladder outlet obstruction, or urodynamic problems. If no correctable problem is identified, particularly if the patient is in the "chronic n'er do well" category, we maintain them on long-term UTI prophylaxis.

Liver transplantation is associated with the highest rate of life-threatening bacterial (and fungal) infections, with major infections reported in 30 to 79% of liver transplant recipients (17–19). Although UTIs occur with a high enough frequency to make prophylaxis worthwhile, most infections are located intra-abdominally and are related to such factors as surgical manipulation of the bowel and biliary tree, intraperitoneal hemorrhage perioperatively, the need for reexploration, and the use of a choledochojejunostomy (rather than a choledochocholedochostomy) as an anastomosis. Some groups report favorable results with the selective bowel decontamination approach used in cancer patients, using nonabsorbable antibacterial agents (gentamicin and polymyxin B combined with nystatin or amphotericin B) orally to eradicate the gram-negative and fungal flora while leaving the anaerobic flora, which confers colonization resistance (18,20), intact. Others have achieved similar results in bacterial prophylaxis with oral quinolones (21). In our own liver transplant program, cefazolin followed by prophylactic TMP/SMX plus clotrimazole or nystatin has been very successful in decreasing the incidence of infection. Although these results are difficult to compare because of differences in technique, immunosuppressive regimens, and evaluations of outcome, it is clear that some form of prophylactic therapy targeted at gram-negative and fungal flora in the bowel decreases the incidence of infection in this patient population. It may be that there are subgroups of patients who benefit from greater amounts of preemptive therapy, such as those with bowel perforation or hepatic infarction perioperatively.

Although the immediately perioperative period is the one with the highest risk for bacterial infection, a high rate of colonization of the biliary tree continues postoperatively, particularly in patients whose anastomosis is a choledochojejunostomy. Common organisms include *Staphylococcus epidermidis*, enterococci, and Enterobacteriaceae. Manipulation of the colonized biliary tract and bile may result in cholangitis or intrahepatic abscess (22). For this reason, we administer preemptive therapy with drugs such as vancomycin and aztreonam whenever liver biopsy is performed or biliary tract manipulation such as a cholangiogram or removal of a T tube is carried out.

The second major category of bacterial infection following transplantation is that acquired through the gastrointestinal tract, including such pathogens as nontyphoidal *Salmonella*, *L. monocytogenes*, and *C. jejuni*. Perhaps the most important prophylactic intervention is counseling avoidance of high-risk foods and cooking practices. We tell all patients to avoid foods containing raw or undercooked eggs, chicken, or meat. In addition, our empiric antimicrobial therapy in solid organ transplant patients with fever and diarrhea includes coverage for these organisms, for example, use of ampicillin/sulbactam. In our experience, the incidence of these infections, as well as infection due to *N. asteroides*, has declined markedly in patients who receive routine UTI prophylaxis, presumably due to the activity of these agents against a variety of bacterial species (1).

The third category of bacterial infection is that caused by mycobacterial species (1,23). Infection due to *M. tuberculosis* is the prototype infection that requires an intact cellular immune response for its control, and it is no surprise that tuberculous disease occurs in renal transplant patients at a rate more than one hundred times that of the general population (24). Most disease represents reactivation in those with prior infection, although primary infection may also occur. As in other immunosuppressed patients, extrapulmonary or disseminated disease is more common, reflecting the inability of the host to keep infection localized to the site of reactivation or primary infection.

Although the incidence of tuberculosis is much higher in transplant patients, most transplant recipients with positive tuberculin tests pretransplant and no other risk factors for reactivation do not develop active tuberculosis. Other risk factors beside the immunosuppressive regimens are those recognized in other populations, including presumed genetic predisposition in Asians, Pacific Islanders, Africans, or African Americans or individual predisposition due to factors such as protein-calorie malnutrition or recent acquisition of infection. A history of active tuberculosis in the past, especially if inadequately treated, and the presence of abnormalities on chest radiographs, particularly parenchymal scars or fibrosis, reflect a larger burden of infection in the past and thus confer higher risk for reactivation. Given the significant risk of hepatotoxicity and drug interaction of cyclosporine with isoniazid or rifampin, in a patient population that already has a high incidence of hepatotoxicity, we do not give antituberculous prophylaxis to all patients with positive tuberculin tests preoperatively, but reserve it for those with other risk factors for disease. Patients who receive prophylaxis receive it for 9 to 12 months. Those who are not given prophylaxis are followed closely for symptoms and have chest radiographs every 6 months.

Antimicrobial Strategies against *Pneumocystis carinii*, *Toxoplasma gondii*, and *Strongyloides stercoralis*

Pneumocystis carinii is included here for historical reasons because it was formerly classified as a protozoa. Now, on the basis of rRNA sequencing, it is classified as a fungus. There is at least a 10% incidence of *P. carinii* pneumonia in organ transplant patients who receive no prophylaxis (1,25). Although most infection can be cured, the first-line therapies have significant toxicities: renal, hematologic, rash, and fever in the case of TMP/SMX and renal and pancreatic in the case of pentamidine. This potential toxicity is added to the significant renal and hematologic toxicities of the medications these patients are already receiving, such as cyclosporine A and azathioprine. In contrast, the low doses of TMP/SMX used for UTI prophylaxis are very effective and much less toxic than therapeutic doses. In patients unable to tolerate this regimen, alternative regimens are used. There is evidence in patients infected with HIV, however, that alternative prophylaxis with dapsone is less effective than TMP/SMX, and aerosol pentamidine less effective still. The optimal duration of prophylaxis is unclear; however, since 80% of the cases of *P. carinii* occur in the first 6 months posttransplantation, we continue prophylaxis for 6 months in renal transplant patients and a year with other solid organ transplants, where higher doses of immunosuppression are used. Prophylaxis is reinstituted at times when the patient will receive a significant increase in the level of immunosuppression for more than a few days. In addition, patients in the "chronic n'er do well" category, who are always on higher doses of immunosuppression, are often maintained on prophylaxis for longer periods of time, sometimes indefinitely.

Heart transplant patients who are seronegative for *T. gondii* but receive an allograft from a toxoplasma-seropositive donor are at high risk for disseminated toxoplasmosis (1,25). Although this may also occur in noncardiac transplant recipients, the incidence appears to be so low that routine prophylaxis is not indicated. In heart transplant patients, sulfadiazine and pyrimethamine (with folinic acid to help prevent hematologic toxicity) provide effective prophylaxis against disseminated toxoplasmosis and also against *P. carinii* infection. However, the hematologic toxicity has required a change in some of our patients, and these have been given successful prophylaxis with pyrimethamine alone, or in combination with new drugs that appear promising for toxoplasmosis, atovaquone (26) or azithromycin (27).

Strongyloides stercoralis is an intestinal nematode that occurs with low frequency in the United States but with higher frequency in the tropics (1,25,28). Asymptomatic infection of the intestinal tract may be present for years or even decades after acquisition, generally causes mild symptoms, and is easily treated with thiabendazole. However, the capacity of *Strongyloides* to persist through a unique autoinfection cycle may lead to massive dissemination in the immunocompromised host, even decades after acquisition of the original infection. Direct tissue invasion or accompanying gram-negative bacillary sepsis or meningitis may be fatal in these patients. Thus, it is important to examine multiple stool samples for ova and parasites in patients from endemic areas (the tropics, southeastern United States) prior to transplantation. In patients with a past history of infection or who are particularly at high risk, small bowel sampling with a device such as the Enterotest (Hedeco, Palo Alto, California) or small bowel biopsy is much more sensitive. However, given the potential morbidity of endoscopic small bowel biopsy, preemptive therapy on the basis of past epidemiologic exposure is probably more practical.

Antimicrobial Strategies against Fungal Infection

Fungal infection in the recipient of a solid organ transplant can be divided into two categories. The first is opportunistic infection with organisms that rarely cause invasive disease in the normal host, such as *Candida* species, *Aspergillus* species, *C. neoformans*, and *Mucor*. The second is infection with one of the fungi causing the endemic mycoses such as histoplasmosis, coccidioidomycosis, or blastomycosis. By far the most common fungal infections are those caused by *Candida* and *Aspergillus* species (1,29).

Candida species are found throughout the gastrointestinal tract, on the skin, and in the vagina. The most common manifestation of infection in the transplant patient is mucocutaneous overgrowth, such as thrush in the oropharynx, vaginitis, or intertrigo. Topical therapy to the skin or orally with nonabsorbable fungal agents such as clotrimazole or nystatin is usually effective in preventing or controlling these. When topical prophylaxis fails, fluconazole is highly effective. We prescribe topical therapy such as oral clotrimazole or nystatin during the first 6 months after transplantation in kidney transplant recipients, for the first year in recipients of other organs, and whenever antibacterial therapy is used, immunosuppression is increased or other factors known to promote fungal infection are present in all transplant patients.

Another common presentation of candidal infection is UTI. This is often iatrogenic, associated with use of urinary catheters. In renal transplant recipients, this may result in ascending infection, pyelonephritis, and fungemia. One mechanism for this is obstructive uropathy due to a "fungal ball" at the ureterovesical junction, particularly in diabetic patients with fungal UTIs. For these reasons, we always treat asymptomatic candiduria preemptively in these patients. We use either 2 weeks of fluconazole, or if the organism is thought not to be susceptible (such as *Candida krusei* and *Torulopsis glabrata*), low-dose (10 mg/d) amphotericin B, sometimes combined with flucytosine.

As mentioned previously, candidal infection in the abdominal cavity and the liver is a major problem in liver transplantation. Bowel decontamination that includes prophylaxis aimed at *Candida* species appears to decrease the incidence of posttransplant candidal infection (18,20,30). Whether optimal decontamination regimens should include nonabsorbable drugs such as nystatin or clotrimazole or systemic therapies such as fluconazole is not yet clear.

Invasive aspergillosis of the lungs and sinuses (1,29,31) is an infection that occurs in solid organ transplant patients after an intense environmental exposure, for example, after construction in a hospital, in the face of excessive immunosuppression, or following infection with immunomodulating viruses, especially CMV. Avoidance of exposures in the hospital, for example, use of masks when traveling off the transplant unit, particularly if construction is going on in the hospital, may help prevent some cases of infection. In addition, we perform fungal as well as bacterial cultures of sputum specimens in patients who are awaiting lung transplant, who are hospitalized for prolonged periods of time, who are immunosuppressed or on broad-spectrum antibiotics pretransplant, or who have other risk factors for *Aspergillus* infection such as preceding CMV infection. We administer preemptive therapy to anyone whose respiratory tract is colonized with *Aspergillus* pre- or posttransplant, as such colonization carries a significant risk of invasion. In our experience, itraconazole appears effective and well tolerated in this setting, although patients should be carefully monitored for increasing cyclosporine levels due to competition of itraconazole and cyclosporine for metabolism by hepatic P-450 enzymes. There may also be a role in some patients for amphotericin B if the itraconazole is unsuccessful.

Antimicrobial Strategies against Viral Infection

Cytomegalovirus is the single most important viral infection in solid organ transplant recipients. It most commonly presents as a nonspecific febrile illness, often associated with leukopenia, thrombocytopenia, and liver function test abnormalities. However, gastrointestinal tract ulcers, frank hepatitis, pneumonia, and later chorioretinitis may also be seen. CMV infection is also associated with profound immune dysregulation and is often followed by other complications: an increased incidence of bacterial and fungal infections and Epstein-Barr virus-associated lymphoma and a higher rate of allograft rejection (7). Thus antimicrobial strategies directed against CMV would be expected to decrease the incidence of other infectious complications in this patient population.

There are three major patterns of CMV infection in organ transplantation. Each may carry a different risk of clinical disease and may thus warrant different preventive strategies (1):

1. *Primary infection (R−/D+).* Here, a CMV-seronegative recipient receives cells latently infected with CMV from a seropositive donor. More than 60% of patients who become primarily infected experience symptomatic disease.

2. *Reactivation infection (R+/D−)* in which seropositive recipients reactivate their own endogenous latent virus. Here, the host recipient has some preexisting immunity and the rate of symptomatic disease is about 20%.

3. *Superinfection (R+/D+).* Here, a seropositive recipient receives an organ from a seropositive donor. In over half of these patients, some or all of the virus that reactivates can be shown to be of donor origin. This group has a higher rate of symptomatic infection than the reactivation group above, ranging from 20 to 40%.

Many prophylactic regimens have been studied for the prevention of disease due to CMV. These include programs using high-dose oral acyclovir (32–35), both CMV hyperimmune (36–38) and standard immunoglobulin (39,40), a combination of these two approaches (41,42) as well as ganciclovir (43,44). Although the data are difficult to compare due to the different patient populations, immunosuppressive regimens, antiviral programs, and measurements of outcome, Table 14.1 provides a summary of the estimated efficacies of

Table 14.1.   Estimated Efficacies of Prophylactic Antiviral Strategies against Cytomegalovirus Infection in Different Forms of Solid Organ Transplantation

Type of Organ	Form of CMV	Antimicrobial Strategy	Efficacy	Reference
Kidney	Primary	CMV hyperimmune globulin	2+	37
		High-dose acyclovir	2+	33, 34, 43
		CMV hyperimmune globulin plus moderate-dose acyclovir	3+	41
	Secondary	High-dose acyclovir	3+	33, 34, 43
		CMV hyperimmune globulin plus moderate-dose acyclovir	3+	41
Heart and/or lung	Primary	High-dose ganciclovir (1 mo)	0	32, 44
	Secondary	High-dose ganciclovir (1 mo)	4+	32, 44
Liver	Primary	CMV hyperimmune globulin	0	38
	Secondary	CMV hyperimmune globulin	3+	38

SOURCE: Modified from Rubin RH, Tolkoff-Rubin NE. Antimicrobial strategies in the care of organ transplant recipients. Antimicrob Agents Chem 1993;37:619–623.

different prophylactic strategies in the available studies. Only semiquantitative estimates of efficacy are given due to the many differences between the studies. Unless otherwise noted, the antiviral regimens were administered for at least 3 months. For the purposes of this summary, no differentiation is made between reactivation or superinfection; therefore all patients seropositive before transplant appear in the category of secondary infection.

Clearly, the most difficult scenario in which to prevent disease is that of primary infection, in which the recipient has no preexisting immunity to CMV. Here, the best results are seen in renal transplant patients, where high-dose oral acyclovir or CMV hyperimmune globulin, given alone or in combination, decrease (though do not eliminate) the incidence of symptomatic disease. The same cannot be said of heart, lung, or liver recipients, where no study has convincingly demonstrated a decrease in primary CMV disease after prophylaxis of any kind.

In the case of renal transplant patients with reactivation, high-dose acyclovir, or CMV hyperimmune globulin and high-dose acyclovir, is even more efficacious than in primary infection. In contrast to primary infection, some regimens also appear effective in nonrenal transplants, such as high-dose ganciclovir in heart or lung transplants or CMV hyperimmune globulin in liver transplants.

In any of these patients, as stated above, increased antirejection therapy markedly decreases the effectiveness of the prophylactic regimens. This is particularly true for the use of antilymphocyte antibody therapy (polyclonal or monoclonal), which increases the incidence of symptomatic disease, for example, up to fivefold in renal transplant recipients (46). This is a scenario in which preemptive therapy would be expected to be effective; indeed, Hibberd et al. (47) administered low-dose ganciclovir preemptively during antilymphocyte antibody therapy and showed a marked decrease in incidence of clinical CMV disease in all patients from greater than 50% to about 15%. This approach also appears to be effective in liver and heart (47) as well as lung (48) transplant recipients.

Although considerable progress has been made in the prevention of CMV disease, still many patients, particularly in the primary infection category, develop disease. The optimal prophylactic regimen to be given to all patients at risk, probably some combination of an antiviral with a polyclonal or monoclonal immune globulin, must be defined. New agents, such as the oral preparation of ganciclovir (currently limited by oral bioavailability) or other antivirals, may play a role in the near future. In addition, preemptive therapy with antivirals will presumably be added at times of maximal risk. Attempts must continue to identify still other subgroups of patients at high risk of disease in whom preemptive therapy may be indicated. One such group may be patients with early evidence of reactivation of virus. This approach has proven effective in a patient population (bone marrow transplant patients) at particular risk of CMV pneumonitis where ganciclovir therapy given after CMV was isolated in bronchoalveolar lavage prevented the development of CMV pneumonia (49). In solid organ transplant patients, quantification of increased levels of virus in the buffy coat by immunocytochemistry (50) or quantative PCR (51) may help define a high risk subgroup of patients.

Infection with EBV in normal hosts may be asymptomatic or may result in the self-limited lymphoproliferative disease infectious mononucleosis. The virus is transmitted through saliva and initiates lytic infection in the epithelial cells of the oropharynx. Subsequently, B lymphocytes trafficking through this lymphoid-rich tissue become infected and B cell proliferation, activation, and immortalization ensue. In nonimmunocompromised individuals, this B cell proliferation is controlled by potent T cell responses. However, immunosuppression markedly impairs these responses. In solid organ transplant patients, EBV infection is associated with a progressive and often fatal syndrome, posttransplant lymphoproliferative disorder (PTLD) (52,53). Unlike other lymphomas, this is primarily an extranodal disease, and most commonly presents with fever and evidence of disease in the gastrointestinal tract, central nervous system, liver, or any other organ, including the allograft. Pathologic analysis of tissues indicates that the B cell tumors causing disease may simply consist of polyclonal aggregates of B cells, or, because the B cell proliferation and activation favor mutational events, of a frank, monoclonal lymphoma (54).

The highest risk of PTLD occurs with primary infection. Because most adults are already seropositive before transplantation, the highest incidence is found in children. The incidence of PTLD has risen in recent years, coincident with the use of more potent immunosuppressive regimens, particularly cyclosporin A and antilymphocyte antibodies. Currently, rates as high as 5 to 15% in heart or heart-lung transplants, 3 to 5% in liver transplants and 1 to 3% in renal transplants are reported (52,53). Multiple interventions have been tried, and decreased immunosuppression and surgical resection when possible appear to have some efficacy. Other modalities such as antivirals (which work on lytic but not the mostly latent, B cell-associated form of EBV), radiation, chemotherapy, and, most recently, monoclonal antibodies to B cell epitopes do not result in a lasting response. Thus, the overall mortality associated with this disorder is between 60 and 80%, and there is a particularly urgent need to focus on prevention rather than treatment of established disease.

At any given time, EBV can be isolated from the pharyngeal secretions of 10 to 20% of normal hosts who are seropositive, up to 50% of transplant patients, and up to 80% of transplant patients on antilymphocyte antibodies. Investigators have wondered if there is a relationship between the amount of EBV shed in the pharynx, the number of infected B cells, and the subsequent risk of PTLD. Preiksaitis et al. measured EBV DNA in oropharyngeal epithelium and showed that lymphoproliferative disease was more likely to develop in the group of patients who had the greatest amount of viral replication (55). These were also the patients on highest doses of immunosuppression and who were likely to have primary infection. One patient who received treatment doses of intravenous ganciclovir for a primary CMV infection and one who received intravenous acyclovir had clearance of detectable oropharyngeal EBV while on therapy. It is tempting to postulate that increased EBV replication in the oropharynx might result in an increased number of infected B cells and confer a higher risk for PTLD. Although these sequential relationships have not yet been examined directly, if such a relationship did exist, a preventive antiviral strategy similar to that used for CMV, with prophylaxis for everyone and preemptive therapy for certain groups during periods of increased immuno-suppression, might decrease the incidence of PTLD.

In addition, Basgoz et al. have recently shown that symptomatic disease with CMV is a significant independent risk factor for the development of subsequent PTLD (56). This could relate to the profound immune dysregulation seen during symptomatic CMV infection (57). Such dysregulation includes effects on cytotoxic and helper T cells as well as on cytokines. Thus, strategies aimed at prevention of CMV could conceivably decrease the incidence of PTLD as well.

The final infections we will discuss are those caused by the hepatotropic viruses, HBV and HCV.

Hepatitis B virus infection may be acquired perioperatively, from the al-lograft itself or from blood products, or may be present before the transplant. It is clear that renal transplant patients who acquire infection at the time of transplant or in the first months thereafter do poorly, with a high rate of fulminant hepatitis but also a very high rate of chronic hepatitis (58). Therefore, it is the practice of all transplant centers to screen for hepatitis B in donors and not to use organs from donors who are hepatitis B carriers (HBsAg positive). Today, the far more common question is what to do with patients with renal failure who are already hepatitis B carriers before transplantation. Although this population has begun to decrease in size as a result of the universal screening of blood products for hepatitis B and the avoidance of transfusion altogether by the use of recombinant erythropoietin, a significant number of patients are still in this category. Although these patients appear to do well in the first year or two after transplantation, subsequently they begin to do poorly (59–62). Increased mortality due to chronic liver disease, cirrhosis, hepatocellu-lar carcinoma, and extrahepatic sepsis is seen. One group reported the risk of death from liver-related complications in renal transplant patients with HBsAg antigenemia was as high as 5% per year. In addition, limited studies show treatment of established HBV infection in these patients is not as effective as even the modest effectiveness observed in nontransplant patients. Based on these and similar studies, many groups now do not transplant these patients at all.

In the case of liver transplantation, donors who are hepatitis B carriers are never used. The more common problem is that of patients who are HBsAg positive before transplant and are likely undergoing transplantation for liver disease due to this virus (63). Nearly all of these patients have evidence of recurrent infection after liver transplantation (64). This is presumably due to the replication of HBV in extrahepatic sites, such as bone marrow, spleen, pancreas, and circulating mononuclear cells (65). This recurrent infection is associated not only with an accelerated course of acute and chronic hepatitis, but with more rapid development of cirrhosis and hepatocellular carcinoma as well (66). Reminiscent of the renal transplant patients, these patients appear to have an increased risk of extrahepatic sepsis, presumably due to impairment of their immune system by the virus (64).

With the recognition that HBV infection often recurs after transplantation, many attempts have been made to identify markers that might predict an increased risk of recurrence of infection and an increased risk of progression to chronic liver disease, cirrhosis, and hepatocellular carcinoma. In general, active HBV replication pretransplantation, as manifested by the presence of HBeAg or HBV DNA, is associated with universal reinfection as well as with a more rapid and more severe course of liver disease (63,64,66). Another factor that may be significant is the presence of chronic hepatitis as opposed to fulminant hepatitis. Patients transplanted for fulminant hepatitis B are not only less likely to become reinfected, but if reinfected may be less likely to develop severe recurrent liver disease (64,67). A small number of reports have looked at the impact of coinfection with the delta hepatitis agent, HDV, on recurrence of HBV and its clinical course. In small numbers of patients, the rate of clearance of HBsAg posttransplant appears substantially higher in patients coinfected with HDV, perhaps reflecting the inhibition of HBV replication that occurs in the presence of HDV (68). Although no better, the liver disease appeared no worse in the patients with HBV/HDV coinfection pretransplant.

Given the morbidity and mortality associated with recurrent hepatitis B infection, especially in the presence of active viral replication, many prophylactic treatments of HBsAg-positive recipients have been tried, mostly with very poor results. Hepatitis B vaccination, interferon, and short-term passive immunization with hepatitis B immunoglobulin or hepatitis B monoclonal antibody have all been disappointing (63). However, Samuel et al. (69) used high-dose, long-term passive immunoprophylaxis with hepatitis B immunoglobulin and reported a significant reduction in HBV reinfection. Patients without evidence of active HBV replication (HBeAg or HBV DNA) before transplantation were more likely to remain uninfected, and this group alone showed improved survival with immunoprophylaxis. However, use of long-term immunoprophylaxis must be weighed against potential side effects as well as the enormous costs, which can run as much as $15,000 to 20,000 annually. Given the cost of recurrent liver disease and retransplantation in this population, it is hoped that some less costly form of immunoprophylaxis or some combination of immunoprophylaxis with future antiviral drugs may yet prove cost effective.

Hepatitis C infection is now known to be the cause of the great majority of cases of posttransfusion non-A, non-B hepatitis. Like hepatitis B, it is associated with chronic liver disease and hepatocellular carcinoma. Also, like hepatitis B, this virus is known to have an extrahepatic reservoir in lymphocytes, and transmission by liver donation as well as donation of extrahepatic organs was known well before the discovery of the agent and the availability of diagnostic assays.

Early attempts to define the epidemiology of hepatitis C in transplantation were hampered by the limitations of the diagnostic tests (70). The first-generation enzyme-linked immunosorbent assay (ELISA) detected antibody to the one viral antigen known at the time and had an unacceptable rate of false negative and false positive results. Although the subsequent second-generation ELISA, which was later combined with a recombinant immunoblot assay (RIBA), significantly improved the sensitivity and specificity of testing, both tests still detected only antibody responses, which can be quite late and variable in normal hosts, and are often absent in immunocompromised hosts.

These antibody tests were primarily used in two different scenarios. The first was to detect transmission of infection from a seropositive donor to a previously seronegative recipient. In these studies, the recipients failed to seroconvert, falsely suggesting that transmission of hepatitis C by solid organ transplantation was a rare event (71). It is now apparent that serologic testing alone is useless to detect transmission of infection in these patients. The serologic tests have met with greater success in the screening of potential organ donors. In a large number of donors, the sensitivity of the first- and second-generation ELISAs appeared excellent, such that if they were applied to potential organ donors, the resulting near perfect negative predictive value would eliminate transmission of HCV (72). Unfortunately, however, even with a specificity for HCV of 97 to 98%, the positive predictive value of the tests in the low-prevalence organ donor population would only be 55%. Organs from 45% of donors testing positive on the second-generation ELISA would thus be unnecessarily discarded.

It was not until the development of technologies for direct detection of HCV RNA in serum, such as the polymerase chain reaction (PCR), that the epidemiology of HCV in organ transplantation could begin to be elucidated, and the questions critical to patient safety and to optimal use of precious organs addressed. These questions include:

1   How many cadaveric donors are HCV antibody or RNA positive?

2   How many recipients become infected and how many develop disease? Can we stratify risks for infection?

3   What is the course of posttransplantation HCV infection?

4   Is it treatable?

5   What is the serostatus of the recipient and what is its role in decision-making?

6   What is the organ needed by the recipient?

What is currently known can be summarized as follows (73). Using the best serologic assays, it is estimated that HCV is present in about 1 to 2% of potential organ donors, although it is higher in some urban centers or populations. As discussed above, all serologic assays significantly underestimated the risk of transmission of infection by organ transplantation. It now appears the majority of kidney transplant recipients and all liver transplant recipients from HCV-infected donors become infected (74,75).

The consequences of posttransplantation HCV infection vary in different small series. Because liver dysfunction may be due to many different causes in this population and different studies use different criteria for clinical hepatitis, it is difficult to determine a true incidence of posttransplant hepatitis C infection. What is clear is that there is a wide spectrum of posttransplant HCV liver disease, both histologically and clinically, from viremia without hepatitis to hepatic failure (74–76). In general, the consequences of HCV appear far less devastating than those of HBV infection. Risk factors for transmission of infection probably include the presence of detectable HCV RNA in the serum (73), a finding that has also recently been reported in a study of risks for vertical transmission of HCV (77). There is also some evidence that the level of pretransplantation viremia, the level of posttransplantation viremia and a higher level of posttransplantation immunosuppression (including use of antilymphocyte globulins) may all be associated with more severe disease and allograft injury (73). Unfortunately, treatment with α-interferon appears quite ineffective in these patients, with the attendant concerns of precipitation of allograft rejection by immune modulation (78).

One way of bypassing these issues in some patients might be to give HCV-seropositive organs to HCV-seropositive recipients. Unfortunately, known information gives one pause in this regard. First, in an experimental setting, chimpanzees who have cleared their viremia can be reinfected and go on to redevelop disease with this same strain (79). Second, different strains have now been described (73). It is hoped that one day we will be able to reliably differentiate seropositive donors who are infectious from seropositive donors who are not, prevent HCV transmission from a seropositive donor, and perhaps successfully treat HCV infection in donor and recipient. Until that time, however, it seems most prudent to limit the use of organs from HCV antibody-positive donors to lifesaving transplants (i.e., liver, heart, or lung), and not for kidney transplants at all.

CONCLUSIONS

Infection has always been a major threat to the solid organ transplant patient on immunosuppressive therapy. Improvements in the prevention and treatment of infections have contributed greatly to the improved outcome in these patients. However, the available information is still incomplete. Further well-designed studies are needed to delineate patients at high risk for infection as well as the optimal types, doses, and durations of prophylactic or preemptive therapy in these patients. It is hoped that the development of new, effective, and less toxic antimicrobial agents will aid in this effort. The underlying principle remains that infection and rejection are always closely linked and that the immunosuppression required to optimize allograft function requires an optimal antimicrobial program to render it as safe as possible. Two principles appear to be united in developing such a program. First, the intensity of antimicrobial therapy, both pharmacologic and environmental, must be matched to the intensity of the immunosuppressive program being used. Second, different time points in the posttransplant course carry a higher risk of different forms of infection, thus necessitating the use of different antimicrobial strategies at different time points.

REFERENCES

1 **Rubin RH.** Infection in the organ transplant recipient. In: Rubin RH, Young LS, eds. Clinical Approach to Infection in the Compromised Host, 3rd ed. New York: Plenum Medical Book Co., 1994.

2 **Rubin RH, Tolkoff-Rubin NE.** The impact of infections on the outcome of transplantation. Transplant Proc 1991;23:2068–2074.

3 **Rubin RH.** Preemptive therapy in immunocompromised hosts. N Engl J Med 1991; 324:1057–1058. (Editorial).

4 **Rubin RH, Wolfson JS, Cosimi AB, Tolkoff-Rubin NE.** Infection in the renal transplant recipient. Am J Med 1981;70: 405–411.

5 **Rubin RH.** The compromised host as sentinel chicken. N Engl J Med 1977;317:1151–1153.

6 **Hopkins C, Weber DJ, Rubin RH.** Invasive aspergillus infection: possible non-ward common source within the hospital environment. J Hosp Infect 1989;12: 19–25.

7 **Rubin RH.** Impact of cytomegalovirus infection on organ transplant recipients. Rev Infect Dis 12(suppl 7):S754–S766.

8 **Tillegard A.** Renal transplant wound infection: the value of prophylactic antibiotic treatment. Scand J Urol Nephrol 1984;18: 215–221.

9 **Townsend TR, Rudolf LE, Westervelt FB Jr.** Prophylactic antibiotic therapy with cefamandole and tobramycin for patients undergoing renal transplantation. Infect Control 1980;1:93–96.

10 **Novick AC.** The value of intraoperative antibiotics in preventing renal transplant wound infections. J Urol 1981;125:151–152.

11 **Ramsey DE, Finch WT, Birtch AG.** Urinary tract infections in kidney transplant recipients. Arch Surg 1979;114:1022–1025.

12 **Martin DC.** Urinary tract infection in clinical renal transplantation. Arch Surg 1969; 99:474–476.

13 **Myerowitz RL, Medeiros AAM, O'Brien TF.** Bacterial infection in renal homotransplant recipients: a study of fifty three bacteremic episodes. Am J Med 1972;53: 308–314.

14 **Nielsen HE, Korsager B.** Bacteremia after renal transplantation. Scand J Infect Dis 1977;9:111–117.

15 **Fox BC, Sollinger HW, Belzer FO, Maki DG.** A prospective, randomized, double-blind study of trimethoprim-sulfamethoxazole for prophylaxis of infection in renal transplantation: clinical efficacy, absorption of trimethoprim-sulfamethoxazole, effects on the microflora, and the cost-benefit of prophylaxis. Am J Med 1990;89:255–274.

16 **Hibberd PL, Tolkoff-Rubin NE, Cosimi AB, et al.** Trimethoprim-sulfamethoxazole compared with ciprofloxacin for the prevention of urinary tract infection in renal transplant recipients: a double-blind, randomized controlled trial. Online J Curr Clin Trials, in press.

17 **Kusne S, Dummer JS, Singh N, et al.** Infection after liver transplantation: an analysis of 101 consecutive cases. Medicine 1988; 67:132–143.

18 **Paya CV, Hermans PE, Washington JA II, et al.** Incidence, distribution, and outcome of episodes of infection in 100 orthotopic liver transplantations. Mayo Clin Proc 1989;64:555–564.

19 **George DL, Arnow PM, Fox AS, et al.** Bacterial infection as a complication of liver transplantation: epidemiology and risk factors. Rev Infect Dis 1991;13:387–396.

20 **Wiesner RH, Hermans PE, Rakela JA, et al.** Selective bowel decontamination to de-

crease gram negative aerobic bacterial and *Candida* colonization and prevent infection after orthotopic liver transplantation. Transplantation 1988;45:570–574.

21 **Cuervas-Mons V, Barrios C, Garrido A, et al.** Bacterial infections in liver transplant patients under selective decontamination with norfloxacin. Transplant Proc 1989;21: 3558–3559.

22 **Bubak ME, Porayko RA, Krom RA, Wiesner RH.** Complications of liver biopsy in liver transplant patients: increased sepsis associated with choledochojejunostomy. Hepatology 1991;14:1063–1065.

23 **Sugar A.** Mycobacterial and nocardial infection in the compromised host. In: Rubin RH, Young LS, eds. Clinical Approach to Infection in the Compromised Host, 3rd ed. New York: Plenum Medical Book Co., in press.

24 **Lichtenstein IH, MacGregor RR.** Mycobacterial infections in renal transplant recipients: report of five cases and review of the literature. Rev Infect Dis 1983;5:216–230.

25 **Fishman J.** Parasitic diseases in the compromised host. In: Rubin RH, Young LS, eds. Clinical Approach to Infection in the Compromised Host, 3rd ed. New York: Plenum Medical Book Co., in press.

26 **Kovacs JA and the NIAID-Clinical Center Intramural AIDS Program.** Efficacy of atovaquone in treatment of toxoplasmosis in patients with AIDS. Lancet 1992;340: 637–638.

27 **Cantin L, Chamberland S.** In vitro evaluation of the activities of azithromycin alone and combined with pyrimethamine against *Toxoplasma gondii.* Antimicrob Agents Chemother 1993;37:1993–1996.

28 **Morgan JS, Schaffner W, Stone WJ.** Opportunistic strongyloidiasis in renal transplant recipients. Transplantation 1986;42:518–524.

29 **Castaldo P, Stratta RJ, Wood RP, et al.** Clinical spectrum of fungal infections after orthotopic liver transplantation. Arch Surg 1991;126:249–256.

30 **Wiesner RH.** The incidence of gram-negative bacterial and fungal infections in liver transplant patients treated with selective decontamination. Infection 1990;18:(suppl 1):S19–S21.

31 **Brems JJ, Hiatt JR, Klein AS, et al.** Disseminated aspergillosis complicating orthotopic liver transplantation for fulminant hepatic failure refractory to corti-

costeroid therapy. Transplantation 1988; 46:479–481.

32 **Bailey TC, Trulock NA, Ettenger GA, et al.** Failure of prophylactic ganciclovir to prevent cytomegalovirus disease in recipients of lung transplants. J Infect Dis 1992; 165:548–552.

33 **Balfour HH Jr, Chace JT, Stapleton RL, et al.** A randomized, placebo-controlled trial of oral acyclovir for the prevention of cytomegalovirus disease in recipients of renal allografts. N Engl J Med 1989;320:1381–1387.

34 **Fletcher CV, Englund JA, Edelman CK, et al.** The pharmacologic basis for high-dose oral acyclovir prophylaxis of cytomegalovirus in renal allograft recipients. Antimicrob Agents Chemother 1991;35: 938–943.

35 **Wong T, Toupance O, Chanard J.** Acyclovir to prevent cytomegalovirus infection after renal transplantation. Ann Intern Med 1991;115:68–75.

36 **Metselaar HJ, Rothbarth PH, Brouer ML, et al.** Prevention of cytomegalovirus-related death by passive immunization; a double-blind, placebo-controlled study in kidney transplant recipients treated for rejection. Transplantation 1989;48:264–266.

37 **Snydman DR, Werner BG, Dougherty NN, et al.** Cytomegalovirus immune globulin prevents serious CMV-associated disease syndromes in orthotopic liver transplantation. Ann Intern Med, in press.

38 **Snydman DR, Werner BG, Heinze-Lacey B, et al.** Use of cytomegalovirus immune globulin to prevent cytomegalovirus disease in renal transplant recipients. N Engl J Med 1987;317:1049–1054.

39 **Steinmuller DR, Graneto D, Swift C, et al.** Use of intravenous immunoglobulin prophylaxis for primary cytomegalovirus infection post living-related donor renal transplantation. Transplant Proc 1989;21: 2069–2071.

40 **Steinmuller DR, Novick AC, Streem SB, et al.** Intravenous immunoglobulin infusions for the prophylaxis of secondary cytomegalovirus infection. Transplantation 1990;49:68–70.

41 **Nicol D, MacDonald AS, Bitter-Suermann H, et al.** Combination prophylaxis therapy with CMV hyperimmune globulin and acyclovir reduces the risk of primary CMV disease in renal transplant recipients. 18th Annual Meeting of the American Society of Transplant Surgeons, 1992. (Abstract E-5).

42 **Stratta RJ, Shaefer MS, Cushin KA, et al.** A randomized, prospective trial of acyclovir and immune globulin prophylaxis in liver transplant recipients receiving OKT3 therapy. Arch Surg 1992;127:55–64.

43 **Balfour HH Jr.** Prevention of cytomegalovirus disease in renal allograft recipients. Scand J Infect Suppl 78:S88–S93.

44 **Merigan TC, Renlund DG, Keay S, et al.** A controlled trial of ganciclovir to prevent cytomegalovirus disease after heart transplantation. N Engl J Med 1992;326:1182–1186.

45 **Rubin RH, Tolkoff-Rubin NE.** Antimicrobial strategies in the care of organ transplant recipients. Antimicrob Agents Chemother 1993;37:619–623.

46 **Hibberd PL, Tolkoff-Rubin NE, Cosimi AB, et al.** Symptomatic cytomegalovirus disease in the cytomegalovirus antibody seropositive renal transplant recipient treated with OKT3. Transplantation 1992; 53:68–72.

47 **Hibberd PL, Tolkoff-Rubin NE, Doran M, et al.** Preemptive therapy with ganciclovir during OKT3 administration—a promising strategy for the prevention of symptomatic cytomegalovirus (CMV) disease in liver and heart transplant recipients. 11th Annual Meeting of the American Society of Transplant Physicians, 1992. (Abstract 57).

48 **Hibberd PL, Wain J, Rubin RH, et al.** Preemptive ganciclovir for the prevention of cytomegalovirus pneumonitis in lung transplant recipients. 13th Annual Meeting of the American Society of Transplant Physicians, 1994. (Abstract).

49 **Goodrich JM, Mori M, Gleaves CA, et al.** Early treatment with ganciclovir to prevent cytomegalovirus disease after allogeneic bone marrow transplantation. N Engl J Med 1991;235:1601–1607.

50 **The TH, van der Bij W, van den Berg AP, et al.** Cytomegalovirus antigenemia. Rev Infect Dis 1990;12(suppl 7):S737–S744.

51 **Hsia K, Spector DH, Lawrie J, Spector SA.** Enzymatic amplification of human cytomegalovirus sequences by polymerase chain reaction. J Clin Microbiol 1989;27: 1802–1809.

52 **Straus SE, moderator.** Epstein-Barr virus infections: biology, pathogenesis and management. Ann Intern Med 1992;118: 45–58.

53 **Cohen JE.** EBV lymphoproliferative disease associated with acquired immunodeficiency. Medicine 1991;70:137–160.

54 **Locker J, Nalesnik M.** Molecular genetic analysis of lymphoid tumors arising after organ transplantation. Am J Pathol 1989; 135:977–987.

55 **Preiksaitis JK, Diaz-Mitoma F, Mirzayans S, et al.** Quantitative oropharyngeal Epstein-Barr virus shedding in renal and cardiac transplant recipients: relationship to immunosuppressive therapy, serological responses, and the risk of post-transplant lymphoproliferative disorder. J Infect Dis 1992;166:986–994.

56 **Basgoz N, Hibberd PL, Tolkoff-Rubin NE, Cosimi AB, Rubin RH.** Possible role of cytomegalovirus disease in the pathogenesis of post-transplant lymphoproliferative disorder. 12th Annual Meeting of the American Society of Transplant Physicians, 1993. (Abstract P-1-50).

57 **Rinaldo CR Jr.** Immune suppression by herpesviruses. Ann Rev Med 1990;41:331–338.

58 **Katkov WN, Rubin RH.** Liver disease in the organ transplant recipient: etiology, clinical impact and clinical management. Transplant Rev 1991;5:200–208.

59 **Rao KV, Andersen RC.** Long-term results and complications in renal transplant recipients. Observations in the second decade. Transplantation 1988;45:45–52.

60 **Huang CC, Lai MK, Fong MT.** Hepatitis B liver disease in cyclosporine-treated renal allograft recipients. Transplantation 1990; 49:540–544.

61 **Rao KV, Kasiske BL, Anderson WR.** Variability in the morphologic spectrum and clinical outcome of chronic liver disease in hepatitis B-positive and B-negative renal transplant recipients. Transplantation 1991;51:391–396.

62 **Parfrey PS, Forbes RD, Hutchinson TA, et al.** The clinical and pathological course of hepatitis B liver disease in renal transplant recipients. Transplantation 1984;37:461–467.

63 **Lake JR, Wright TL.** Liver transplantation for patients with hepatitis B: What have we learned from our results? Hepatology 1991;13:796–799. (Editorial).

64 **Todo S, Demetris AJ, Van Thiel D, et al.** Orthotopic liver transplantation for patients with hepatitis B virus-related liver disease. Hepatology 1991;13:619–626.

65 **Yoffe B, Burns DK, Bhatt HS, et al.** Extrahepatic hepatitis B virus DNA sequences in patients with acute hepatitis B infection. Hepatology 1990;12:187–192.

66 **Demetris AJ, Todo S, Van Thiel DH, et al.** Evolution of hepatitis B virus liver disease after hepatic replacement: practical and theoretical considerations. Am J Pathol 1990;137:667–676.

67 **Emond JC, Aran PP, Whitington PF, et al.** Liver transplantation in the management of fulminant hepatic failure. Gastroenterology 1989;96:1583–1588.

68 **Colledan M, Grendele M, Gridelli B, et al.** Long-term results after liver transplantation in B and delta hepatitis. Transplant Proc 1989;21:2421–2423.

69 **Samuel D, Bismuth A, Mathieu D, et al.** Passive immunoprophylaxis after liver transplantation in HBsAg-positive patients. Lancet 1991;337:813–815.

70 **Houghton M, Weiner A, Han J, et al.** Molecular biology of the hepatitis C viruses: implications for diagnosis, development and control of viral disease. Hepatology 1991;14:381–388.

71 **Roth D, Fernandez JA, Babischin S, et al.** Detection of hepatitis C virus infection among cadaver organ donors: evidence for low transmission of disease. Ann Intern Med 1992;117:470–475.

72 **Pereira BJG, Wright TL, Schmid C, et al.** Clinical characteristics and prevalence of markers of hepatitis C infection in cadaver organ donors—a status report of a U.S. National Collaborative Study. 12th Annual Meeting of the American Society of Transplant Physicians, 1993. (Abstract 1).

73 **Wright TL.** Liver transplantation for chronic hepatitis C infection. Adv Liver Transplant 1993;22:231–241.

74 **Pereira BJG, Milford EL, Kirkman RL, Levey AS.** Transmission of hepatitis C virus by organ transplantation. N Engl J Med 1991;325:454–460.

75 **Gretch DR, de la Rosa C, Perskin J, et al.** HCV infection in liver transplant recipients: chronic reinfection is universal, de novo acquisition rare. Hepatology 1992;16:45–49.

76 **Ferrell LD, Wright TL, Roberts J, et al.** Pathology of hepatitis C viral infection in liver transplant recipients. Hepatology 1992;16:865–876.

77 **Ohto H, Terazawa S, Sasaki N, et al.** Transmission of hepatitis C virus from mothers to infants. N Engl J Med 1994;330:744–750.

78 **Wright TL, Gavaler JS, van Thiel DH.** Preliminary experience with alpha-2b-interferon therapy of viral hepatitis in liver allograft recipients. Transplantation 1992;53:121–124.

79 **Farci, Alter HJ, Govindarajan S, et al.** Lack of protective imunity against reinfection with hepatitis C virus. Science 1992;258:135–140.

Index